Charting

made **Incredibly Easy!**®

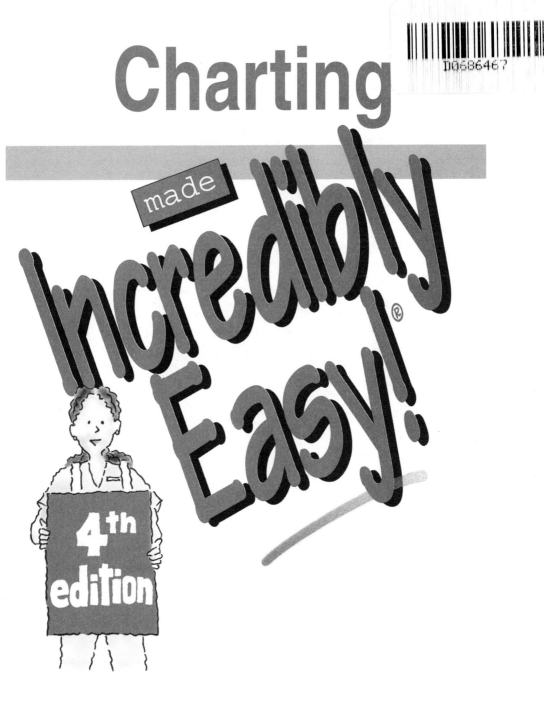

4th edition

⊞ Wolters Kluwer | Lippincott Williams & Wilkins
Health

Philadelphia • Baltimore • New York • London
Buenos Aires • Hong Kong • Sydney • Tokyo

Staff

Executive Publisher
Judith A. Schilling McCann, RN, MSN

Clinical Director
Joan M. Robinson, RN, MSN

Art Director
Elaine Kasmer

Clinical Project Managers
Diane Hines, RN, BSN; Jennifer Meyering, RN, BSN, MS, CCRN

Editors
Margaret Eckman, Diane Labus, Liz Schaeffer

Copy Editor
Jerry Altobelli

Illustrator
Bot Roda

Design Assistant
Kate Zulak

Associate Manufacturing Manager
Beth J. Welsh

Editorial Assistants
Karen J. Kirk, Jeri O'Shea, Linda K. Ruhf

Printed in the United States of America.

CHMIE4010509—021110

Library of Congress Cataloging-in-Publication Data

Charting made incredibly easy. — 4th ed.
   p. ; cm.
Includes bibliographical references and index.
ISBN 978-1-60547-196-9
1. Nursing records. I. Lippincott Williams & Wilkins.
[DNLM: 1. Nursing Records. 2. Documentation.
WY 100.5 C486 2010]
RT50.C483 2010
610.73 — dc22

               2009010577

Contents

Contributors and consultants

Katrina D. Allen, RN, MSN, CCRN
Nursing Faculty
Faulkner State Community College
Bay Minette, Ala.

Cheryl L. Brady, RN, MSN
Assistant Professor
Kent State University
Salem, Ohio

Marie O. Brewer, RN, LNC
Vice President
Clinical Services and Corporate Compliance
Tender Loving Care Home Health Services, Inc.
Hortense, Ga.

Joy L. Herzog, RN
Director of Nursing Services
LifeQuest Nursing Center
Quakertown, Pa.

Roseanne Hanlon Rafter, RN, MSN, GCNS-BC
Director, Professional Nursing Practice
Chestnut Hill Hospital
Philadelphia, Pa.

Susan M. Kilroy, RN, MS
Clinical Nurse Specialist
Massachusetts General Hospital
Boston, Mass.

Donna Ratcliff, RN, MSN
Director, Nursing Education
North Oakland Medical Centers
Pontiac, Mich.

Lauren R. Roach, LPN, HCS-D
Nurse Support Coordinator
Good Samaritan Home Care Services, LLC
Vincennes, Ind.

Marilyn D. Sellers, RN-BC, MS, FNP-BC
Family Nurse Practitioner
VAMC
Hampton, Va.

Leigh Ann Trujillo, RN, BSN
Nurse Educator
St. James Hospital and Health Center
Olympia Fields, Ill.

Not another boring foreword

If you're like me, you're too busy caring for your patients to have the time to wade through a foreword that uses pretentious terms and umpteen dull paragraphs to get to the point. So let's cut right to the chase! Here's why this book is so terrific:

1. It will teach you all the important things you need to know about charting. (And it will leave out all the fluff that wastes your time.)
2. It will help you remember what you've learned.
3. It will make you smile as it enhances your knowledge and skills.

Don't believe me? Try these recurring logos on for size:

 Case in point — Describes the nursing implications of real-life court cases in which documentation was key

 Advice from the experts — Offers tips, pointers, and guidelines galore to help make charting precise, patient-focused, and litigation-proof

 Art of the chart — Illustrates filled-in forms to help you understand exactly how to chart and why

 That's a wrap — Re-examines the key chapter points in a succinct, quick-review format

 Memory jogger — Reinforces learning through easy-to-remember anecdotes and mnemonics

See? I told you! And that's not all. Look for me and my friends in the margins throughout this book. We'll be there to explain key concepts, provide important care reminders, and offer reassurance. Oh, and if you don't mind, we'll be spicing up the pages with a bit of humor along the way, to teach and entertain in a way that no other resource can.

I hope you find this book helpful. Best of luck throughout your career!

Joy

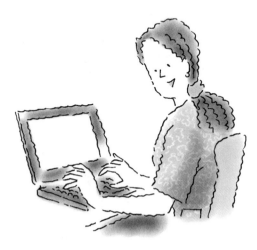

Part I Charting in contemporary health care

Understanding charting

Just the facts

In this chapter, you'll learn:

♦ the importance of charting

♦ the components of a medical record

♦ types of medical records.

A look at charting

Charting—or documentation—is the process of preparing a complete record of a patient's care. Accurate, detailed charting shows the extent and quality of the care you've provided, the outcome of that care, and treatment and education that the patient still needs.

Charting is a vital tool for communication among health care team members. Commonly, decisions, actions, and revisions related to the patient's care are based on charting from various team members. A well-prepared medical record shows the high degree of collaboration among health care team members.

You reach a wide audience

The information that's documented by team members must be easily retrievable and readable because a patient's medical record may be read by a wide audience, including:
• other members of the health care team
• reviewers from accrediting, certifying, and licensing organizations
• performance-improvement monitors
• peer reviewers
• Medicare and insurance company reviewers
• researchers and teachers
• lawyers and judges.

> Wow! Great charting! I can tell right away that the patient received thorough, high-quality care.

One of the most compelling reasons for you to develop good charting practices is to document that you've fulfilled your professional responsibility by meeting the standards of care.

A short history of charting

In the past, charting consisted of cursory observations, such as *patient ate well* or *patient slept well*. The chief purpose of these documents was to show that the doctor's orders and the facility's policies had been followed and that the patient had received the proper care.

In the 19th century, the British nurse Florence Nightingale paved the way for modern nursing documentation. In the book, *Notes on Nursing*, she stressed the importance of training nurses to gather patient information in a clear, concise, organized manner. As her theories gained acceptance, nurses' perceptions and observations about patient care gained credence and respect. More than a century later, in the 1970s, nurses began creating their own vocabulary for documentation based on nursing diagnoses.

The history of charting dates back to Florence Nightingale.

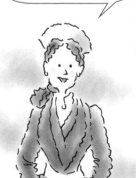

Role of charting

Accurate nursing documentation is important for many reasons:

- It's a mode of communication among health care professionals.
- It's checked in health care evaluations.
- It's legal evidence that protects you.
- It's used to aid research and education.
- It helps facilities obtain accreditation and licensure.
- It's used to justify reimbursement requests.
- It's used to develop improvements in the quality of care.
- It indicates compliance with the state nurse practice act.
- It establishes professional accountability.

Communication

Patients are cared for by many people who work different shifts, and these various caregivers may speak with each other infrequently. The medical record is the main source of information and communication among nurses, doctors, physical therapists, social workers, and other caregivers. Today, nurses are commonly considered managers of care as well as practitioners, and nurses usually document the most information. Everyone's notes are important, however, because together they present a complete picture of the patient's care.

A growing team

As health care facilities continue to streamline and redesign care delivery systems, tasks that were historically performed by nurses are now being assigned to multiskilled workers. To deliver highly specialized care, each caregiver must provide accurate, thorough information and be able to interpret what others have written about a patient. Then each can use this information to plan future patient care.

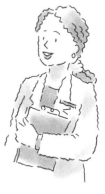

As nurses, we usually document the most information.

Health care evaluation

When health care is evaluated by reviewers, insurance companies, Medicare representatives, lawyers, or judges, accurate documentation is one way to prove that you're providing high-quality care. Complete documentation is a record of what you do for your patient and written evidence that this care is necessary. It's also a record of your patient's response to your care and any changes you make in his care plan.

Legal protection

On the legal side, accurate documentation shows that the care you provide meets the patient's needs and expressed wishes. It also proves that you're following the accepted standards of nursing care mandated by the law, your profession, and your health care facility.

The evidence speaks for itself

Proper documentation communicates crucial clinical information to caregivers so they make fewer errors. How and what you document can determine whether you or your employer wins or loses a legal dispute. Medical records are used as evidence in cases involving disability, personal injury, and mental competency. Poor documentation is the pivotal issue in many malpractice cases.

Just think, my charting may go to trial.

Research and education

Documentation also provides data for research and continuing education. For example, researchers and nurse-educators may study medical records to determine the effectiveness of care. Their scrutiny may also reveal ways to improve documentation, such as by revising existing computerized forms or creating more efficient forms. The need for simple, accurate point-of-care documentation encourages researchers to develop new technologies to improve communication between health care providers, improve patient safety, and optimize a nurse's time.

A reciprocal relationship

Researchers also review medical records to gauge how patient teaching affects compliance and how well the patient followed the treatment regimen. As a result, they may identify the need for patient teaching materials that are written more simply and clearly for those with limited formal education.

Accreditation and licensure

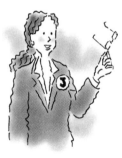

For a facility to remain accredited, caregivers must document care that reflects the care standards set by national organizations, such as the American Nurses Association and The Joint Commission. Some states also require facilities to be licensed; licensing laws, in turn, require each facility to establish policies and procedures for operation.

A facility's accreditation and licensure may be jeopardized by substandard documentation. Besides being complete and accurate, documentation must also be readable. (This requirement has driven many facilities to develop computerized systems.) When a facility is cited for having poor documentation or for not meeting set standards, a warning is given and a target date is set for the facility to make necessary changes and corrections. A facility may lose its license if these changes aren't accomplished.

Quality is key

In effect, accreditation is evidence that a facility provides quality care and is qualified to receive federal funds. The federal government works with state accrediting organizations to make sure facilities are eligible to receive Medicare reimbursement. Accreditation and reimbursement eligibility require documentation that accurately reflects the care provided to patients. Good charting demonstrates that facility and state nursing policies have been followed.

Getting what they deserve

How do officials of accrediting organizations decide if a facility should be accredited? They look at the facility's structure and function. They also conduct surveys and audits of patient records and medical records to see if care meets the required standards.

Track with a tracer

To conduct their survey, The Joint Commission surveyors use an evaluation method called *tracer methodology*. They select a patient and use that patient's record to evaluate the organization's compliance with required standards. As part of the process, they interview the patient and caregivers about the care the patient received on this visit as well as previous visits. The patient's self-reports of care are then compared to nursing and other clinical documentation. Patient-reported care must match clinician-documented care.

Charting clinical competence

Furthermore, surveyors use the medical record to determine whether the patient received competent care from all clinicians, including nurses. During the evaluation process, the surveyor seeks to identify any performance or system level issues that affected patient care.

Is that safe?

Patient safety and medical errors are a national concern. The first National Patient Safety Goals (NPSGs) were approved by The Joint Commission in July 2002. Effective January 1, 2008, accredited hospitals must show that the NPSGs are implemented in daily care. (See *2008 National Patient Safety Goals for hospitals*, page 8.)

Quality and consistency

Officials review charts and files to ensure good charting. For example, in a case where physical restraints were used, officials may ask, "Is there a form for charting the need for restraints and their correct use?" and "Does the documentation in the charts show that restraints were used correctly?" Proper charting reflects the quality of care provided and the facility's accountability.

Accrediting organizations also regularly survey and audit records to make sure the standard of care is consistent throughout a facility. For example, a woman who's recovering from anesthesia after a cesarean birth should expect to receive the same monitoring in the labor and delivery suite as she would in the postanesthesia care unit. The Joint Commission inspectors review the documentation of both departments to ensure that a uniform standard of care is given and documented. Most accrediting organizations have similar standards for documentation. (See *What's in a medical record?*, page 9)

> My charting reflects the quality of my patient care.

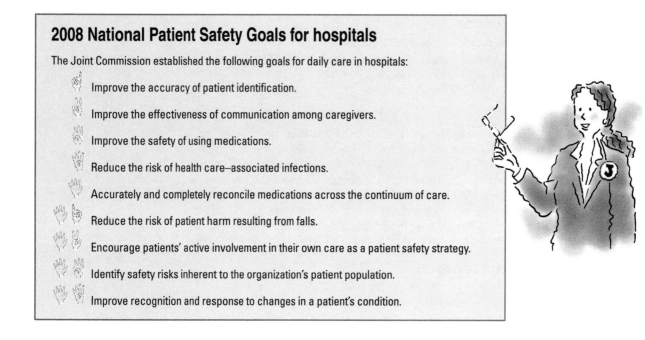

2008 National Patient Safety Goals for hospitals

The Joint Commission established the following goals for daily care in hospitals:

Improve the accuracy of patient identification.

Improve the effectiveness of communication among caregivers.

Improve the safety of using medications.

Reduce the risk of health care–associated infections.

Accurately and completely reconcile medications across the continuum of care.

Reduce the risk of patient harm resulting from falls.

Encourage patients' active involvement in their own care as a patient safety strategy.

Identify safety risks inherent to the organization's patient population.

Improve recognition and response to changes in a patient's condition.

Reimbursement

Reimbursement from Medicare and insurance companies depends heavily on accurate nursing documentation. For example, many hospitals today use elaborate electronic dispensing carts to keep track of supplies. Nursing documentation has to justify the use of these supplies to be reimbursed for them.

It's payback time...or is it?

Charting is also used to determine the amount of reimbursement a facility receives for care provided. The federal government, for example, uses a prospective payment system based on diagnosis-related groups (DRGs) to determine Medicare reimbursements. In other words, they pay a fixed amount for a particular diagnosis. For a facility to receive payment, the patient's medical record at discharge must contain the correct DRG codes and show that he received the proper care, including appropriate patient teaching and discharge planning.

Likewise, most insurance companies base reimbursements on a prospective payment system, and they usually don't reimburse for unskilled nursing care. They pay for skilled medical and nursing care only. For example, they compensate nurse practitioners and home health care nurses for skilled care, which includes

What's in a medical record?

Accrediting organizations require many of the same standards for documentation. For example, each patient's medical record must contain:
• identification data
• medical history, which includes the patient's chief complaint; details of his present illness; relevant past, social, and family histories; and a body-system assessment
• nursing assessment form
• assessment and summary of the patient's psychosocial and cultural identification needs as appropriate to the patient's age
• report of relevant physical examination findings
• statement of the impressions drawn from the admission history and physical examination
• the care plan

• diagnostic and therapeutic orders
• evidence of informed consent
• information on advanced directives
• clinical observations, including the effects of treatment
• progress notes
• consultation reports, if applicable
• reports of operative and other invasive procedures and tests and their results, if appropriate
• reports of diagnostic and therapeutic procedures, such as radiology and nuclear medicine examinations
• records of donation and receipt of transplants or implants, if applicable
• final diagnosis
• discharge summaries and instructions
• results of autopsy, when performed.

assessing a patient's condition, creating a care plan, and following a strict treatment regimen.

Examinations aren't just for patients

Before reimbursing, an examiner studies the patient's medical record to decide whether he needed and received skilled nursing care. The examiner may request copies of the patient's monthly bills and look at documented progress notes, especially if the intensity, frequency, and cost of the care increased.

Examiners also check for inconsistencies in charting, such as a discrepancy between the treatment ordered and the one provided. If the discrepancy isn't explained adequately, the insurer may deny payment.

Keeping the proper care going

In addition to keeping a facility from getting reimbursed, faulty documentation can keep patients from getting the care they need. For example, an insurer might deny payment to a home health care agency if the nurse's charting doesn't prove that home visits were necessary. If that happens, home health care may be discontinued prematurely.

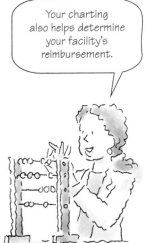

Your charting also helps determine your facility's reimbursement.

Performance improvement

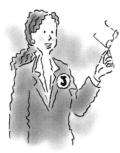

Individual states and The Joint Commission require all health care facilities to regularly monitor, evaluate, and seek ways to improve the quality of care for their patients. In each facility, a committee of doctors, nurses, pharmacists, administrators, and other employees gets together to develop performance improvement measures. Committee members then implement the measures, analyze the improvements, and report their findings to the facility's board of trustees.

Multidisciplinary committee members also develop methods to assess the structure, process, and outcome of patient care. One way to implement these methods is to monitor and evaluate the content of medical records.

Up to snuff?

What if the care described in a medical record doesn't meet an established standard? Performance improvement committee members must then decide how to correct this problem. They may assign a focus group to investigate ways to do this.

The focus group may recommend changes in the facility's policies, procedures, or documentation forms in an effort to improve patient care. For example, many facilities have been cited in court for lack of documentation when physical restraints were used. As a result, some facilities have developed forms to document restraint orders from doctors, which may be used in court as proof that the facility's policy was followed and that restraints were needed.

Nurse practice acts

Nurse practice acts are state laws spelling out what duties nurses can perform in that state. State nurse practice acts are revised frequently; when nurse practice acts change, charting requirements usually change as well. With laws and regulations in a constant state of flux, you must be especially meticulous about charting your care to show compliance with standards.

Accountability

Accurate nursing documentation is evidence that you acted as required or ordered. Accountability means you comply with the charting requirements of your health care facility, professional organizations, and state law.

Types of medical records

Medical records are kept for virtually every person who steps through the door of a health care facility. That's a lot of assessment forms, flow sheets, and lists to fill out. How can nurses deal with this responsibly?

An insightful record

Many nurses try to create order in medical records by organizing patient data by category. However, this practice emphasizes form instead of content. Remember, a medical record isn't just a summary of illness and recovery. It's an insightful record of a patient's care and potential patient care problems.

Forms are your friends

You can think of the medical record as an ally in your organization efforts. It's a place to organize your thoughts about patient care and record your actions. Used properly, it can help you save time, identify problem areas, plan better patient care, and avoid litigation. (See *Tips for fast, faultless charting*.)

Although every medical record provides evidence of the quality of patient care, not all records are alike. Some are organized by a source-oriented narrative method, some by a problem-oriented method, and others by variations of these two.

Tips for fast, faultless charting

When you document, you must record information quickly without sacrificing accuracy. Here are some actions you can take to help you accomplish these two goals:
- Follow the nursing process.
- Use nursing diagnoses.
- Use flow sheets.
- Document at the bedside.
- Individualize your charting.
- Don't repeat information (which could lead to errors).
- Sign off with your name and credentials.
- Don't document for other caregivers.
- Use computerized documentation.

Source-oriented narrative method

With the source-oriented narrative method, caregivers (the source) from each discipline record information in a separate section of the medical record.

Missing the complete picture?

This traditional method of documentation has several serious drawbacks: Because charting is done in various parts of the record, information is disjointed, topics aren't always clearly identified, and information is difficult to retrieve. These issues keep team members from getting a complete picture of the patient's care and cause breakdowns in communication.

Get on the same page

Collaboration among team members who use source-oriented narrative charting is more easily documented if everyone writes on the same progress notes. For example, doctors', nurses', and respiratory therapists' progress notes can be combined into what may be called patient progress notes. These notes serve as the primary source of reference and communication among health care team members.

Problem-oriented method

A problem-oriented medical record (POMR) contains baseline data obtained from all departments involved in a patient's care. The problem-oriented charting method is based on the patient's chief complaint. Data include:
• patient's health history, including his medical, social, and emotional status
• other initial assessment findings
• diagnostic test results.
    The POMR also contains:
• problem list
• care plan for each problem
• progress notes.
    The problem list is distilled from baseline data and used to construct a care plan. (See *Got a problem?*)

Focusing on each problem

The care plan in a POMR addresses each of the patient's problems, which are routinely updated in the plan and the progress notes. (See *A close look at a medical record*, page 14.)

Art of the chart

Got a problem?

The chart below shows a nursing problem list for a patient with acute pancreatitis.

#	Date	Problem statement	Initials	Resolved
1	9/4/09	Deficient fluid volume related to vomiting	C.B.	
2	9/4/09	Acute pain related to physiologic factors	C.B.	
3	9/4/09	Imbalanced nutrition: Less than body requirements related to inability to digest nutrients	C.B.	
4	9/4/09	Ineffective tissue perfusion (GI) related to decreased cellular exchange	C.B.	
5	9/4/09	Ineffective coping related to situational crisis	B.A.	

Other medical record formats

Some facilities modify the source-oriented or problem-oriented method of documentation to suit their needs. If your facility does this, you're in a position to influence the type and style of documentation you use in medical records.

Designer documentation

For example, home health care nurses have created many specialized documentation forms — including an initial assessment form, problem list, day-visit sheet, and discharge summary — to reflect the unique services and the essential quality of care they provide. These forms meet their charting needs while complying with state and federal laws and other regulations. (See *Specialized forms,* page 15.)

> Whatever format you use, charting should reflect the quality of nursing care you deliver.

A close look at a medical record

Although each health care facility has its own system for keeping medical records, most records contain the documents described here:

• face sheet—first page of the medical record; contains the patient's name, birth date, social security number, address, marital status, closest relative or guardian, food and drug allergies, admitting diagnosis, and attending doctor

• general consent-to-treat form

• advance directives—living will, medical power of attorney, do-not-resuscitate order, and end-of-life decisions

• medical history and physical examination—completed by the doctor; contains the initial medical examination and evaluation data

• doctor's order sheet—a record of the doctor's medical orders

• initial nursing assessment form—contains nursing data, including health history, physical assessment findings, and cultural and psychosocial needs

• integrated assessment form—assessment form used by all members of the health care team

• problem or nursing diagnosis list—lists the patient's problems; used with problem-oriented medical records

• nursing care plan—based on information gathered during patient assessment; specifies patient care needs, planned interventions, and the patient's progress toward meeting goals and objectives

• graphic form—flow sheet that tracks the patient's temperature, pulse, respiratory rate, blood pressure and, possibly, daily weight; also may include skin care, blood glucose levels, urinalysis results, neurologic assessment data, and patient intake and output; the nurse dates, initials, or checks off the appropriate column to show a task was completed

• medication administration record—lists medications the patient receives, including dosage, administration route, site, date, and time

• nurse's progress notes—details patient care information, nursing interventions, and patient responses

• doctor's progress notes—contains doctors' observations, notes on the patient's progress, and treatment data

• diagnostic findings—contains diagnostic and laboratory data

• health care team records—includes information from the physical therapist, the respiratory therapist, the social worker, and other team members

• consultation sheets—includes evaluations by specialists consulted for diagnostic and treatment recommendations

• discharge plan and summary—presents a brief account of the patient's time in the facility and care plans after discharge.

Computerized charting

Computerized charting is popular for completing medical records from admission through discharge. Some of the benefits of computerized documentation are listed here:

• It promotes standardization.

• Legibility problems that accompany handwritten entries are eliminated.

Art of the chart

Specialized forms

The form shown below is an example of a specialized form that may be developed by registered nurses, licensed practical nurses, and mental health technicians to target the essential elements of charting on their unit.

Behavioral Services Department　　　　　　　　　　　　**Patient Stamp**

SIP _I _II _III
[ ] Pt suicidal
[ ] Pt has plan
[ ] Pt is homicidal
[ ] Pt has plan
Affect _____ *flat* _____
ADLs __ good __ fair _✓_ poor
[✓] Pt made contact
　[ ] did not make contact
[✓] Pt attended groups
　[ ] did not attend groups
　[✓] attended some groups
[ ] Pt compliant with SA program
[ ] Pt socializing with peers
[ ] Pt seclusive/withdrawn
[✓] Pt select interacting
[ ] Pt hostile
[✓] Pt ate breakfast _10%_
[✓] Pt ate lunch _____ _25%_
[ ] Pt ate snack
[✓] Pt had BM
　[ ] No BM _____ days
　[ ] action taken_____
[✓] Dual diagnosis track
[ ] Compliant with SA groups
[✓] Med. seeking
[ ] Consultation completed

NURSE'S NOTES

Date: *9/11/09*

72 hr notice
Time _____
Dr. notified _____
Notice rescinded _____

> This checklist targets key assessment and evaluation parameters.

7-3 SHIFT　　　　☐ **Admission Note**　　　☑ **Nursing Problem**

9/11/09 0930. Ineffective coping related to alcohol abuse and wife leaving him.
Denies that alcohol is a problem. States, "I only drank more lately because she left me.
I drink because I want to, not because I have to." ——————— M. Carson, rn
9/11/09 1400. Went to 1100 A.A. meeting. Stated, "I don't want to be with other
people now." Went to room to rest. ——————— M. Carson, RN

- Fewer errors may be made.
- It leads to decreased recording time and costs.
- Communication among team members is aided.
- It allows easier access to medical data for education, research, and performance improvement.

They even have good bedside manners

Information filed on computers includes nursing care plans, progress notes, medication records, records of vital signs, intake and output sheets, and patient classifications. Some facilities even have bedside computers for quick data entry and access. (See *Super-successful automated charting.*)

One of the drawbacks of computerized charting is the potential for unauthorized personnel to access confidential medical records. However, the electronic security provisions of the Health Insurance Portability and Accountability Act of 1996 (HIPAA) are meant to prevent this from occurring. These provisions prohibit clinicians from using facility computers for recreation, shopping, or other pursuits not related to patient care. Refraining from these activities will help safeguard computers from computer viruses that could allow unauthorized access to confidential information.

For more information about computerized documentation, see chapter 5, *Computerized charting.*

Now, you're supposed to make charting easier.

That's a wrap!

Review of charting basics

Roles of charting
- Serves as a medium of communication for the health care team
- Can be used in health care evaluations
- Serves as legal evidence
- Can be used to aid research and education
- Helps facilities obtain accreditation and licensure
- Provides justification for reimbursement
- Is used to develop improvements in the quality of care
- Indicates compliance with your state's nurse practice act
- Establishes professional accountability

Types of medical records
- Source-oriented — has separate sections for each discipline's documentation, which keeps team members from getting the complete picture and breaks down communication
- Problem-oriented — is based on the patient's chief complaint and contains baseline data from all departments

Computerized charting
- Promotes standardization
- Eliminates legibility problems
- Leads to decreased recording time and costs
- Aids team communication
- Allows easier access to medical data

Advice from the experts

Super-successful automated charting

To be effective, an automated charting system must:
- record and send data to the appropriate department
- adapt easily to the health care facility's needs
- display highly selective information on command
- provide easy access and retrieval for all trained personnel.

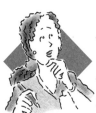

Quick quiz

1. The main drawback to source-oriented narrative records is that they:
    A.   are problem oriented.
    B.   require a baseline assessment.
    C.   require each discipline to record information on a separate section of the record.
    D.   require nurses to chart in the same section as other disciplines.

Answer: C. This type of charting causes communication breakdowns because information is disjointed and hard to retrieve, topics aren't always clearly identified, and team members can't easily get a complete picture of the patient's care.

2. One benefit of computerized charting is that:
    A.   it minimizes the number of forms to be completed.
    B.   it promotes individualization of the medical record.
    C.   it improves legibility.
    D.   it increases cost.

Answer: C. Computers eliminate legibility problems that accompany handwritten entries.

3. The Joint Commission regulates standards of care to:
    A.   make sure that all nurses use the same charting system.
    B.   ensure quality patient care.
    C.   ensure subjective documentation.
    D.   make sure insurance companies get paid correctly.

Answer: B. To meet The Joint Commission standards, facilities must uphold certain levels of quality in patient care.

4. Nursing documentation as we know it today was first used in what time period?
    A.   1970s
    B.   19th century
    C.   18th century
    D.   17th century

Answer: B. Florence Nightingale established modern nursing documentation in the 19th century.

5. Which part of the medical record can be used as evidence in court?

    A.   The care plan
    B.   The medical orders
    C.   The entire record
    D.   Nursing notes

Answer: C. The entire medical record is a legal document that's admissible in court.

Scoring

☆☆☆ If you answered all five questions correctly, fantastic! You're clear, concise, and consistent — a charting champion.

☆☆ If you answered four questions correctly, dandy! Your documentation definitely deserves to be accredited.

☆ If you answered fewer than four questions correctly, don't worry! With a little review, your recording will reap regular reimbursement.

The nursing process

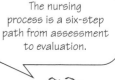

Just the facts

In this chapter, you'll learn:

♦ guidelines for performing an assessment based on the nursing process

♦ methods for formulating a nursing diagnosis

♦ ways to write nursing care plans with expected outcomes and appropriate interventions

♦ evaluation and documentation of nursing interventions and outcomes.

A look at the nursing process

The nursing process is a problem-solving approach to nursing care. It's a systematic method for determining the patient's health problems, devising a care plan to address them, implementing the plan, and evaluating the effectiveness of the care provided.

The nursing process emerged in the 1960s, as team health care came into wider practice and nurses were increasingly called on to define their specific roles. The roots of the nursing process can be traced to World War II, however, when technology, medical advances, and a growing need for nurses began to change the nursing profession.

Going through the phases

The nursing process consists of six distinct phases:

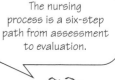 assessment

nursing diagnosis

> The nursing process is a six-step path from assessment to evaluation.

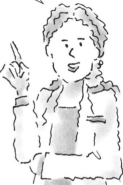

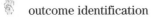 outcome identification

planning care

implementation

evaluation.

These six phases are dynamic and flexible, and they commonly overlap. Together, they resemble the steps that many other professions take to identify and correct problems.

Assessment

The first step in the nursing process—assessment—begins when you first see a patient. Assessment continues throughout the patient's hospitalization as you obtain more information about his changing condition.

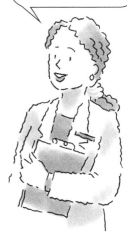

The assessment data that I collect establish the basis for the rest of the nursing process.

Getting the whole picture

During assessment, you collect relevant information from various sources and analyze it to form a complete picture of your patient. As you collect this information, you need to document it accurately for two reasons:
• It guides you through the rest of the nursing process, helping you formulate nursing diagnoses, expected outcomes, and nursing interventions.
• It serves as a vital communication tool for other team members and as a baseline for evaluating a patient's progress.

The information that you gather at the first patient contact may indicate that the patient needs a broader or more detailed assessment such as a nutritional assessment. (See *Assessing nutritional status.*)

Further assessment depends on the:
• patient's diagnosis
• care setting
• patient's consent to treatment
• care the patient is seeking
• patient's response to previous care.

First impressions

In your initial assessment, consider the patient's immediate and emerging needs, including not only his physical needs but also his psychological, spiritual, and social concerns. The initial assessment helps you determine what care the patient needs and sets the stage for further assessments. Remember that a patient's family, culture, and religion are important factors in the patient's response to illness and treatment.

Begin your assessment by collecting a health history and conducting a physical examination.

Health history

The health history includes physical, psychological, cultural, spiritual, and psychosocial data. It's the main source of information about the patient's health status and guides the physical examination that follows.

A nursing history is different from a medical history. A medical history guides diagnosis and treatment of illness; a nursing history focuses holistically on the human response to illness.

The nursing history you collect helps you:
• plan health care
• assess the impact of illness on the patient and members of his family
• evaluate the patient's health education needs
• initiate discharge planning.

Getting started

Although nurses conduct health histories in different ways, all interviews must progress in a logical sequence and the nurse must record the patient's response in an organized way.

Before conducting the health history, consider the patient's ability to participate. If he's sedated, confused, hostile, angry, dyspneic, or in pain, ask only the most essential questions. Then perform an in-depth interview later. In the meantime, ask family members or close friends to provide some information.

Get off on the right foot by finding a quiet, private space where the patient feels as comfortable and relaxed as possible. Ask another nurse to cover your other patients so you won't be interrupted. This reassures the patient that you're interested in what he says and that you'll keep the information confidential. (See *Health history lessons*, page 22.)

Making the most of your time

Finding time to conduct a thorough patient history can be hard. However, a few strategies can help you keep interview time to a minimum without sacrificing quality. (See *Health history in a hurry*, page 23.)

Sometimes an interview isn't even necessary — you can simply ask the patient to complete a questionnaire about his past and present health status. Then you can quickly and easily document the

---

Assessing nutritional status

As part of the admission assessment, the answers to some questions automatically call for another discipline to be consulted. An example is in the nutrition section.

With the following questions, one "no" requires a nutritional consult:
• Do you have sufficient funds to buy food?
• Do you have access to a food market?
• Can you shop, cook, and feed yourself?

With the following questions, one "yes" requires a nutritional consult:
• Do you have an illness or condition that made you change the amount or kind of food you eat?
• Do you have dental or mouth problems that make it difficult for you to chew or swallow food?
• Do you need help getting to a food market?
• Have you lost or gained 10 lb within the last 6 months without trying?

patient's health history by reviewing the information on the questionnaire and filing it in the patient's chart.

This method is most successful for patients who are to undergo short or elective procedures. The questionnaire can be completed before the patient's admission, which can save you time.

In some acute care settings, modified questionnaires are used to evaluate language or reading problems the patient may have. The nurse then reviews sections that are completed by the patient.

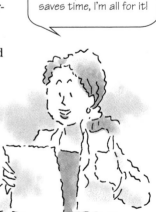

If a questionnaire saves time, I'm all for it!

Physical examination

The second half of the assessment process involves performing a physical examination. Use the following techniques to conduct the examination:
- inspection
- palpation

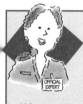

Advice from the experts

Health history in a hurry

When you're pressed for time, use the following tips to speed up health history documentation:

• Before the interview, fill in as much information as you can from admission forms, transfer summaries, and the medical history to avoid duplicating efforts. If information isn't clear, ask the patient for more details. For instance, you might say, "You told Dr. Brown that you sometimes feel like you can't catch your breath. Can you tell me more about when this happens?"

• Check your facility's policy on who may gather assessment data. Maybe you can have an unlicensed nursing assistant or technician collect routine information, such as allergies and past hospitalizations. Remember, however, that reviewing and verifying the information is your responsibility.

• Begin by asking about the patient's chief complaint. Then, even if the interview is interrupted, you'll still be able to write a care plan.

• Use your facility's nursing assessment documentation form only as a guide to organize information. Ask your patient only pertinent questions from the form.

• Take only brief notes during the interview, so you don't interrupt the flow of conversation. Write detailed notes as soon as possible after the interview. You can always go back to the patient if you need to clarify or verify information.

• Record your findings in concise, specific phrases.

• Use only approved abbreviations, symbols, and acronyms. Review your facility's policy and The Joint Commission's "do not use" abbreviation list. (See chapter 6, pages 117 to 120, for more information.)

 • percussion
 • auscultation.

The objective data you gather during the physical examination may be used to confirm or rule out health problems that were suggested or suspected during the health history. You rely on these findings when you develop a care plan and when you conduct patient teaching. For example, if the patient's blood pressure is high, he may need a sodium-restricted diet and instruction on how to control hypertension.

It's in the details

How detailed should your examination be? That depends on the patient's condition, the clinical setting, and the policies and procedures established by your health care facility. The main components of the physical examination include:
 • height
 • weight
 • vital signs
 • review of the major body systems. (See *Rapid review of the physical assessment,* page 24.)

Advice from the experts

Rapid review of the physical assessment

During a physical examination, your main task is to record the patient's height, weight, and vital signs and review the major body systems. Here's a typical body system review for an adult patient.

Respiratory system

Note the rate and rhythm of respirations, and auscultate the lung fields. Watch for flaring or retractions as the patient breathes. Inspect the lips, mucous membranes, and nail beds. Also inspect the sputum, noting color, consistency, and other characteristics.

Cardiovascular system

Note the color and temperature of the extremities, and assess the peripheral pulses. Check for edema and hair loss on the extremities. Inspect the neck veins and auscultate for heart sounds and regularity.

Neurologic system

Assess the patient's level of consciousness, noting his orientation to time, place, and person and his ability to follow commands. Also assess pupillary reactions. Check the extremities for movement and sensation.

Eyes, ears, nose, and throat

Assess the patient's ability to see objects with and without corrective lenses. Assess his ability to hear spoken words clearly. Inspect the eyes and ears for discharge and the nasal mucous membranes for dryness, irritation, and blood. Inspect the teeth, gums, and condition of the oral mucous membranes and palpate the lymph nodes in the neck.

GI system

Auscultate for bowel sounds in all quadrants. Note abdominal distention or ascites. Gently palpate the abdomen for tenderness. Note whether the abdomen is soft, hard, or distended. Assess the condition of the mucous membranes around the anus.

Musculoskeletal system

Assess the range of motion of major joints. Look for swelling at the joints, contractures, muscle atrophy, or obvious deformity. Assess muscle strength of the trunk and extremities.

Genitourinary and reproductive systems

Note any bladder distention or incontinence. If indicated, inspect the genitalia for rashes, edema, or deformity. (Inspection of the genitalia may be waived at the patient's request or if no dysfunction was reported during the interview.) If indicated, inspect the genitalia for sexual maturity. Also examine the breasts, noting any abnormalities.

Integumentary system

Note any sores, lesions, scars, pressure ulcers, rashes, bruises, discoloration, or petechiae. Also note the patient's skin turgor.

The Joint Commission standards

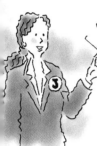

Under the standards of The Joint Commission, your initial assessment of the patient should consider:
- *physical factors*
- *psychological, social, and cultural factors*
- *nutritional and hydration status*
- *environmental factors*
- *self-care capabilities*
- *learning needs*
- *discharge planning needs*
- *input from the patient's family and friends when appropriate.*

Physical factors

Physical factors include the physical examination findings from your review of the patient's major body systems.

Psychological, social, and cultural factors

The patient's fears, anxieties, and other concerns about hospitalization are psychological, social, and cultural factors. (See *Identifying your patient's cultural needs*, pages 26 to 28.)

Family matters

Find out what support systems the patient has by asking such questions as, "How does being in the hospital affect your home situation or financial needs?" A patient who's worried about his family or finances might be less able or willing to comply with treatment. Also, find out if being in the hospital is disrupting the patient's religious or cultural practices.

Environmental factors

The patient's home environment affects care needs during hospitalization and after discharge. Factors to ask about may include:
- where he lives and the type of housing (house or apartment)
- whether he has adequate heat, ventilation, hot water, and bathroom facilities
- how many flights of stairs he has to climb
- whether the layout of his home poses any hazards
- whether his home is convenient to stores and doctors' offices.

Is the patient well-equipped?

In addition, ask if he uses equipment that isn't available in the hospital when he performs activities of daily living (ADLs) at home. Tailor your questions to his condition.

(Text continues on page 29.)

Identifying your patient's cultural needs

A transcultural assessment tool can help promote cultural sensitivity in any nursing setting. Consult your facility's policy on the use of such forms, or incorporate the information included in this sample form when developing your patient's care plan.

Date _5/1/09_ **Time** _1015_ **Pt name** _Claudette Valiente_ **Age** _34_ ☐ M ☑ F
Medical dx: _36 weeks pregnant, states "high sugar in my blood"_

Communication (language, voice quality, pronunciation, use of silence and nonverbals)
Subjective data
Can you speak English? ☑ Yes ☐ No
Can you read English? ☑ Yes ☐ No _with difficulty_
Are you able to read lips? ☐ Yes ☑ No
Native language? _Creole_
Do you speak or read any other language? _No_
How do you want to be addressed? ☐ Mr. ☐ Mrs. ☐ Ms. ☑ First name ☐ Nickname

Objective data
How would you characterize the nonverbal communication style? _Very open_
Eye contact: ☐ Direct ☑ Peripheral gaze or no eye contact preferred during interactions
Use of interpreter: ☐ Family ☐ Friend ☐ Professional ☐ Other ☑ None
Overall communication style: ☑ Verbally loud and expressive ☐ Quiet, reserved ☐ Use of silence
Meaning of common signs—O.K., got ya nose, index finger summons, V sign, thumbs up
   Understands above signs except "got ya nose"
Determine any familial colloquialisms used by individuals or families that may impact on assessment, treatment, or
other interventions. _None noted_

Social orientation (culture, race, ethnicity, family role function, work, leisure, church, and friends)
Subjective data
Country of birth? _Haiti_ Years in this country? _3_
(If an immigrant or a refugee, how long has the patient lived in this country? —You are not questioning citizen status.)
What setting did you grow up in? ☐ Urban ☐ Suburban ☑ Rural
What is your ethnic identity? _Haitian_
Who are the major support people? ☑ Family members ☐ Friends ☐ Other
Who are the dominant family members? _Husband, grandparents_
Who makes major decisions for the family? _A family meeting is held_
Occupation in native country? _None_ Present occupation? _None_
Education? _Finished 6th grade_
Is religion important to you? _Yes_
What is your religious affiliation? _Catholic_ Would you like a chaplain visit? ☐ Yes ☑ No
Any cultural/religious practices/restrictions? If yes, describe _Balancing "hot" and "cold," believes in some_
voodoo passed down from mother and grandmother

Identifying your patient's cultural needs (continued)

Social orientation (continued)

Objective data

Interaction with family/significant other — describe   *Animated, physically close, frequent touch, eye contact with family members*

Age and life cycle factors must be considered in interactions with individuals and families (for example, high value placed on the decision of elders, the role of the eldest man or woman in the family or roles and expectation of children within the family).   *Elders highly respected, children expected to be obedient and respectful*

Religious icons on person or in room?   *Wearing cross*

Space (comfort in conversation, proximity to others, body movement, perception of space)

Subjective data

Do you have any plans for the future?   *No, believes God will guide her*

What do you consider a proper greeting?   *Kissing and touch with family*

Objective data

☑ Tactile relationships, affectionate & embracing

☐ Non-contact

Personal space   *Very close with family, maintains 2–3 foot distance from RN*

Biological variations (skin color, body structure, genetic and enzymatic patterns, nutritional preferences and deficiencies)

Subjective data

What type of food do you prefer?   *Rice, beans, plantains*

What type of food do you dislike?   *Yogurt, cottage cheese*

What do you believe promotes health?   *Good spiritual habits, balancing "hot" and "cold," and eating well*

Family history of disease?   *Malaria, high blood pressure, "sugar"*

Objective data

Skin color   *Deep brown*   Hair type   *Coarse*

Environmental control (health practices, values, definitions of health and illness)

Subjective data

What do you think caused your problem?   *"Ate wrong foods."*

Do you have an explanation for why it started when it did?   *"No."*

What does your sickness do to you; how does it work?   *"I don't think anything is wrong, but the doctor does."*

How severe is your sickness? How long do you expect it to last?   *"It will go away soon."*

(continued)

Identifying your patient's cultural needs *(continued)*

Environmental control *(continued)*

Subjective data *(continued)*

What problems has your sickness caused you? *"The doctor says my baby is big. But, a big baby is a strong baby."*

What fears do you have about your sickness? *"I have no fear. I will have a healthy baby."*

What kind of treatment do you think you should receive? *"Eating healthy."*

What are the most important results you hope to receive from this treatment? *"A healthy baby."*

What are the health and illness beliefs and practices of the family? *Uses home remedies such as herbs to treat sickness*

What are the most important things you do to keep healthy? *"Eat well."*

Any concerns about health and illness? *"No."*

What types of healing practices do you engage in (hot tea and lemon for cold, copper bracelet for arthritis, magnets)? *"Avoiding spices because they bother the baby, balancing hot and cold"*

Objective data

Describe patient's appearance and surroundings *Patient is clean and neatly groomed. Appears slightly overweight.*

What diseases/disorders are endemic to the culture or country of origin? *Intestinal problems, malnutrition, STDs, TB, sickle cell anemia, htn, cancer, AIDs*

What are the customs and beliefs concerning major life events? *Pregnant women are treated as special. Father of the baby doesn't participate in the birth experience; this is "women's business."*

Time (use of measures, definitions, social and work time, time orientation — past, present, and future)

Subjective data

Preventative health measures? ☐ Yes ☑ No

Objective data

Time orientation ☐ Present ☑ Past

History of noncompliance, missed appointments *Often misses appts or arrives late*

Art of the chart

Discharge assessment questions

The sample discharge assessment form below is one section of the nursing admission assessment form.

Discharge planning needs

Living arrangements/caregiver:_____ *Sara Smith (patient's daughter)*_____

Type of dwelling: Apartment _____ House _✓_ Nursing home _____ Boarding home _____ Other _____

Physical barriers in home: No _____ Yes _✓_ Explain: *12-step flight of stairs to bathroom and bedroom*

Access to follow-up medical care: Yes _✓_ No _____ Explain: _____

Ability to carry out ADLs: Self-care _____ Partial assistance _____ Total assistance _✓_

Needs help with: Bathing _✓_ Eating _✓_ Ambulation _✓_ Other_____

Anticipated discharge destination: Home _____ Rehab _____ Nursing home _✓_ Skilled nursing facility _____

Boarding home _____ Other _____

Self-care capabilities

A patient's ability to perform ADLs affects how well he complies with therapy before and after discharge. Assess your patient's ability to eat, wash, dress, use the bathroom, turn in bed, get out of bed, and get around. Some facilities use an ADL checklist to indicate if a patient can perform these tasks independently or if he needs assistance.

Learning needs

Deciding early what your patient needs to know about his condition leads to effective patient teaching. During the initial assessment, evaluate your patient's knowledge of the disease process, self-care, diet, medications, lifestyle changes, treatment measures, and limitations caused by the disease or treatment.

No yes-or-no answers, please

One way to evaluate your patient's learning needs is to ask open-ended questions, such as "What do you know about the medicine you take?" His response will tell you if he understands and complies with his medication regimen or if he needs more teaching.

Learning obstacles

You should also assess factors that can hinder learning, which can result from the patient's:
- illness, injury, or physical disability
- health beliefs
- religious beliefs
- educational level
- cognitive disorder
- developmental disability
- sensory deficits such as hearing problems
- language barriers
- stress level
- age
- pain or discomfort
- cultural norms (may affect who the patient will take instruction from).

Discharge planning needs

Discharge planning should also start as soon as possible (in some cases, even before admission), especially if the patient needs help after discharge. Find out where the patient will go after discharge. Is follow-up care accessible? Is there a caregiver who will be available to assist the patient? Are community resources, such as visiting nurse services and Meals On Wheels, available where he lives? If not, you need time to help the patient make other arrangements. (See *Discharge assessment questions*, page 29.)

Prioritize, prioritize, prioritize

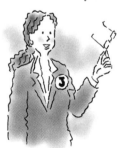

Because inpatient lengths of stay have become shorter and patient care has become increasingly complex, nurses must prioritize their assessment data. (See *Establishing priorities for patient assessment.*)

Input from family and friends

Another Joint Commission requirement is that you obtain assessment information from the patient's family and friends, when appropriate. When you interview someone other than the patient, be sure to document the nature of the relationship. If the interviewee isn't a family member, ask about and record the length of time the person has known the patient.

Advice from the experts

Establishing priorities for patient assessment

After completion of an initial assessment, The Joint Commission requires nurses to use the gathered information in prioritizing their care decisions. To systematically set priorities, follow these steps:
- Identify the patient's problems.
- Identify the patient's risk of injury.
- Identify the patient's need for help with self-care in the hospital and following discharge.
- Identify the educational needs of the patient and members of his family.

Nursing diagnosis

Your assessment findings form the basis for the next step in the nursing process: the nursing diagnosis. According to NANDA International (NANDA-I), a nursing diagnosis is a clinical judgment about individual, family, or community responses to actual or potential health problems or life processes. Nursing diagnoses are used in selecting nursing interventions to achieve outcomes for which the nurse is accountable.

Diagnosing a diagnosis

Each nursing diagnosis describes an actual or potential health problem that a nurse can legally manage. A diagnosis usually has three components:

☝ the human response or problem — an actual or potential problem that can be affected by nursing care

✌ related factors — factors that may precede, contribute to, or be associated with the human response

🖖 signs and symptoms — defining characteristics that lead to the diagnosis.

One patient, two types of treatment

When you become familiar with nursing diagnoses, you'll clearly see how nursing practice and medical practice differ. Although problems are identified in nursing and medicine, medical and nursing treatment approaches are very different.

The main difference is that doctors are licensed to diagnose and treat illnesses, and nurses are licensed to diagnose and treat the patient's *response* to illness. Nurses can also diagnose the need for patient education, offer comfort and counsel to patients and families, and care for patients until they're physically and emotionally ready to provide self-care.

Emergencies get top billing

Whenever you develop nursing diagnoses, you must prioritize them. Then begin your care plan with the highest priority. *High-priority* diagnoses involve emergency or immediate physical care needs. *Intermediate-priority* diagnoses involve nonemergency needs, and *low-priority* diagnoses involve peripheral needs or those related to enhanced functioning or wellness. Maslow's hierarchy of needs can help you set priorities in your care plan. (See *Maslow's pyramid*, page 32.)

Maslow's pyramid

To formulate nursing diagnoses, you must know your patient's needs and values. Maslow's pyramid (shown below) illustrates those needs. Of course, physiologic needs—represented by the base of the pyramid in the diagram below—must be met first.

Self-actualization
Recognition and realization of one's potential, growth, health, and autonomy

Self-esteem
Sense of self-worth, self-respect, independence, dignity, privacy, self-reliance

Love and belonging
Affiliation, affection, intimacy, support, reassurance

Safety and security
Safety from physiologic and psychological threat, protection, continuity, stability, lack of danger

Physiologic needs
Oxygen, food, elimination, temperature control, sex, movement, rest, comfort

Outcome identification

The goal of your nursing care is to help your patient reach his highest functional level with minimal risk and problems. If he can't recover completely, your care should help him cope physically and emotionally with his impaired or declining health.

Keeping it real

With this goal in mind, you should identify realistic, measurable expected outcomes and corresponding target dates for your patient. Expected outcomes are goals the patient should reach as a result of planned nursing interventions. Sometimes, a nursing diagnosis requires more than one expected outcome.

An outcome can specify an improvement in the patient's ability to function—for example, an increase in the distance he can walk—or it can specify the correction of a problem such as a reduction of pain. In either case, each outcome calls for the maximum realistic improvement for a particular patient.

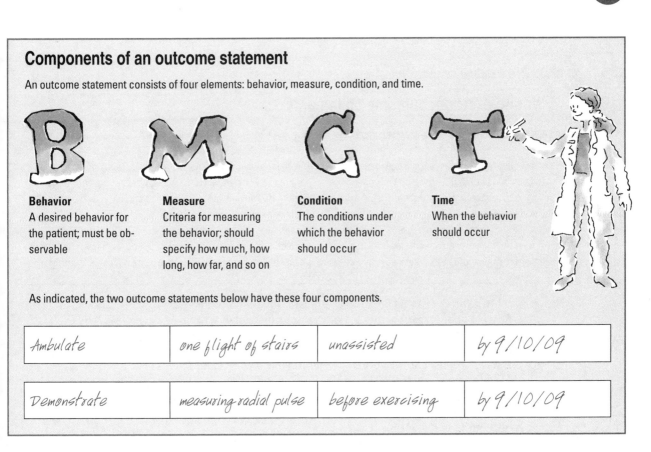

Components of an outcome statement

An outcome statement consists of four elements: behavior, measure, condition, and time.

Behavior
A desired behavior for the patient; must be observable

Measure
Criteria for measuring the behavior; should specify how much, how long, how far, and so on

Condition
The conditions under which the behavior should occur

Time
When the behavior should occur

As indicated, the two outcome statements below have these four components.

| Ambulate | one flight of stairs | unassisted | by 9/10/09 |
| Demonstrate | measuring radial pulse | before exercising | by 9/10/09 |

Four-part format

An outcome statement consists of four parts:

1. specific behavior that shows the patient has reached his goal

2. criteria for measuring that behavior

3. conditions under which the behavior should occur

4. when the behavior should occur. (See *Components of an outcome statement.*)

Writing outcome statements

Save time when writing outcome statements by choosing your words carefully and being clear and concise. (See *Writing excellent outcome statements*, page 34.)

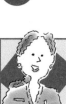

Advice from the experts

Writing excellent outcome statements

The following tips will help you write clear, precise outcome statements:

• When writing expected outcomes in your care plan, always start with a specific action verb that focuses on your patient's behavior. By telling your reader how your patient should *look, walk, eat, drink, turn, cough, speak,* or *stand,* for example, you give a clear picture of how to evaluate progress.

• Avoid starting expected outcome statements with *allow, let, enable,* or similar verbs. Such words focus attention on your own and other health team members' behavior—not on the patient's.

• With many documentation formats, you won't need to include the phrase *The patient will...* with each expected outcome statement. You will, however, have to specify which person the goals refer to when family, friends, or others are directly concerned.

• Include realistic target dates for outcomes to help the patient and all health care team members track the patient's progress.

Here are some tips for writing efficient outcome statements:

• Avoid unnecessary words—For example, instead of writing *Pt will demonstrate correct wound-care technique by 11/1,* drop the first two words. Everyone knows you're talking about the patient.

• Use accepted abbreviations—Refer to your facility's and The Joint Commission's official "Do Not Use" abbreviation lists. If it uses relative dates (describes the patient's stay in day-long intervals), use abbreviations such as *HD1* for hospital day 1 or *POD 2* for postoperative day 2.

• Make your statements specific—*Understand relaxation techniques* doesn't tell you much; how do you observe a patient's understanding? Instead, *Practice progressive muscle relaxation techniques unassisted for 15 minutes daily by 4/9* tells you exactly what to look for when assessing the patient's progress.

• Focus on the patient—Outcome statements should reflect the patient's behavior, not your intervention. *Medication brings chest pain relief* doesn't say anything about behavior. A correct statement would be *Express relief of chest pain within 1 hour of receiving medication.*

• Let the patient help you—A patient who helps write his outcome statements is more motivated to achieve his goals. His input, along with family member input, can help you set realistic goals.

• Consider medical orders—Don't write outcome statements that ignore or contradict medical orders. For example, before writing *Ambulate 10' unassisted twice a day by 11/9,* make sure that the medical orders don't call for more restricted activity, such as bed rest.

• Adapt the outcome to the circumstances—Consider the patient's coping ability, age, education, cultural influences, family support, living conditions, socioeconomic status, and anticipated

> These guidelines will help you write great outcome statements.

Advice from the experts

Tips for top-notch care plans

Use either a traditional or standardized method for recording your care plan. A traditional care plan is written from scratch for each patient. A standardized care plan saves time because it's predetermined, based on the patient's diagnosis.

No matter which method you use, follow these tips to write a plan that's accurate and useful:

• Write in ink, sign your name, and include the date.
• Use clear, concise language, not vague terms or generalities.
• Use standard abbreviations to avoid confusion.
• Review all your assessment data *before* selecting an approach for each problem. If you can't complete the initial assessment, immediately write *insufficient information* on your records.
• Write an expected outcome and a target date for each problem you identify.

• Set realistic initial goals.
• When writing nursing interventions, consider what to watch for and how often, what nursing measures to take and how to perform them, and what to teach the patient and family before discharge.
• Make each nursing intervention specific.
• Avoid duplicating or restating existing medical or nursing interventions.
• Make sure your interventions match the resources and capabilities of the staff.
• Be creative; include a drawing or an innovative procedure if this makes your directions more specific.
• Record all of the patient's problems and concerns so they won't be forgotten.
• Make sure your plan is implemented correctly.
• Evaluate the results of your plan and discontinue nursing diagnoses that have been resolved. Select new approaches, if necessary, for problems that haven't been resolved.

length of stay. Also consider the health care setting. For example, *Ambulates outdoors with assistance for 20 minutes t.i.d. by 11/9* is probably unrealistic in a large city hospital.

Planning care

The fourth step of the nursing process is planning. The nursing care plan is a written plan of action designed to help you deliver quality patient care. The care plan is based on problems identified during the patient's admission interview. The plan consists of:
• nursing diagnoses
• expected outcomes
• nursing interventions.

The care plan becomes a permanent part of the patient's record and is used by all members of the nursing team. Remember, patients' problems and needs change, so review your care plan often and modify it if necessary.

Take three giant steps

Writing a care plan involves these three steps:

1. assigning priorities to the nursing diagnoses

2. selecting appropriate nursing interventions to accomplish expected outcomes

3. documenting the nursing diagnoses, expected outcomes, nursing interventions, and evaluations. (See *Tips for top-notch care plans*, page 35.)

Implementation

Now you're ready to select interventions and implement them, the fifth step of the nursing process. Nursing interventions are actions that you and your patient agree will help him reach the expected outcomes. Base these interventions on the second part of your nursing diagnosis, the related factors.

For example, with a nursing diagnosis of *Impaired physical mobility related to arthritic morning stiffness*, select interventions that reduce or eliminate the patient's stiffness, such as mild stretching exercises. Write at least one intervention for each outcome statement.

Divine intervention

How do you come up with interventions? There are several ways. First, consider interventions that you or your patient have successfully tried before. For example, if the patient is having trouble sleeping in the hospital and he tells you that a glass of warm milk helps him get to sleep at home, this could work as an intervention for the expected outcome *Sleep through the night without medication by 11/9.*

You can also pick interventions from standardized care plans, ask other nurses about interventions they've used successfully, or check nursing journals for evidence-based interventions. If these methods don't work, try brainstorming with other nurses.

Writing interventions

To help you write interventions clearly and correctly, follow these guidelines:

• Clearly state the necessary action — Note how and when to perform the intervention, and include special instructions. *Promote comfort* doesn't say what specific action to take, but *Administer ordered analgesic ½ hour before dressing change* says exactly what to do and when to do it.

• Make interventions fit the patient — Consider the patient's age, condition, developmental level, environment, and values. For instance, if he's a vegetarian, don't write an intervention that requires him to eat lean meat to gain extra protein for healing.

• Keep the patient's safety in mind — Consider the patient's physical and mental limitations. For instance, before teaching a patient how to give himself medication, make sure he's physically able to do it and that he can remember and follow the regimen.

• Follow your facility's rules — For example, if your facility allows only nurses to administer medications, don't write an intervention calling for the patient to *Administer hemorrhoidal suppositories as needed.*

• Consider other health care activities — Adjust your interventions when other activities interfere with them. For example, you might want your patient to get plenty of rest on a day when he has several diagnostic tests scheduled.

• Use available resources — If your patient needs to learn about his cardiac problem, use your facility's education department, literature from the American Heart Association, and local support groups. Write your intervention to reflect the use of these resources.

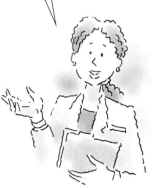

When writing interventions, clearly state the necessary action.

Charting interventions

After you've performed an intervention, record the nature of the intervention, the time you performed it, and the patient's response. Also record other interventions that you performed based on his response and the reasons you performed them. Doing so makes your documentation *outcome-oriented*.

Tailor your style (and format) to policy

Where do you document interventions? That depends on your facility's policy. You can document them on graphic records, on a patient care flow sheet that integrates all nurses' notes for a 1-day period, on integrated or separate nurses' progress notes, on specialized documentation forms such as the medication administration record, and in electronic patient records.

Your facility's policies also dictate the style and format of your documentation. You should record interventions when you give routine care, give emergency care, observe changes in the patient's condition, and administer medications.

Evaluation

The current emphasis on evaluating your interventions has changed nursing documentation. Traditional documentation didn't always reflect the end results of nursing care, but today your progress notes must include an evaluation of your patient's progress toward the expected outcomes you've established in the care plan.

Charting changes

The most commonly used charting method is expected outcomes and evaluation documentation. It focuses on the patient's response to nursing care and helps you provide high-quality, cost-effective care. It's replacing narrative charting and lengthy, handwritten care plans. (See *Effective evaluation statements.*)

A tough transition

The transition to outcome documentation has been difficult for some nurses. In outcome documentation, the nurse is expected to record nursing judgments, not just nursing interventions. Unfortunately, nurses have traditionally been trained not to make judgments. Today, nurses are being asked to gather and interpret data, refer and prioritize care, and document their findings.

The belief that hands-on care is more important than documentation is one reason nurses commonly focus more on nursing interventions than on documenting patient responses. However, worthwhile interventions lead to a desired outcome. Outcomes and evaluation documentation compels nurses to focus on patient responses. When you evaluate the results of your interventions, you help ensure that your plan is working.

The value of evaluation

Evaluation of care gives you a chance to:
- determine if your original assessment findings still apply
- uncover complications
- analyze patterns or trends in the patient's care and his response to it
- assess the patient's response to all aspects of his care, including medications, changes in diet or activity, procedures, unusual incidents or problems, and teaching

---

Effective evaluation statements

The evaluation statements below clearly describe common outcomes. Note that they include specific details of the care provided and objective evidence of the patient's response to care.
- *Can describe the signs and symptoms of hyperglycemia* (response to patient education)
- *States leg pain decreased from 9 to 6 (on a scale of 1 to 10) 30 minutes after receiving PCA morphine* (response to pain medication within 1 hour of administration)
- *Can ambulate to chair with a steady gait, approximately 10', unassisted* (tolerance of change or increase in activity)
- *Can't tolerate removal of O_2; became dyspneic on room air even at rest* (tolerance of treatments)

- determine how closely care conforms to established standards
- measure how well you have cared for the patient
- assess the performance of other members of the health care team
- identify opportunities to improve the quality of your care.

Whenever within sight

Evaluation itself is an ongoing process that takes place whenever you see your patient. However, how often you're required to make evaluations depends on several factors, including where you work.

If you work in an acute care setting, your facility's policy may require you to review care plans every 24 hours. If you work in a long-term care facility, the required interval between evaluations may be as long as 30 days. In either case, you should evaluate and revise the care plan more often if warranted.

Evaluating expected outcomes

Evaluation includes gathering reassessment data, comparing findings with the outcome criteria, determining the extent of outcome achievement (whether the outcome was met, partially met, or not met), writing evaluation statements, and revising the care plan.

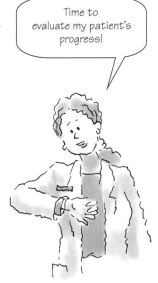

Time to evaluate my patient's progress!

Not resolved? Revise...

Revision starts with determining whether the patient has achieved the outcomes. If outcomes haven't been fully met and you decide that the problem is resolved, the plan can be discontinued. If the problem persists, continue the plan with new target dates until the desired status is achieved. If outcomes are partially met or unmet, identify interfering factors, such as misinterpreted information, unrealistic patient outcomes, or a change in the patient's status, and revise the plan accordingly.

Revision may involve:
- clarifying or amending the database to reflect new information
- reexamining and correcting nursing diagnoses
- establishing outcome criteria that reflect new information and new or amended nursing strategies
- adding the revised nursing care plan to the original document
- recording the rationale for the revision in the nurses' progress notes.

Documenting evaluation

Evaluation statements should indicate whether expected outcomes were achieved and should list evidence supporting this conclusion. Base these statements on outcome criteria

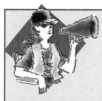

That's a wrap!

Nursing process review

Nursing process basics
- Problem-solving approach to nursing care
- Emerged in 1960s but its roots began in World War II (when the nursing profession began to change)
- Includes six steps: assessment, nursing diagnosis, outcome identification, planning care, implementation, and evaluation

Assessment
- Guides the nursing process and communicates information to the health care team about the patient's condition
- Begins with a health history and physical examination
- Should follow The Joint Commission standards:
  – physical factors
  – psychological, social, and cultural factors
  – environmental factors
  – self-care capabilities
  – learning needs
  – discharge planning needs
  – input from the patient's family and friends when appropriate

Nursing diagnosis
- Consists of the human response or problem, related factors, and signs and symptoms
- Must be formulated, prioritized, and then used to guide the care plan

Outcome identification
- Consists of four parts: behavior, measure, condition, and time
- Should be concise, specific, realistic, measurable, and patient focused

Planning care
- May be traditional or standardized
- Consists of nursing diagnoses, expected outcomes, and nursing interventions
- Used by all members of the health care team
- Involves assigning priorities, selecting nursing interventions, and documenting diagnoses, outcomes, interventions, and evaluations
- Should be modified if patient's condition changes

Implementation
- Involves interventions, which help the patient reach his expected outcomes and should be formulated with the patient's input
- Should be documented properly (interventions that clearly state the action, are individualized, address patient safety, adhere to facility policy, consider other heath care activities, and use available resources)

Evaluation
- Consists of outcomes that include specific details about patient care and evidence of the patient's response to this care
- Includes gathering reassessment data, comparing findings, determining outcome achievement, writing evaluation statements, and revising the care plan, if necessary

from the care plan, and use action verbs, such as *demonstrate* or *ambulate*.

Get specific

Include the patient's response to specific treatments, such as medication administration or physical therapy, and describe the condition under which the response occurred or failed to occur. Document patient teaching and palliative or preventive care as well.

After evaluating the outcome, be sure to record it in the patient's chart with clear statements that demonstrate his progress toward meeting the expected outcomes.

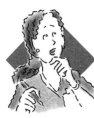

Quick quiz

1. The nursing health history is most accurately described as:
    A. a tool to guide diagnosis and treatment of the illness.
    B. a follow-up to the medical history.
    C. an interview that focuses holistically on the human response to illness.
    D. a care plan.

Answer: C. A nursing health history focuses on responses, whereas a medical health history focuses on diagnosis and treatment.

2. The primary source of assessment information is:
    A. the patient.
    B. past medical records.
    C. the patient's family members.
    D. the patient's friends.

Answer: A. The patient should be your primary source of assessment information. However, if the patient is sedated, confused, hostile, angry, dyspneic, or in pain, you may have to rely initially on family members or close friends to supply information.

3. Expected outcomes are defined as:
    A. goals the patient should reach as a result of planned nursing interventions.
    B. goals the patient and family ask you to accomplish.
    C. goals that are set slightly higher than what the patient can realistically achieve to help motivate him.
    D. goals that are set little lower than expected to help motivate the patient.

Answer: A. Expected outcomes are realistic, measurable goals and their target dates.

4. A good way to come up with interventions is by:
    A. asking the doctor.
    B. asking the patient what has worked for him before.
    C. reviewing past medical records.
    D. reviewing doctor's orders and using them.

Answer: B. You can also ask other nurses, check nursing journals, pick interventions from standardized care plans, or brainstorm.

Scoring

☆☆☆   If you answered all four questions correctly, chalk one up to success! You're an avid assessment aficionado.

☆☆   If you answered three questions correctly, document your diligence! You're a dedicated diagnosis devotee.

☆   If you answered fewer than three questions correctly, keep striving for excellence! Soon you'll be an expert evaluation enthusiast.

Care plans

Just the facts

In this chapter, you'll learn:

♦ reasons for writing a care plan

♦ differences between traditional and standardized care plans

♦ functions and parts of a patient-teaching plan

♦ components of critical pathways and their uses.

A look at the nursing care plan

The nursing care plan is a vital part of documentation. To the health care team, the nursing care plan is a principal source of information about the patient's problems, needs, and goals. It contains detailed instructions for achieving the goals established for the patient and is used to direct care. It also includes suggestions for solving the patient's problems and dealing with unexpected complications.

There are five aspects to writing a care plan:

establishing care priorities based on assessment data

identifying expected outcomes

developing nursing interventions to attain these outcomes

evaluating the patient's responses

documenting the plan in the format required by your facility.

Now a part of the permanent record

Until 1991, a care plan wasn't a required part of a patient's permanent record. It was used by the nursing staff and, in some facilities, it was discarded when a patient was discharged. *Now, The*

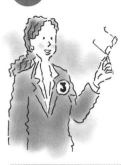

Joint Commission requires that the care plan be permanently integrated into the medical record by written or electronic means.

The Joint Commission policy changes have also led to greater flexibility when writing care plans. The commission no longer specifies the format for documenting patient care, so new methods have emerged that can make planning faster and easier.

Types of care plans

You may write your care plans in one of two styles, *traditional* or *standardized*. Whatever approach you use, your care plan should cover all nursing care from admission to discharge.

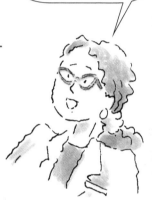

What's your style, traditional or standardized?

Traditional care plans

Also called an *individually developed care plan*, the traditional plan is written from scratch for each patient. After you analyze your assessment data for a patient, you either write the plan by hand or enter it into a computer. (See *It's traditional.*)

Good form

The basic form for the traditional care plan varies, depending on the function of this important document in your facility or department. Most forms have four main columns:
• one for nursing diagnoses
• a second for expected outcomes
• a third for interventions
• a fourth for outcome evaluations.

There may be other columns for the dates when you initiated the care plans, target dates for expected outcomes, and the dates for review, revisions, and resolutions. Most forms also have a place for you to sign or initial whenever you make an entry or a revision.

Looking toward an outcome

What should you include on the forms? This information varies, too. Because shorter hospital stays are more common today, in most health care facilities, you're expected to write only short-term outcomes that the patient can reach by the time he's discharged.

However, some facilities—especially long-term care facilities—also want you to chart long-term outcomes for the patient's maximum functioning level. These facilities commonly provide forms with separate spaces for short- and long-term outcomes.

Art of the chart

It's traditional

Here's an example of a traditional care plan. It shows how these forms are typically organized. Remember that a traditional plan is written from scratch for each patient.

Date	Nursing diagnosis	Expected outcomes	Interventions	Outcomes evaluation (initials and date)
1/15/09	Ineffective breathing pattern R/T pain as evidenced by c/o pain with deep breaths or coughing	Respiratory rate stays within 5 of baseline ABG levels remain normal Achieves comfort without depressing respirations Demonstrates correct use of incentive spirometry Auscultation reveals no adventitious breath sounds States understanding of the importance of taking deep breaths periodically Reports ability to breathe comfortably	Assess and record respiratory status q4h. Assess for pain q3h. Give pain medication as ordered p.r.n. Assist the patient to a comfortable position. Assist the patient in using incentive spirometry. Teach the patient how to splint chest while coughing. Perform chest physiotherapy to aid in mobilizing and removing secretions. Provide rest periods. Encourage the patient to use incentive spirometry. Provide oxygen as ordered.	

Nursing diagnoses, expected outcomes, interventions, and outcomes evaluations are key elements of traditional care plans.

Review dates				
Date	Signature			Initials
1/16/09	M. Hopper, RN			MH

Personal, visual, clear

The traditional method has several advantages:
- It provides a personalized plan for each patient.
- The format allows health care team members and the patient to easily visualize the plan.
- Columns for outcomes evaluations are clearly delineated.

Time isn't on its side

The main disadvantage of the traditional method is that it's time-consuming to read and write because it requires lengthy documentation.

Standardized care plans

Standardized care plans are more commonly used. They eliminate the problems associated with traditional plans by using preprinted information. This saves documentation time. (See *Why stand on tradition? Use a standardized plan.*)

Some standardized plans are classified by medical diagnoses or diagnosis-related groups (DRGs); others, by nursing diagnoses. The preprinted information included in a standardized care plan includes interventions for patients with similar diagnoses and, usually, root outcome statements.

Insist on individuality

Early versions of standardized care plans didn't allow for differences in patients' needs. However, current versions require you to explain how you have individualized the plan for each patient by adding the following information:
• "related to" (R/T) statements and signs and symptoms for a nursing diagnosis — If the form provides a root diagnosis, such as "Acute pain R/T _____," you might fill in *inflammation, as exhibited by grimacing and other expressions of pain.*
• time limits for the outcomes — To a root statement of the goal *Perform postural drainage without assistance,* you might add *for 15 minutes immediately upon awakening in the morning, by 11/12.*
• frequency of interventions — To an intervention such as *Perform passive range-of-motion exercises,* you might add *twice per day: once in the morning and in the evening.*
• specific instructions for interventions — For the standard intervention *Elevate the patient's head,* you might specify *before sleep, on three pillows.*

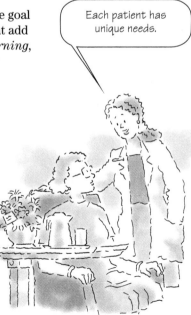

Each patient has unique needs.

Computers make combos less cumbersome

When a patient has more than one diagnosis, you must combine standardized care plans, which can make records long and cumbersome. However, if your facility uses computerized plans, you can extract only the parts you need from each plan and then combine them to make one manageable plan. Some computer programs

Art of the chart

Why stand on tradition? Use a standardized plan

The standardized care plan below is for a patient with a nursing diagnosis of *Impaired tissue integrity*. To customize it to your patient, complete the diagnosis—including signs and symptoms—and fill in the expected outcomes.

Date ___1/15/09___

Nursing diagnosis
Impaired tissue integrity _related to arterial insufficiency_

Target date ___1/17/09___

Expected outcomes
Attains relief from immediate symptoms: _pain, ulcers, edema_
Voices intent to change aggravating behavior: _will stop smoking immediately_
Maintains collateral circulation: _palpable peripheral pulses, extremities warm and pink with good capillary refill_
Voices intent to follow specific management routines after discharge: _foot care guidelines, exercise regimen as specified by physical therapy department_

> Standardized plans require a lot less writing.

Date ___1/15/09___

Interventions
- Provide foot care. Administer and monitor treatments according to facility protocols.
- Encourage adherence to an exercise regimen as tolerated.
- Educate the patient about risk factors and prevention of injury. Refer the patient to a stop-smoking program.
- Maintain adequate hydration. Monitor I/O _q8h_
- To increase arterial blood supply to the extremities, elevate head of bed _6" to 8"_
- Additional interventions: _inspect skin integrity q8h_

Date _____

Outcomes evaluation
Attained relief of immediate symptoms: ─────────────
Voiced intent to change aggravating behavior: ─────────────
Maintained collateral circulation: ─────────────
Voiced intent to follow specific management routines after discharge: ─────────────

provide a checklist of interventions from which you can select to build your own plan.

Although standardized plans usually include only essential information, most provide space for you to write additional nursing diagnoses, expected outcomes, interventions, and outcomes evaluations.

These advantages come standard

Standardized care plans offer many advantages because they:
• require far less writing than traditional plans
• are more legible
• are easier to duplicate
• make compliance with a facility's policy easier for all members of the health care team, including experts, novices, and ancillary staff
• guide you in creating the plan and allow you the freedom to adapt it to your patient.

Is it individualized?

This method has one main drawback: If you simply check off items on a list or fill in the blanks, you might not individualize the patient's care or document your findings adequately.

Patient-teaching plan

A patient-teaching plan serves several important functions:
• It pinpoints what the patient needs to learn and how he'll be taught.
• It sets criteria for evaluating how well the patient learns.
• It helps all caregivers coordinate their teaching.
• It serves as legal proof that the patient received appropriate instruction and satisfies the requirements of regulatory agencies such as The Joint Commission.

Pointers for the perfect plan

To make sure that your teaching plan is as effective as possible, consider carefully what the patient needs to learn, how you'll teach him, and how you'll measure the results. Work closely with the patient, members of his family, and other health care team members to create realistic and attainable goals for your plan. Also provide for follow-up teaching at home if appropriate.

Be sure to keep your plan flexible. Allow for factors that may interfere with effective teaching, such as a patient's unreceptiveness because of a poor night's sleep or your own daily time constraints.

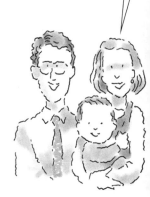

Make sure that you include us in your teaching plan.

Parts of the teaching plan

The patient-teaching plan is divided into six sections:

✌ the patient's learning needs

✌ expected learning outcomes

- teaching content
- teaching methods
- teaching tools
- evaluation of teaching effectiveness.

Learning needs

The first step in developing a teaching plan is to identify what your patient needs to learn. Consider what you, the doctor, and other health care team members expect him to learn as well as what he expects to learn.

Learning outcomes

After you identify the patient's learning needs, you can establish expected learning outcomes, sometimes called *learning objectives*. Beginning with your assessment findings, list the topics and strategies that the patient must learn to reach the maximum level of health and self-care.

An integrated approach

Like other patient care outcomes, expected learning outcomes should focus on the patient and be easy to measure. Learning behaviors and the outcomes you develop fall into three categories:

- cognitive — relating to understanding
- affective — dealing with attitudes and feelings
- psychomotor — involving manual skills.

For example, for a patient who's learning to give himself subcutaneous injections, identifying an injection site is a *cognitive outcome*, coping with the need for injections is an *affective outcome*, and giving the injection is a *psychomotor outcome*. (See *Penning precise learning outcomes*, page 50.)

Which evaluation techniques are most valuable?

To develop precise, measurable outcomes, decide which evaluation techniques best reveal the patient's progress. For cognitive learning, you might use questions and answers; for psychomotor learning, you might use return demonstration.

To measure affective learning — which can be difficult because changes in attitude develop slowly — you can use several evaluation techniques. For example, to determine whether a patient has overcome his anxiety about giving himself an injection, try asking him

Penning precise learning outcomes

Learning behaviors fall into three categories: cognitive, psychomotor, and affective. Keeping these categories in mind will help you write clear, concise learning outcomes. Remember that your outcomes should clarify what you plan to teach, what behavior you expect to see, and what criteria you'll use for evaluating the patient's learning.

Compare the following two sets of learning outcomes.

Well-phrased learning outcomes	Poorly phrased learning outcomes
Cognitive domain	
The patient with heart failure will be able to:	The patient with heart failure will be able to:
• state when to take each prescribed drug	• remember his medication schedule
• describe symptoms of heart failure.	• recognize when his respiratory rate is increased.
Affective domain	
The patient with heart failure will be able to:	The patient with heart failure will be able to:
• report feeling comfortable when breathing	• adjust successfully to the limitations of the disease
• demonstrate willingness to comply with therapy by keeping scheduled doctor appointments.	• realize the importance of seeing his doctor.
Psychomotor domain	
The patient with heart failure will be able to:	The patient with heart failure will be able to:
• demonstrate diaphragmatic pursed-lip breathing	• take his respiratory rate
• demonstrate skill in conserving energy while carrying out activities.	• bring in a sputum specimen for laboratory studies.

if he still feels anxious. You also can assess his willingness to perform the procedure and observe whether he hesitates or shows other signs of stress while doing it.

Then write the outcome statement based on the selected evaluation technique. For example, if you select return demonstration as your evaluation technique, an appropriate outcome statement might be *Demonstrates skill in giving a subcutaneous injection.*

Content

Next, select what to teach the patient to help him achieve the expected outcomes. Be sure to consult with the patient, members of his family, and other caregivers before deciding what to teach. Even if the patient is learning to care for himself, you should still teach a family member how to provide physical and emotional support or how to help the patient remember his care.

Start simple

After you have decided what to teach, organize your instruction to begin with the simplest concepts and work toward the more complex ones. Doing so is especially helpful when teaching a patient who has little education, a learning disability, or anxiety.

Methods

Now, select the appropriate teaching methods. Most of your teaching can probably be done one-on-one. Teaching one-on-one allows you to learn about your patient, build a relationship with him, and individualize your teaching to his needs.

Taking different paths to learning

Many different teaching methods work well along with, or instead of, one-on-one teaching. For instance, try incorporating demonstration, practice, and return demonstration in your teaching plan. Role playing can increase your patient's involvement in the plan, as can case studies, which require him to evaluate how someone else with his disorder responds to different situations.

Other methods include self-monitoring, which requires the patient to assess his situation and determine which aspects of his environment or behavior need correction. You also can conduct group lectures and discussions if several patients require similar instruction, such as with childbirth or diabetes education.

Tools

Finally, decide what teaching tools will help enhance patient education. When choosing your tools, focus on what will work best for your patient. For instance, if your patient learns best by watching how something is done, use a videotape of a procedure or a closed-circuit television demonstration. (See *Tools for tuning up teaching.*)

If the patient prefers a hands-on approach, let him handle the equipment he'll use. If he likes to work interactively at his own pace, try an interactive, computerized patient-teaching program. If he learns best by reading, provide written materials.

Tracking down teaching tools

To get the tools you need, consult unit-based staff instructors, your facility's educational resource center, electronic teaching modules, and staff specialists. If you can't find what you need, call pharmaceutical and medical supply companies in your community. Also, contact national associations and foundations such as the American Cancer Society. These organizations usually have many patient education materials written for the layperson. They also provide pamphlets and brochures in several languages.

Tools for tuning up teaching

This list includes teaching materials and methods you can use to optimize your patient's learning.

Teaching materials
Teaching materials include:
- brochures and pamphlets
- DVDs and videotapes
- closed-circuit television
- computer programs
- equipment being used for patient care (for example, syringes, needles, and pumps).

Teaching methods
Teaching methods include:
- one-on-one teaching
- role playing
- return demonstration
- self-monitoring
- group lecture.

Keep the patient's abilities and limitations in mind as you choose teaching tools. For example, before giving him written materials, such as brochures and pamphlets, make sure that he can read and understand them. Keep in mind that the average adult reads at only a seventh-grade level.

Break down language barriers

Likewise, make sure you're aware of any language barriers between you and your patient. Use appropriate communication—including interpreter and translation services; bilingual aids, such as cards and pamphlets; and assistive listening devices—to overcome these barriers.

Evaluation

Evaluate the effectiveness of your teaching by using the technique you used for your expected learning outcomes. Document the patient's progress by documenting the patient's learning behaviors and indicating if the patient has met the expected learning outcomes.

Documenting the patient-teaching plan

The patient-teaching plan is a key part of the patient's care plan. By reading it, health care team members can see at a glance what the patient learned and what he still needs to learn. The health care facility also uses it to show what quality improvement measures are in progress.

Give it time...and thought

Constructing individual teaching plans requires time and thought. Ideally, health care team members collaborate to create these plans. However, because nurses typically spend more time with patients than other team members, they're usually responsible for individualizing standard teaching plans to meet each patient's needs.

Forms, forms, and more forms

There are several different forms for documenting your patient-teaching plan. Many of these incorporate the nursing process as it applies to patient education. (See *Go with the flow sheet.*)

Just your type

Patient-teaching plans also come in two basic types that are similar to traditional and standardized care plans. The traditional type begins with the nursing diagnosis statement *Deficient knowledge* and an individualized *related to* statement—for example, *Deficient*

(Text continues on page 54.)

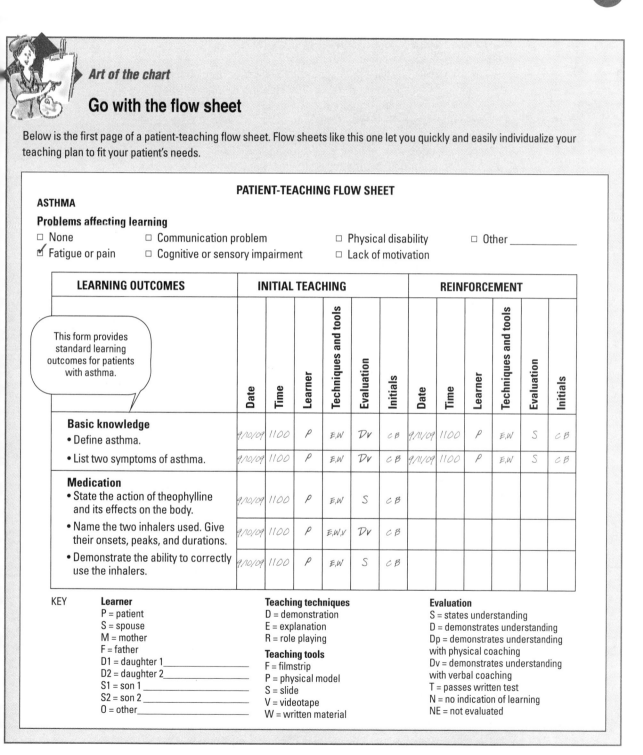

Art of the chart

Go with the flow sheet

Below is the first page of a patient-teaching flow sheet. Flow sheets like this one let you quickly and easily individualize your teaching plan to fit your patient's needs.

PATIENT-TEACHING FLOW SHEET

ASTHMA

Problems affecting learning

☐ None   ☐ Communication problem   ☐ Physical disability   ☐ Other _____
☑ Fatigue or pain   ☐ Cognitive or sensory impairment   ☐ Lack of motivation

LEARNING OUTCOMES	INITIAL TEACHING						REINFORCEMENT					
This form provides standard learning outcomes for patients with asthma.	Date	Time	Learner	Techniques and tools	Evaluation	Initials	Date	Time	Learner	Techniques and tools	Evaluation	Initials
Basic knowledge • Define asthma.	9/10/09	1100	P	E,W	Dv	C B	9/11/09	1100	P	E,W	S	C B
• List two symptoms of asthma.	9/10/09	1100	P	E,W	Dv	C B	9/11/09	1100	P	E,W	S	C B
Medication • State the action of theophylline and its effects on the body.	9/10/09	1100	P	E,W	S	C B						
• Name the two inhalers used. Give their onsets, peaks, and durations.	9/10/09	1100	P	E,W,V	Dv	C B						
• Demonstrate the ability to correctly use the inhalers.	9/10/09	1100	P	E,W	S	C B						

KEY

Learner
P = patient
S = spouse
M = mother
F = father
D1 = daughter 1_____
D2 = daughter 2_____
S1 = son 1 _____
S2 = son 2 _____
O = other_____

Teaching techniques
D = demonstration
E = explanation
R = role playing

Teaching tools
F = filmstrip
P = physical model
S = slide
V = videotape
W = written material

Evaluation
S = states understanding
D = demonstrates understanding
Dp = demonstrates understanding with physical coaching
Dv = demonstrates understanding with verbal coaching
T = passes written test
N = no indication of learning
NE = not evaluated

knowledge related to low-sodium diet. It provides only the format and requires you to come up with the plan.

The standardized type allows you to check off or date steps as you complete them and add or delete information to individualize the plan. It's best suited for patients who need extensive teaching.

Some plans include space for documenting problems that could hinder learning, for comments and evaluations, and for dates and signatures, or you may need to include this information in your progress notes. No matter which teaching plan you use, this information becomes a permanent part of the patient's medical record.

Critical pathways

A critical pathway is an interdisciplinary care plan that describes assessment criteria, interventions, treatments, and outcomes for specific health-related conditions (usually based on a DRG) across a designated time line.

Accomplished a goal? Check it off!

Think of the pathway as a predetermined checklist describing the tasks you and the patient need to accomplish. In this way, it's similar to a standardized care plan. However, unlike a care plan, its focus is multidisciplinary, covering all of the patient's problems, not just those identified during a nursing assessment.

Critical pathways go by many different names: *clinical pathways, critical paths, interdisciplinary plans, anticipated recovery plans, care maps, interdisciplinary action plans,* and *action plans.*

A collaborative effort

Members of the health care team involved in providing care should collaborate to develop each critical pathway. The goals of the critical pathway include:
• achieving expected patient and family outcomes
• promoting professional collaborative practice and care
• ensuring continuity of care
• ensuring appropriate use of resources
• reducing the cost and length of stay
• establishing a framework for instituting and monitoring performance improvement.

Practical when predictable

Critical pathways are most useful in specific types of patient care situations. They work well with high-volume cases (meaning the facility cares for a lot of patients with this particular problem) and in situations that have relatively predictable outcomes. Complex situations with unpredictable outcomes normally aren't managed with critical pathways.

It's simple: A critical pathway is a critical tool...

A critical pathway is a permanent part of the medical record. It provides a consistent assessment and documentation tool for third-party payers. It's also used to compare the diagnoses of patients and determine their needs.

Critical pathways cover the key events that must occur before the patient's target discharge date. These events include:
- consultations
- diagnostic tests
- treatments
- medications
- procedures
- activities
- diet
- patient teaching
- discharge planning
- achievement of anticipated outcomes.

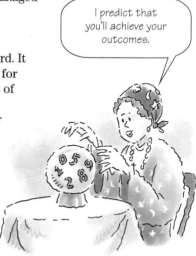

I predict that you'll achieve your outcomes.

Charting the path

A critical pathway is usually organized according to categories, such as activity, diet, treatments, medications, patient teaching, and discharge planning. Appropriate categories are determined based on the patient's medical diagnosis. The medical diagnosis also dictates expected length of stay, daily care guidelines, and expected outcomes. Care guidelines are listed under appropriate categories.

The structure of a critical pathway and the categories it contains vary among facilities. Within a facility, the structure and content of critical pathways may vary depending on the specific DRG. (See *Take the critical pathway*, pages 56 and 57.)

Some facilities use nursing diagnoses as the basis for critical pathways, but this use is controversial. Critics argue that this format interferes with communication and the coordination of care among nonnursing members of the health care team.

A bundle of benefits

Critical pathways are mostly a benefit to nurses. Here's why:
- They eliminate duplicate charting. You must write narrative notes when a standard on the pathway remains unmet or when the patient needs care that's different than what's written on the

(Text continues on page 58.)

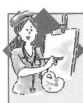

Art of the chart

Take the critical pathway

At any point in a treatment course, a glance at the critical pathway allows you to compare the patient's progress and your performance as a caregiver with standards. The standard critical pathway below outlines care for a patient with a colon resection.

CRITICAL PATHWAY: COLON RESECTION WITHOUT COLOSTOMY				
	Patient visit	**Presurgery day 1**	**Day 0 O.R. day**	**Postoperative day 1**
Assessments	History and physical with breast, rectal, and pelvic examinations Nursing assessment	Nursing admission assessment	Nursing admission assessment on TBA patients in holding area Postoperative review of systems assessment*	Review of systems assessment*
Consults	Social service consult Physical therapy consult	Notify referring doctor of impending admission		
Labs and diagnostics	Complete blood count (CBC) PT/PTT Electrocardiogram Chest X-ray (CXR) Chemistry profile CT scan ABD w/wo contrast CT scan pelvis Urinalysis Barium enema and flexible sigmoidoscopy or colonoscopy Biopsy report	Type and screen for patients with Hg level less than 10	Type and screen for patients in holding area with Hg level less than 10	C
Interventions	Many or all of the above labs and diagnostics will have already been done. Check all results and fax to the sur-	Admit by 8 a.m. Check for bowel preparation orders Bowel preparation* Antiembolism stockings Incentive spirometry Ankle exercises* I.V. access* Routine VS* Pneumatic inflation boots	Shave and prepare in operating room NG tube maintenance* I/O VS per routine* Indwelling urinary catheter care Incentive spirometry* Ankle exercises* I.V. site care* HOB 30° Safety measures* Wound care* Mouth care*	NG tube maintenance* I/O* VS per routine* Indwelling urinary catheter care Incentive spirometry* Ankle exercises* I.V. site care* HOB 30°* Safety measures* Wound care* Mouth care* Antiembolism stockings
I.V.s		I.V. fluids, $D_5 \frac{1}{2}$ NSS	I.V. fluids, D_5LR	I.V. fluids, D_5LR
Medication	Prescribe GoLYTELY or NuLYTELY 10a-2p Neomycin at 2p, 3p, and 10p Erythromycin at 2p, 3p, and 10p	GoLYTELY or NuLYTELY 10a-2p Erythromycin at 2p, 3p, and 10p Neomycin at 2p, 3p, and 10p	Preoperative ABX in holding area Postoperative ABX × 2 doses PCA (basal rate 0.5 mg) subcutaneous heparin	
Diet/GI	Clears presurgery day NPO after midnight	Clears presurgery day NPO after midnight	NPO/NG tube	
Activity			4 hours after surgery ambulate with abdominal binder* Discontinue pneumatic inflation boots once patient ambulates	Ambulate t.i.d. with abdominal binder* May shower Physical therapy b.i.d.
KEY: *= NSG Activities **V = Variance** **N = No Var.** **Signatures:**	1. 2. 3. V V V Ⓝ N N 1. _C. Molloy, RN_ 2. _____ 3. _____	1. 2. 3. V V V Ⓝ Ⓝ Ⓝ 1. _M. Connel, RN_ 2. _J. Smith, RN_ 3. _R. Joseph, RN_	1. 2. 3. V V V Ⓝ Ⓝ Ⓝ 1. _L. Singer, RN_ 2. _J. Smith, RN_ 3. _P. Joseph, RN_	1. 2. 3. V V V Ⓝ Ⓝ Ⓝ 1. _L. Singer, RN_ 2. _J. Smith, RN_ 3. _P. Joseph, RN_

> The pathway designates a specific time frame for patient care activities.

> The pathway is organized into categories based on the patient's medical diagnosis.

> The pathway lists tasks that the patient and caregivers must accomplish.

Take the critical pathway *(continued)*

CRITICAL PATHWAY: COLON RESECTION WITHOUT COLOSTOMY			
	Postoperative day 2	**Postoperative day 3**	**Postoperative day 4**	**Postoperative day 5**
Assessments	Review of systems assessment*	Review of systems assessment*	Review of systems assessment	Review of systems assessment*
Consults		Dietary consult		Oncology consult if indicated (Dukes B2 or C or high risk lesion) (or to be done as outpatient)
Labs and diagnostics	Electrolyte 7 (EL-7) CXR	CBC EL-7	Pathology results on chart	CBC EL-7
Interventions	Discontinue nasogastric (NG) tube if possible* (per guidelines) Intake and output (I/O)* VS per routine* Discontinue indwelling urinary catheter Ambulating* Incentive spirometry* Ankle exercises* I.V. site care* Head of bed (HOB) 30°* Safety measures* Wound care* Mouth care* Antiembolism stockings	I/O* VS per routine* Incentive spirometry* Ankle exercises* I.V. site care* Safety measures* Wound care* Antiembolism stockings	I/O* VS per routine* Incentive spirometry* Ankle exercises* I.V. site care* Safety measures* Wound care* Antiembolism stockings	Consider staple removal Replace with adhesive strips Assess that patient has met discharge criteria* Discontinue saline lock
I.V.s	I.V. fluids $D_5\frac{1}{2}$ NSS+ MVI	I.V. convert to saline lock	Continue saline lock	Discontinue saline lock
Medication	PCA (0.5 mg basal rate)	Discontinue PCA P.O. analgesia Resume routine home meds	P.O. analgesia Preoperative meds	P.O. analgesia Preoperative meds
Diet/GI	Discontinue NG tube per guidelines: (Clamp tube at 8 a.m. if no N/V and residual < 200 ml, discontinue tube at 12 noon)* (Check with doctor first)	Clears if+bm/flatus Advance to postoperative diet if tolerating clears (at least one tray of clears)	House	House
Activity	Ambulate q.i.d. with abdominal binder* May shower Physical therapy b.i.d.	Ambulate at least q.i.d. with abdominal binder* May shower Physical therapy b.i.d.	Ambulate at least q.i.d. with abdominal binder* May shower Physical therapy b.i.d.	
Teaching	Reinforce preoperative teaching* Patient and family education p.r.n.* Re: family screening	Reinforce preoperative teaching* Patient and family education p.r.n.* Re: family screening Begin discharge teaching	Reinforce preoperative teaching* Patient and family education p.r.n.* Discharge teaching re: reportable s/s, follow-up, and wound care*	Review all discharge instructions and Rx including:* follow-up appointments: with surgeon within 3 weeks with oncologist within 1 month if indicated
KEY: *= NSG Activities **V = Variance** **N = No Var.** **NSG care performed:** **Signatures:**	1. 2. 3. V V V Ⓝ Ⓝ Ⓝ 1. _A. McCarthy, RN_ 2. _R. Moyer, RN_ 3. _M. Koller, RN_	1. 2. 3. V V V Ⓝ Ⓝ Ⓝ 1. _A. McCarthy, RN_ 2. _R. Moyer, RN_ 3. _M. Koller, RN_	1. 2. 3. V V V Ⓝ Ⓝ Ⓝ 1. _L. Singer, RN_ 2. _J. Smith, RN_ 3. _L. Joseph, RN_	1. 2. 3. V V V Ⓝ Ⓝ N 1. _L. Singer, RN_ 2. _J. Smith, RN_ 3. _____

> The pathway also lists key events that must occur before the patient's discharge date.

form. Most pathways provide a place to document care alterations.

• With standardized orders or protocols, you can advance the patient's activity level, diet, and treatment without waiting for a doctor's order. Nurses have more freedom to make care decisions.

• Communication improves between members of the health care team because everyone works from the same plan. That's why problems are called *collaborative problems*. All members of the team work together to achieve the desired outcome.

• Quality of care improves because of shared accountability for patient outcomes.

• Patient teaching and discharge planning improve. When critical pathways are adapted and given to patients, patients are less anxious and more cooperative because they know what to expect and what's expected of them. Some patients even recover and go home sooner than anticipated.

• Pathways help team members determine the best and most effective treatment methods.

Yippee! Critical pathways improve my performance!

Here's where it gets complicated...

Even so, critical pathways are less effective for patients who have several diagnoses or who have complications. Establishing a time line for these patients is more difficult. For example, treatment progress is usually predictable for a patient who has a cholecystectomy and is otherwise healthy. However, if a patient has diabetes and coronary artery disease, the treatment course is fairly unpredictable, and the care plan is likely to change, resulting in lengthy, fragmented documentation.

Choosing the right path

When using pathways, review them periodically to evaluate their usefulness and to ensure that the interventions and timelines are appropriate. Revise them as needed. Remember, shortened hospital stays can compromise or compress critical pathways.

Priorities in the pathway

Just as you prioritize nursing diagnoses, you must prioritize collaborative problems in the critical pathway. For example, if your patient needs whirlpool treatments by the physical therapist and nebulizer treatments from a respiratory therapist, you must coordinate these activities according to the patient's current status and needs. If every team member plans carefully and pays attention to the patient's response to treatments, you should be able to carry out your respective activities for the patient's benefit.

That's a wrap!

Care plans review

Five aspects to writing care plans
- Establishing care priorities
- Identifying expected outcomes
- Developing nursing interventions to attain these outcomes
- Evaluating the patient's response
- Documenting

Types of plans
Traditional
- Advantages
- Provides a personalized plan for each patient
- Allows the health care team and patient to visualize the plan
- Is clearly organized
- Disadvantage
- Is time-consuming to read and write

Standardized
- Advantages
- Uses preprinted information organized by diagnosis, which saves documentation time and facilitates adherence to facility standards
- Requires less writing, which makes it easier to read
- Is easier to duplicate
- Guides care while allowing adaptability
- Disadvantage
- May not be individualized properly if the nurse overlooks this important step

Patient-teaching plan
- Can be traditional or standardized
Functions
- To pinpoint what the patient needs to learn and how he'll be taught
- To establish criteria for patient-learning evaluation
- To help caregivers coordinate teaching
- To prove that the patient received appropriate instruction

Parts of the teaching plan
- Learning needs
- Expected learning outcomes
- Content
- Methods
- Tools
- Evaluation

Critical pathway
Basics
- Includes a predetermined checklist of tasks you and your patient must accomplish
- Provides daily care guidelines and expected outcomes
- Dictates the length of stay
Goals
- To achieve expected patient and family outcomes
- To promote professional collaborative practice and care
- To ensure continuity of care
- To ensure appropriate use of resources
- To reduce the cost and length of stay
- To establish a framework for instituting and monitoring continuous quality improvement
- To determine, over time, the most effective treatment
Advantages
- Eliminates duplicate charting
- Gives nurses more freedom in making care decisions
- Improves communication between members of the health care team
- Improves quality of care
- Improves patient teaching and discharge planning
Disadvantage
- Is less effective for patients with multiple diagnoses and those who experience complications

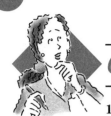

Quick quiz

1. Before 1991, the nursing care plan was commonly:
   A.   discarded when the patient was discharged.
   B.   part of the patient's permanent record.
   C.   used by doctors as well as nurses.
   D.   a vital part of documentation.

Answer: A. In 1991, The Joint Commission began requiring that the care plan be permanently integrated into the patient's medical record.

2. People with access to the care plan include:
   A.   all caregivers, the patient, and members of his family.
   B.   the nursing staff only.
   C.   just nurses and doctors.
   D.   doctors only.

Answer: A. In addition to caregivers, the patient and members of his family should use the care plan and make recommendations and evaluations.

3. Compared with a standardized care plan, a traditional care plan is:
   A.   easier to duplicate.
   B.   easier to adapt to recent policy changes by The Joint Commission.
   C.   easier to adapt to the individual patient.
   D.   more legible.

Answer: C. The traditional care plan is written from scratch to meet the needs of an individual patient. Standardized care plans are preprinted and based on interventions for patients with similar diagnoses.

Scoring

☆☆☆ If you answered all three questions correctly, wow! You might be nominated for the Pulitzer Prize in Outstanding Outcomes.

☆☆ If you answered two questions correctly, wonderful! Your plans are more than precise, they're poetic. You excel in traditional, standardized, and free-verse formats.

☆ If you answered fewer than two questions correctly, practice more planning! The critics will soon be raving about your crafted critical pathways.

Charting systems

Just the facts

In this chapter, you'll learn:

♦ different types of charting systems and how to use them

♦ advantages and disadvantages of each type of system

♦ criteria to consider when choosing a charting system.

A look at charting systems

Different health care facilities set their own requirements for documentation and evaluation but all must comply with legal, accreditation, and professional standards. A nursing department also may select a documentation system as long as it adheres to those standards.

Narrative or alternative?

Depending on your facility's policy, you'll use one or more documentation systems to record your nursing interventions and evaluations and the patient's response. Some facilities use traditional narrative charting systems. Others choose alternative systems.

Each documentation system includes specific policies and procedures for charting, so make sure you understand the documentation requirements for the system your facility uses. Understanding and adhering to these requirements will help you to document care systematically and accurately. (See *Comparing charting systems*, page 62.)

Comparing charting systems

The table below compares elements of the different charting systems used today. Note that the second column provides information on which systems work best in which settings.

System	Useful settings	Parts of record	Assessment	Care plan	Outcomes and evaluations	Progress notes format
Narrative	• Acute care • Long-term care • Home care • Ambulatory care	• Progress notes • Flow sheets to supplement care plan	• Initial: history and admission form • Ongoing: progress notes	• Care plan	• Progress notes • Discharge summaries	• Narration at time of entry
Problem-oriented medical record (POMR)	• Acute care • Long-term care • Home care • Rehabilitation • Mental health facilities	• Database • Problem list • Care plan • Progress notes • Discharge summary	• Initial: Database and care plan • Ongoing: progress notes	• Database • Nursing care plan based on problem list	• Progress notes (section E of SOAPIE and SOAPIER)	• SOAP, SOAPIE, SOAPIER
Problem-intervention-evaluation (PIE)	• Acute care	• Assessment flow sheets • Progress notes • Problem list	• Initial: Assessment form • Ongoing: assessment form every shift	• None; included in progress notes (section P)	• Progress notes (section E)	• Problem • Intervention • Evaluation
FOCUS	• Acute care • Long-term care	• Progress notes • Flow sheets • Checklists	• Initial: patient history and admission assessment • Ongoing: assessment form	• Nursing care plan based on problems or nursing diagnoses	• Progress notes (section R)	• Data • Action • Response
Charting by exception (CBE)	• Acute care • Long-term care	• Care plan • Flow sheets, including patient-teaching records and patient discharge notes • Graphic record • Progress notes	• Initial: database assessment sheet • Ongoing: nursing and medical order flow sheets	• Nursing care plan based on nursing diagnoses	• Progress notes (section E)	• SOAPIE or SOAPIER
Flow sheet, assessment, concise, timely (FACT)	• Acute care • Long-term care	• Assessment sheet • Flow sheets • Progress notes	• Initial: baseline assessment • Ongoing: flow sheets and progress notes	• Nursing care plan based on nursing diagnoses	• Flow sheets (section R)	• Data • Action • Response
Core (with DAE)	• Acute care • Long-term care	• Kardex • Flow sheets • Progress notes	• Initial: baseline assessment • Ongoing: progress notes	• Care plan	• Progress notes (section E)	• Data • Action • Evaluation
Computerized	• Acute care • Long-term care • Home care • Ambulatory care	• Progress notes • Flow sheets • Nursing care plan • Database • Teaching plan	• Initial: baseline assessment • Ongoing: progress notes	• Database • Care plan	• Outcome-based care plan	• Evaluative statements • Expected outcomes • Learning outcomes

Traditional narrative

Narrative charting is a chronological account of:
- the patient's status
- the nursing interventions performed
- the patient's responses.

No longer going it alone

Today, few facilities rely on the narrative charting system alone. Instead, they combine it with other systems, especially the source-oriented record.

Using narrative charting

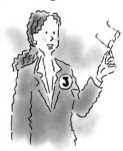

In the traditional narrative system, the nurse usually records data as progress notes, with flow sheets supplementing the narrative notes. Knowing when and what to document and how to organize the data are the key elements of effective narrative charting in the progress notes. (See *The full story on narrative charting*, page 64.)

The Joint Commission requires all health care facilities to establish policies on the frequency of patient reassessment. So assess your patient at least as often as required by your facility's policy, and then document your findings.

Documentation mania!

If you find yourself writing repetitious, meaningless notes, you may be documenting too often. If so, double-check your facility's policy. You may be following a time-consuming, unwritten standard initiated by staff members, not by your facility. To guard against this, review the policy at least every 6 months.

Observe and take note

In addition to documenting according to facility policy, be sure to write specific and descriptive narrative in the progress notes whenever you observe:
- a change in the patient's condition, such as progression, regression, or new problems — for example, write *Patient can ambulate with a walker for 3 minutes before feeling tired.*
- a patient's response to a treatment or medication — for example, write *Patient states that abdominal pain is relieved 1 hour after receiving medication. He's smiling and can turn in bed without difficulty.*
- a lack of improvement in the patient's condition — for example, write *No change in size or condition of sacral*

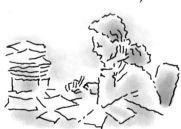

This is beginning to look all too familiar, not to mention meaningless. Am I documenting too much?

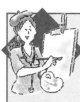

Art of the chart

The full story on narrative charting

This progress note is one example of narrative charting.

Date	Time	Notes
5/26/09	2245	Pt 4 hours postoperative: awakens easily; oriented x 3 but groggy. Incision site in front of Ⓛear extending down and around ear and into neck - approximately 6" in length - without dressing. No swelling or bleeding; bluish discoloration below Ⓛear noted, sutures intact. Jackson Pratt drain in Ⓛneck below ear with 20 ml bloody drainage measured. Drain remains secured in place with suture and anchored to Ⓛanterior chest wall with tape. Pt denied pain but stated she felt nauseated and promptly vomited 100 ml of clear fluid. Pt attempted to get OOB to ambulate to bathroom with assistance but felt dizzy upon standing. Assisted to lie down in bed. Voided 200 ml clear, yellow urine in bedpan. Pt encouraged to deep-breathe and cough qh and turn frequently in bed. Antiembolism pads applied to both lower extremities. Explanations given re: these preventive measures. Pt verbalized understanding. ——————————— *Bridget Smith, RN*
5/26/09	2255	Pt continues to feel nauseated. Reglan 10 mg I.M. given in Ⓡgluteus maximus. ——————————— *Bridget Smith, RN*
5/26/09	2335	Pt states she is no longer nauseated, remains pain-free. No further vomiting. Pt demonstrated taking deep breaths and coughing effectively. —— *Bridget Smith, RN*

> Be sure to record the date and time of each entry.

> Entries should be in chronological order.

> Remember to sign each entry.

pressure ulcer after 6 days of treatment. Dimensions and condition remain as stated in 1/20/09 note.

- a patient's or family member's response to teaching—for example, write *The patient was able to demonstrate walking with crutches using the proper technique.*

One thought leads to another

Before you write anything, organize your thoughts so your paragraphs flow smoothly. If you have trouble deciding what to write, refer to the patient's care plan to review:
- unresolved problems
- prescribed interventions
- expected outcomes.

Then write down your observations of the patient's progress in these areas. (See *Put your thoughts in order.*)

A narrative with a happy story

Narrative charting has a lot going for it. After all, this charting format:
- is the most flexible of all the charting systems and is suitable in any clinical setting
- strongly conveys your nursing interventions and your patients' responses
- is ideal for presenting information that's collected over a long period
- combines well with other documentation devices, such as flow sheets, which cuts down on charting time

---

Advice from the experts

Put your thoughts in order

If you have trouble organizing your thoughts, use this sequence of questions to order your entry:
- How did I first become aware of the problem?
- What has the patient said about the problem that's significant?
- What have I observed that's related to the problem?
- What's my plan for dealing with the problem?
- What steps have I taken to intervene?
- How has the patient responded to my interventions or medical regimen?

A paragraph for each problem

To make your notes as coherent as possible, discuss each of the patient's problems in a separate paragraph; don't lump them together. Alternatively, use a head-to-toe approach to organize your information.

Doctor's orders

Be sure to notify the doctor of significant changes that you observe. Then document this communication, the doctor's responses, and any new orders to be implemented.

AIR: A fresh narrative format

A charting format called AIR may help you to organize and simplify your narrative charting. AIR is an acronym for:

• **A**ssessment
• **I**ntervention
• **R**esponse.

The AIR format synthesizes major nursing events and avoids repetition of information found elsewhere in the medical record. Combined with nursing flow sheets and the nursing care plan, the AIR format can be used to document the care you provide clearly and concisely.

Here's how AIR is used to document nursing care.

Assessment

Summarize your physical assessment findings. Begin by specifying each issue that you address, such as nursing diagnosis, admission note, and discharge planning. Rather than simply describing the patient's current condition, document trends and record your impression of the problem.

Intervention

Summarize your actions and those of other caregivers in response to the assessment data. The summary may include a condensed nursing care plan or plans for additional patient monitoring.

Response

Summarize the outcome or the patient's response to nursing interventions. Because a response may not be evident for hours or even days, this documentation may not immediately follow the entries. In fact, it may be recorded by another nurse, which is why titling each of your assessments and interventions is so important.

• uses narration, the most common form of writing, so training new staff members can usually be done quickly
• places its narrative notes in chronological order, so other team members can review the patient's progress daily.

The narrative takes a turn for the worse...

On the other hand, narrative charting has the following disadvantages:

• You have to read the entire record to find the patient outcome. Even then, you may have trouble determining the outcome of a problem because the same information may not be consistently documented.
• For the same reason, you may have trouble tracking problems and identifying trends in the patient's progress.
• Narrative charting offers no inherent guide to what's important to document, so nurses commonly document everything, resulting in a lengthy, repetitive record.
• Narrative charting doesn't always reflect the nursing process.

• Narratives may contain vague or inaccurate language, such as "appears to be bleeding" or "small amount."

You may be able to avoid some disadvantages of narrative charting by organizing the information you record. (See *AIR: A fresh narrative format,* page 66.)

Problem-oriented medical record

The problem-oriented medical record (POMR) focuses on specific patient problems and aids communication among team members. It was originally developed by doctors and later adapted by nurses. The POMR is most effective in acute care and long-term care settings.

A multidiscipline approach

In this charting system, you describe each problem in multidisciplinary patient progress notes (not on progress notes with only nursing information).

Five-part format

The POMR is divided into five parts:

 database

 problem list

 initial plan

 progress notes

 discharge summary.

A five-star knowledge

In POMR charting, you record your interventions and evaluations in the progress notes and discharge summary only. However, to really understand POMR, review all five parts.

Database

Usually completed by a nurse, the database, or *initial assessment,* is the foundation for the patient's care plan. A collection of subjective and objective information about the patient, the database includes the reason for hospitalization, medical history, allergies, medication regimen, physical and psychosocial findings, self-care abilities, educational needs, and other discharge planning concerns. The database is the basis for a problem list.

Problem list

After analyzing the database, various caregivers list the patient's current problems in chronological order according to the date when each is identified—not in the order of acuteness or priority. This list provides an overview of the patient's health status.

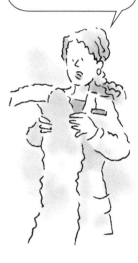

My database forms the basis for a problem list.

Dividing the diagnoses

Originally, POMR called for one interdisciplinary problem list. Although this may still be done, nurses and doctors usually keep separate lists with problems stated as either nursing diagnoses or medical diagnoses.

It's as easy as 1, 2, 3, 4, 5...

As you list the patient's problems, number them so they correspond to the problems in the rest of the POMR. Have every entry on the patient's initial plan, progress notes, and discharge summary correspond to a number. File the numbered problem list at the front of the patient's chart. Keep the list current by adding new numbers as new problems arise. When writing notes, be sure to identify the problem you're discussing by the appropriate number.

When you have resolved a problem, draw a line through it, or show that it's inactive by retiring the problem number and highlighting the problem with a colored felt-tip pen. Don't use the number again for the same patient.

Initial plan

After constructing the problem list, write an initial plan for each problem. This plan includes:
- expected outcomes
- plans for further data collection, if needed
- patient care
- teaching plans.

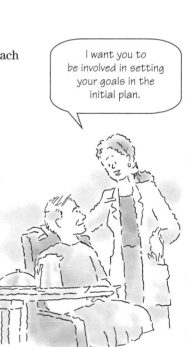

I want you to be involved in setting your goals in the initial plan.

Plan on patient participation

Involve the patient in goal setting as you construct the initial plan. Doing so fosters the patient's compliance and is essential to the effectiveness of your interventions.

Progress notes

One of the most prominent features of the POMR is the structured way that narrative progress notes are written by all team members using the SOAP, SOAPIE, or SOAPIER format. (See *SOAP, SOAPIE, SOAPIER charting.*)

SOAP, SOAPIE, SOAPIER charting

To use the SOAP format in problem-oriented medical record charting, document the following information for each problem:
- **S**ubjective data: Information the patient or family members tell you, such as the chief complaint and other impressions.
- **O**bjective data: Factual, measurable data you gather during assessment, such as observed signs and symptoms, vital signs, and laboratory test values.
- **A**ssessment data: Conclusions based on the collected subjective and objective data and formulated as patient problems or nursing diagnoses. This dynamic and ongoing process changes as more or different subjective and objective information becomes known.
- **P**lan: Your strategy for relieving the patient's problem. This plan should include both immediate or short-term actions and long-term measures.

It's getting SOAPIE.

Some facilities use the SOAPIE format, adding the following to SOAP:
- **I**ntervention: Measures you take to achieve an expected outcome. As the patient's health status changes, you may need to modify your interventions. Be sure to document the patient's understanding and acceptance of the initial plan in this section of your notes.
- **E**valuation: An analysis of the effectiveness of your interventions.

It's even SOAPIER.

The SOAPIER format adds a revision section for the documentation of alternative interventions. If your patient's outcomes fall short of expectations, use the evaluation process called for in SOAPIE as a basis for developing revised interventions, then document these changes:
- **R**evision: Document any changes from the original care plan in this section. Interventions, outcomes, or target dates may need to be adjusted to reach a previous goal.

Usually, you must write a complete note in one of these formats every 24 hours whenever a problem is unresolved or the patient's condition changes.

A clean SOAP or SOAPIE component

You don't need to write an entry for each SOAP or SOAPIE component every time you document. If you have nothing to record for a component, either omit the letter from the note or leave a blank space after it, depending on your facility's policy. (See *Problem-oriented progress notes*, page 70.)

Discharge summary

The discharge summary — the last part of POMR — covers each problem on the list and notes whether it was resolved. This is the place in your SOAP or SOAPIE note to discuss unresolved problems and outline your plan for dealing with the problem after

(Text continues on page 71.)

Art of the chart

Problem-oriented progress notes

The chart below is an example of progress notes as they appear in a problem-oriented medical record.

> No problem!

Date	Time	Notes
		Number each problem for easy reference.
2/1/09	0645	#1 Acute pain
		S: Pt states, "I am having severe back pain again and I'm nauseated."
		O: Pt states pain is #9 on 0-to-10 scale; skin is warm, pale, moist. Pt is restless, pacing in room, holding Ⓡ flank area with his hand.
		A: Pt in severe pain, needs medication for relief.
		P: Check orders for analgesia; check for any allergies; take VS; if within normal limits, give analgesia as ordered. Recheck pt in 30 minutes for response. Monitor pt for adverse reactions to drug. Observe pt for pain frequently; offer medication as ordered before pain becomes severe. —————— Ann Davis, RN
2/1/09	0651	#1 Acute pain
		S: Pt states, "The pain is less and I'm not nauseated."
		O: Pt states his pain is now a #2 on 0-to-10 scale. Skin warm and dry; color normal. Pt sitting on bed, watching the news.
		A: Pt has improved.
		P: Continue to monitor for pain and other symptoms.
		I: BP 158/84, P 104, RR 24 — morphine 4 mg I.V.
		E: Medication was effective. —————— Ann Davis, RN
2/1/09	0130	#2 Anxiety
		S: Pt states, "I am worried about the surgery and being out of work."
		O: Pt wringing his hands, eyes downcast.
		A: Pt is anxious regarding upcoming surgery and its impact on his job.
		P: Encourage verbalization of feelings and concerns. Offer emotional support. Involve family to discuss his concerns if agreeable to pt. —————— Ann Davis, RN
2/1/09	0130	#3 Deficient knowledge
		S: Pt states, "I never had surgery before."
		O: Pt is unsure about what to expect.
		A: Pt needs preoperative and postoperative education.
		P: Teach pt about events before and after surgery, for example, I.V. insertion; teach about the need for coughing and deep breathing, moving frequently in bed, and early ambulation after surgery. Explain why these are important. Evaluate pt's response to the teaching, and document. —————— Ann Davis, RN

> Progress notes are in SOAPIE format.

discharge. Also, record communications with other facilities, home health agencies, and the patient.

POMR pros...

The POMR charting system has several advantages:
• Information about each problem is organized into specific categories that all caregivers can understand. This organization eases data retrieval and communication between disciplines.
• Continuity of care is shown by combining the care plan and progress notes into a complete record of care that's planned and care that's delivered. The caregiver addresses each problem or nursing diagnosis in the nurses' notes.
• It encourages nurses to document the nursing process, chart more consistently, and chart only essential data.
• It can be used effectively with standardized care plans and is an integrated medical record.

...and cons

The POMR system also has some disadvantages, including:
• The emphasis on the chronology of problems, rather than their priority, may cause caregivers to disagree about which problems to list.
• Trends may be hard to analyze if information is buried in the daily narrative.
• Assessments and interventions apply to more than one problem, so charting of these findings is repetitious, especially with the SOAPIE format. This repetition makes documentation time-consuming to perform and read.
• The format emphasizes problems, so routine care may be left undocumented unless flow sheets are used.
• The format doesn't work well in settings with rapid patient turnover, such as a postanesthesia care unit, a short procedure unit, or an emergency department.
• Problems may arise if caregivers don't keep the problem list current or if they're confused about which problems to list.
• Considerable time and cost are needed to train people to use the SOAP, SOAPIE, and SOAPIER method.

PIE system

The problem-intervention-evaluation (PIE) system organizes information according to patients' problems and was devised to simplify the documentation process. This system requires you to keep a daily patient assessment flow sheet and to write structured progress notes. Integrating the care plan into the nurses' progress notes eliminates the need for a separate care plan. The idea is to provide a concise, efficient record of patient care that has a nursing focus. (See *Easy as PIE*.)

Using the PIE system

To use the PIE system, first assess the patient and document your findings on a daily patient assessment flow sheet.

Pieces of PIE

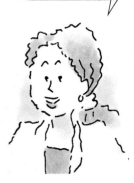

The daily assessment flow sheet lists defined assessment terms under major categories (such as respiration) along with routine care and monitoring measures (such as providing ventilation and monitoring breath sounds). The flow sheet generally includes space to record pertinent treatments.

On the flow sheet, initial only the assessment terms that apply to your patient and mark abnormal findings with an asterisk. Record detailed information in your progress notes.

Next, chart:

- the patient's problems
- your interventions
- your evaluations of the patient's responses.

Problem

After performing and documenting an initial assessment, use the collected data to identify pertinent nursing diagnoses. These form the *problem* piece of PIE. Use the list of nursing diagnoses accepted by your facility, which usually corresponds to the diagnoses approved by NANDA International.

Got a problem with that?

If you can't find a nursing diagnosis on an approved list, write the problem statement yourself using accepted criteria. Make sure you don't use medical diagnoses.

Keeping track

In the progress notes, document all nursing diagnoses or problems, labeling each as *P* and numbering it. For example, the first nursing diagnosis is labeled *P#1*. This way, you can later refer to a specific problem by its label only, without having to redocument the problem statement. Some facilities also use a separate problem-list form to keep a convenient running account of the nursing diagnoses for each patient.

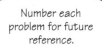

Number each problem for future reference.

Intervention

To chart the *intervention* piece of PIE, document the nursing actions you take for each nursing diagnosis. Write them on the progress sheet, labeling each as *I* and assigning the appropriate problem number. For example, to refer to an intervention for the first nursing diagnosis, write *IP#1*.

Evaluation

After charting your interventions, document the patient's responses in your progress notes. These form the *evaluation* piece of PIE. Use the label *E* followed by the assigned problem number. For example, to identify each evaluation write *EP#1*.

Reevaluate and review

Make sure that you or another nurse evaluates each problem at least once every 8 hours. After every three shifts, review the notes from the previous 24 hours to identify the patient's current problems and responses to interventions.

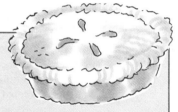

Art of the chart

Easy as PIE

This sample chart shows how to write progress notes using the problem-intervention-evaluation (PIE) system.

Date	Time	Notes
2/20/09	1300	P#1: Sudden onset of generalized itching and hives possibly related to an allergic reaction.
		IP#1: Note extent of symptoms; take VS; assess breath sounds for wheezing. Notify doctor immediately.
		Administer medications as ordered, including I.V. access. Reassure pt.
		EP#1: Symptoms abate; pt maintains adequate respiratory and hemodynamic status; pt verbalized understanding of treatments and need to report further symptoms. ——————— Mary Smith, RN
2/20/09	1300	P#2: Ineffective breathing pattern related to possible allergic reaction.
		IP#2: Take VS frequently and monitor breath sounds and pulse oximetry. Notify doctor for abnormal pulse oximetry or wheezing. Give medications as ordered. Teach pt signs of respiratory distress and the need to report these immediately. ——————— Mary Smith, RN
		EP#2: Pt has no wheezing or dyspnea; pt verbalized understanding of need to notify nurse of changes in breathing patterns. ——————— Mary Smith, RN

This stands for evaluation of problem # 1.

Document continuing problems daily, along with relevant interventions and evaluations. Once resolved and documented as such, a problem doesn't require further documentation.

Reasons to give PIE a try

The PIE format has many attractive features, including:
• ensuring that your documentation includes all the necessary pieces: nursing diagnoses (problems), related interventions, and evaluations
• providing ongoing documentation of current problems
• encouraging you to meet The Joint Commission requirements by providing an organized framework for your thoughts and writing
• simplifying documentation by combining the care plan and progress notes and using the flow sheet for assessment and patient care data
• improving the quality of your progress notes by highlighting interventions and requiring a written evaluation of the patient's response to them.

Problems with PIE

Don't take a "pie-in-the-sky" attitude to this charting system. Here's why:
• Staff members may need in-depth training before they can use it.
• It requires you to reevaluate each problem once every shift, which is time-consuming, usually unnecessary, and leads to repetitive entries.
• It omits documentation of the planning step in the nursing process. This step, which addresses expected outcomes, is essential in evaluating the patient's responses.
• It doesn't incorporate multidisciplinary charting.
• It isn't suitable for long-term care patients.

FOCUS system

Nurses who found the SOAP format awkward developed the FOCUS system of charting. This system is organized into patient-centered topics, or *foci*. It encourages you to use assessment data to evaluate these concerns. FOCUS charting works best in acute care settings and on units where the same care and procedures are repeated frequently.

Coming into FOCUS

To implement FOCUS documentation, you use a progress sheet with columns for the date, time, focus, and progress notes. You can identify the foci by reviewing your assessment data. (See *Focus on FOCUS charting*, page 76.)

In FOCUS charting, you typically write each focus as a nursing diagnosis, such as *Risk for infection* or *Deficient fluid volume*. However, the focus also may refer to:

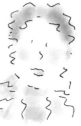
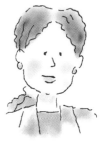

• sign or symptom—such as purulent drainage or chest pain
• patient behavior—such as an inability to ambulate
• special need—such as a discharge need
• acute change in the patient's condition—such as loss of consciousness or increase in blood pressure
• significant event—such as surgery.

Writing FOCUS progress notes

In the progress notes column, identify and divide the information into three categories:

data (D), which include subjective and objective information describing the focus

action (A), which includes immediate and future nursing actions based on your assessment of the patient's condition as well as changes to the care plan as necessary, based on your evaluation

response (R), which describes the patient's response to nursing or medical care.

Lights, camera, data, action, response!

Using all three categories guarantees complete documentation based on the nursing process. Be sure to record routine nursing tasks and assessment data on your flow sheets and checklists.

DAR-e to succeed?

FOCUS charting has several strong points:
• It's flexible enough to adapt to any clinical setting.
• It centers on the nursing process, and the data-action-response format encourages you to record in a process-oriented way.
• Information on a specific problem is easy to find because the FOCUS statement is separate from the progress note. This promotes communication between health care team members.
• It encourages regular documentation of patient responses to nursing and medical care and ensures adherence to The Joint Commission requirements.

Art of the chart

Focus on FOCUS charting

> Progress notes are divided into data, action, and response.

The chart below is an example of progress notes using the FOCUS system.

> This focus is written as a nursing diagnosis.

> The foci zoom in on the topics of major concern.

Date	Time	Focus	Progress notes
2/3/09	1000	Deficient knowledge R/T diagnosis	D: Pt states she does not understand what her diagnosis means.
			A: Illness explained to pt according to her level of understanding. Pt taught symptoms she may expect and why she is having current symptoms. Treatments and procedures explained. Questions answered. Pt encouraged to verbalize need for further instruction or information.
			R: Pt verbalized better understanding of her illness. ———————— Donna Jones, RN
2/3/09	1000	Risk for deficient fluid volume	D: Pt states her period just began and she is passing a large amount of clots.
			A: Amount of bleeding assessed. Pt saturated 2 sanitary napkins in the past hour, currently large amount of bright red clots noted. BP 114/10 P 98 RR 20. Pt status reported to Dr. T. Smith. Orders received. 20G I.V. catheter started, labs drawn; 1,000 ml NSS hung; macro tubing; at 100 ml per hr. Pt tolerated procedures well. Will continue to monitor vital signs and bleeding. Pt taught how to assess amount of vaginal drainage.
			R: Pt verbalizes correct amount of drainage and type. Pt understands procedures. Donna Jones, RN
2/3/09	1000	Anxiety	D: Pt states, "I'm afraid of all this blood."
			A: Emotional support provided. Encouraged verbalization. Explanations given regarding treatments and procedures. Family in to provide support.
			R: Pt observed talking and laughing with family. States she feels less anxious. Donna Jones, RN

• You can use this format to document many topics in addition to those on the problem list or care plan.
• It helps you organize your thoughts and document succinctly and precisely.
• It helps you identify areas in the care plan that need revising as you document each entry.

DAR downers

FOCUS charting also has weaknesses:
• Staff members, especially those who are more familiar with other systems, may need in-depth training before they can use it.
• You have to use many flow sheets and checklists, which can cause inconsistent documentation and problems tracking a patient's problems.

- If you forget to include the patient's response to interventions, FOCUS charting resembles a long narrative, like that seen in progress notes.

Charting by exception

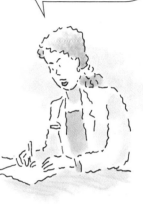

The patient's condition is unchanged, EXCEPT she reports less pain!

The system called charting by exception (CBE) was designed to eliminate lengthy and repetitive notes, poorly organized information, difficult-to-retrieve data, errors of omission, and other long-standing charting problems.

To avoid these pitfalls, the CBE format radically departs from traditional systems by requiring documentation of significant or abnormal findings only.

CBE guidelines

To use CBE effectively, you must adhere to established guidelines for nursing assessments and interventions and follow written standards of practice that identify the nurse's basic responsibilities. Facilities using CBE must have critical pathways or interdisciplinary care plans that address every possible patient problem.

Document deviations

Guidelines for each body system are printed on CBE forms. For example, care standards for patient hygiene might specify a complete linen change every 3 days or sooner, if necessary. Having the standards clearly and concisely written eliminates the need to chart routine nursing care or any other care outlined in the standards; all you document are deviations from the standards.

Get your guidelines here

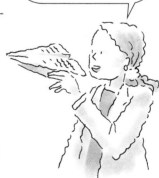

Guidelines for flying straight with the CBE system come from many sources.

Guidelines for interventions used in the CBE system come from these sources:
- *nursing diagnosis–based standardized care plans*, which identify patient problems, desired outcomes, and interventions
- *patient care guidelines*, which are standardized intervention plans created for specific patients, such as those with a nursing diagnosis of *Acute pain* or *Chronic pain*, that outline the nursing interventions, treatments, and time frames for repeated assessments
- *doctor's orders*, which are prescribed medical interventions
- *incidental orders*, which are usually one-time, miscellaneous nursing or medical orders or interdependent interventions related to a protocol or a piece of equipment

• *standards of nursing practice*, which define the acceptable level of routine nursing care for all patients and may describe the essential aspects of nursing practice for a specific unit or for all clinical areas.

CBE format

The CBE format includes a standardized care plan based on the nursing diagnosis and several types of flow sheets. These flow sheets include:
• nursing and medical order flow sheets
• graphic forms
• patient-teaching records
• patient discharge notes.

Making progress?

Sometimes you may need to supplement your CBE documentation by using nurses' progress notes.

Standardized care plans

When using the CBE format for charting, you fill out a preprinted care plan for each nursing diagnosis.

Fill in the blanks

Preprinted care plans have blank spaces so you can individualize them as needed. For example, include expected outcomes and major revisions in your care plan. Place the completed forms in the nurses' progress notes section of the clinical record.

Nursing and medical order flow sheets

Use nursing and medical order flow sheets to document your assessments and interventions. Each flow sheet covers a 24-hour period of care for one patient.

The top part of the flow sheet contains the doctor's orders for assessments and interventions. Each nursing order includes a corresponding nursing diagnosis, labeled *ND#1*, *ND#2*, and so on; doctor's orders are labeled *DO*. (See *Using a nursing and medical order flow sheet.*)

Checks, asterisks, and arrows

In addition to the abbreviations, *ND* for nursing diagnosis and *DO* for doctor's orders, use these symbols when you record care on flow sheets:
• a check mark (✔) to indicate a completed medical order or nursing assessment with no abnormal findings

> *Art of the chart*

Using a nursing and medical order flow sheet

Here are the typical features of a nursing and medical order flow sheet.

NURSING AND MEDICAL ORDER FLOW SHEET

Date 4/22/09

ND #/DO	Assessments and interventions	Time
ND 1	Wound assessment	0100* 1500*
ND 2	Range of motion assessment	
DO	Ancef 2g I.V. stat for one dose	0645✔
Initials		CF CF

> An asterisk indicates an abnormal assessment finding.

Key		
DO = doctor's orders	➔ = no change in condition	
ND = nursing diagnosis	✶ = abnormal or significant finding	
✔ = normal findings	(see Comments section)	

ND #/DO	Time	Comments	Initials
ND 1	0800	® leg wound with yellow drainage, inflammation around border. Dr. T. Smith notified. No complaint of pain.	CF
ND 1	0830	Pt able to move both lower extremities 1" off bed.	CF
ND 1	1100	No drainage on ® leg dressing	CF
ND 2	1100	Pt rates pain decreased to a 3/10	CF
Initials CF		**Signature** Cary Filiaano, RN	

> Explain your findings in the Comments section.

- an asterisk (✶) to indicate an abnormal finding on an assessment or an abnormal response to an intervention
- an arrow (➔) to indicate that the patient's status hasn't changed since the previous entry.

After completing an assessment, compare your findings with the printed guidelines on the back of the form. If a finding is within normal parameters, place a check mark in the appropriate box. If a finding isn't within the normal range, put an asterisk in the box. Then explain your findings in the comments section on the form.

> In CBE, an arrow indicates that the patient's status hasn't changed.

Note normalcy

An assessment finding that isn't defined in the guidelines may be normal for a particular patient. For example, unclear speech may be normal in a patient with a long-standing tracheostomy. Reference this type of note by nursing diagnosis number or doctor's order and time. If the patient's condition hasn't changed from the last assessment, draw a horizontal arrow from the previous category box to the current one.

Make more marks

Document interventions similarly. Use a check mark to indicate a completed intervention and an expected patient response. Indicate significant findings or abnormal patient responses with an asterisk, and write an explanation in the comments section. When the patient's response is unchanged, use an arrow.

After you document an entire column in the assessments and interventions section, initial it at the bottom. Also initial all your entries in the comments section and sign the form at the bottom of the page.

Care-ful combinations

Some facilities use a special nursing care flow sheet that combines all the necessary forms, such as the graphic record, the daily activities checklist, and the patient care assessment section. (See *It flows together: Using a combined nursing care flow sheet.*)

Graphic form

The graphic form section of a flow sheet is used to document trends in the patient's vital signs, weight, intake and output, and stool, urination, appetite, and activity levels.

More checks and asterisks

As with the nursing and medical order flow sheet, use check marks to indicate expected findings and asterisks to indicate abnormal ones. Record information about abnormalities in the nurses' progress notes or on the nursing and medical order flow sheet.

In the box labeled "routine standards," check off the established nursing care interventions you performed such as providing hygiene. Don't rewrite these standards as orders on the nursing and medical order flow sheet. Refer to the guidelines on the back of the graphic form for complete instructions.

Patient-teaching record

Use the patient-teaching form (or section) to identify the information, psychomotor skills, and social or behavioral measures that your patient or his caregiver must learn by a predetermined date.

(Text continues on page 84.)

Art of the chart

It flows together: Using a combined nursing care flow sheet

This sample shows a portion of a nursing care flow sheet that combines a graphic record, a daily nursing care activities checklist, and a patient care assessment form.

> The graphic record makes it easy to spot trends.

Name		Maureen Gallen											
Date				2/29/09									
Hour		0700	0800	0900	1000	1100	1200	1300	1400	1500	1600	1700	1800
Temperature													
°C	°F												
40.6	105												
40	104												
39.4	103												
38.9	102												
37.8	100												
37.2	99												
36.7	98												
36.1	97												
35.6	96												
Pulse		84	80	82	78	76	78	78	82	84	82	80	78
Respiration		16	20	20	22	24	24	18	20	22	20	18	24
BP	Lying												
	Sitting	136/82	130/80	126/74	132/82	132/80	140/82	136/74	130/70	138/78	140/80	132/78	136/76
	Standing												
Intake	Oral		240					360					120
	Tube												
	I.V.												
	Blood												
8-hour total		—	—	—	—	—	—	—	—	600	—	—	—
Output			400				450						
Other													
8-hour total		—	—	—	—	—	—	—	—	850	—	—	—
Teaching		dressing changes, s/s of infection											
Signature		Mary Murphy, RN						Ann Burns, RN					
		0700 - 1500						1500 - 2300					

(continued)

It flows together: Using a combined nursing care flow sheet (continued)

This section enables efficient documentation of daily activities.

Hour		0700	0800	0900	1000	1100	1200	1300	1400	1500	1600	1700
ACTIVITY	Bed rest	MM							→	AB	—	→
	OOB											
	Ambulate (assist)											
	Ambulatory											
	Sleeping											
	Bathroom privileges											
	HOB elevated	MM							→	AB	—	→
	Cough, deep-breathe, turn		MM							AB		
	ROM Active/Passive		MM							AB		
HYGIENE	Bath		MM									
	Shave		MM									
	Oral		MM									
	Skin care											
	Peri care											
NUTRITION	Diet	House										
	% eating			15%			60%					15%
	Feeding											
	Supplemental											
	S-Self, A-Assist, F-Feed		A				A					A
BLADDER	Catheter	indwelling urinary #18 Fr.										
	Incontinent											
	Voiding	clear, yellow urine										
	Intermittent catheter											
BOWEL	Stools (occult blood + or -)											
	Incontinent											
	Normal	large formed brown stool										
	Enema											
SPECIAL TREATMENTS	Special mattress	Low-pressure airflow mattress applied 0900										
	Special bed											
	Heel and elbow pads											
	Antiembolism stockings											
	Traction: + = on, - = off											
	Isolation type											

It flows together: Using a combined nursing care flow sheet *(continued)*

ASSESSMENT FINDINGS

Findings marked by an asterisk must be documented.

KEY: ✔ = normal findings
      ✻ = significant findings

	Day	Evening	Night	
Neurologic	✻ MM	✔ AB		0800 Limited ROM ® shoulder. Pt. states, "I have arthritis and my shoulder is always stiff."
Cardiovascular	✔ MM	✔ AB		
Respiratory	✔ MM	✻ AB		1800 Shallow breathing with poor inspiratory effort at 1700
GI	✔ MM	✔ AB		
Genitourinary	✔ MM	✔ AB		
Surgical dressing and incision	✻ MM	✔ AB		0930 Incision reddened; dime-sized area of serous sanguineous drainage on old dressing
Skin integrity	✔ MM	✔ AB		
Psychosocial	✔ MM	✔ AB		
Educational	✻ MM	✔ AB		0945 Taught pt incisional care and dressing change, and s/s of infection. Pt. able to return demonstration of incisional care.
Peripheral vascular	✔ MM	✔ AB		

NORMAL ASSESSMENT FINDINGS

Neurologic assessment:
- Alert and oriented to time, place, and person.
- Speech clear and understandable.
- Memory intact.
- Behavior appropriate to situation and accommodation.
- Active range of motion (ROM) of all extremities, symmetrically equal strength.
- No paresthesia.

Cardiovascular assessment:
- Regular apical pulse.
- Palpable bilateral peripheral pulses.
- No peripheral edema.
- No calf tenderness.

Pulmonary assessment:
- Resting respirations 10 to 20 per minute, quiet and regular.
- Clear sputum.
- Pink nail beds and mucous membranes.

Gastrointestinal assessment:
- Abdomen soft and nondistended.
- Tolerates prescribed diet without nausea or vomiting.
- Bowel movements within own normal pattern and consistency (as described in Patient Profile).

Genitourinary assessment:
- No indwelling catheter in use.
- Urinates without pain.
- Undistended bladder after urination.
- Urine is clear, yellow to amber color.

Surgical dressing and incision assessment:
- Dressing dry and intact.
- No evidence of redness, increased temperature, or tenderness in surrounding tissue.
- Sutures, staples, or adhesive strips intact.
- Wound edges well-approximated.
- No drainage present.

Skin integrity assessment:
- Skin color normal.
- Skin warm, dry, and intact.
- Moist mucous membranes.

Psychosocial assessment:
- Interacts and communicates in an appropriate manner with others (family, significant others, health care personnel).

Educational assessment:
- Patient or significant others communicate understanding of the patient's health status, care plan, and expected response.
- Patient or significant others demonstrate ability to perform health-related procedures and behaviors as taught.
- Items taught and expected performance must be specifically described in Significant Findings Section.

Peripheral vascular assessment:
- Affected extremity is pink, warm, and movable within average ROM.
- Capillary refill time less than 3 seconds.
- Peripheral pulses palpable.
- No edema, sensation intact without numbness or paresthesia.
- No pain on passive stretch.

A lot to learn? Use more forms...

This record includes teaching resources, dates of patient achievements, and other pertinent observations. If the patient has multiple learning needs, you can use more than one form.

Patient discharge note

Like other discharge forms, the patient discharge note is a flow sheet for documenting ongoing discharge planning. To chart discharge planning, follow the instructions printed on the back of the form. A typical discharge note includes patient instructions, appointments for follow-up care, medication and diet instructions, signs and symptoms to report, level of activity, wound care, and patient education.

Progress notes

Use the progress notes to document revisions in the care plan and interventions that don't lend themselves to the nursing and medical order flow sheet. Because the CBE format allows you to document most assessments and interventions on the nursing and medical order flow sheet, your progress notes usually contain little assessment and intervention data.

It's exception-al!

The CBE format has several important benefits:
• It eliminates documentation of routine care through the use of nursing care standards. This stops redundancies and clearly identifies abnormal data.
• CBE is easily adapted to documentation on critical pathways.
• Information that has already been recorded isn't repeated. For instance, you don't have to write a long entry each time you assess a patient whose condition has stayed the same.
• The use of well-defined guidelines and standards of care promotes uniform nursing practice.
• The flow sheets let you track trends easily.
• Guidelines are printed on the forms for ready reference. Abnormal findings are highlighted to help you quickly pinpoint significant changes and trends in a patient's condition.
• Patient data are immediately written on the permanent record. Because you don't need to keep temporary notes and then transcribe them in the patient's chart later, all caregivers always have access to the most current data, which decreases charting time.
• Assessments are standardized so all caregivers evaluate and document findings consistently.

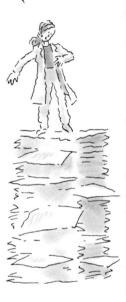

If your patient has multiple learning needs, you can use more than one form. Yikes!

With CBE, I don't waste time charting routine care.

• All flow sheets are kept at the patient's bedside, where they serve as a ready reference. This encourages immediate documentation.

CBE shortcomings

Nothing is perfect, including the CBE system. Here are the drawbacks:

• The development of clear guidelines and standards of care is time-consuming. For legal reasons, these guidelines and standards must be written and understood by all nurses before the system can be implemented.

• This system takes a long time for people to learn, accept, and use correctly and consistently.

• Duplicate charting occurs with CBE; nursing diagnoses on a problem list are also written on the care plan.

• Narrative notes and evaluations of patients' responses may be brief and sketchy in facilities that use multiple forms instead of one combination form.

• This system was developed for RNs. Before LPNs can use it, it must be evaluated and modified to meet their scope of practice.

FACT documentation system

The computer-ready FACT documentation system incorporates many CBE principles. It was developed to help caregivers avoid the documentation of irrelevant data, repetitive notes, and inconsistencies among departments and to reduce the amount of time spent charting.

Using the FACT system

In this system, you document only exceptions to the norm or significant information about the patient.

That's a FACT

The FACT format uses:
• assessment and action flow sheet
• frequent assessment flow sheet
• progress notes.

    The content of flow sheets and notes may be individualized to some extent. The flow sheets cover a 24- to 72-hour time span, and you'll need to date, time, and sign all entries. (See *Face facts with FACT charting*, pages 86 and 87.)

Memory jogger

FACT is an acronym for the four key elements of this charting system. Here's how to remember these elements:
Flow sheets individualized to specific services
Assessment features standardized with baseline parameters
Concise, integrated progress notes and flow sheets documenting the patient's condition and responses
Timely entries recorded when care is given.

(Text continues on page 88.)

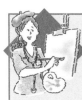

Art of the chart

Face facts with FACT charting

This sample shows portions of an assessment flow sheet and a postoperative flow sheet using the FACT format.

ASSESSMENT RECORD

> Assessment parameters for each body system are on the form.

> Only document exceptions to the norm or significant information about the patient.

	Date	3/18/09	3/18/09	3/18/09
	Time	0100	0500	0900
Neurologic Alert and oriented to time, place, and person. PERLA. Symmetry of strength in extremities. No difficulty with coordination. Behavior appropriate to situation. Sensation intact without numbness or paresthesia.		✓		✔
Orient patient.				
Refer to neurologic flow sheet.				
Pain No report of pain. If present, include patient statements about intensity (0 to 5 scale), location, description, duration, radiation, precipitating and alleviating factors.		1 - Neck pain	✓	4- Neck pain "It hurts."
Location		Cervical spine area		Cervical spine area
Relief measures		Pt repositioned		Percocet p.o.
Pain relief: Yes/No		Y		Y
Cardiac Apical pulse 60 to 100. S_1 and S_2 present. Regular rhythm. Peripheral (radial, pedal) pulses present. No edema or calf tenderness. Extremities pink, warm, movable within patient's ROM.		✓	✔	✓
I.V. solution and rate		D_5 1/2 NSS @ 30 ml per hr	D_5 1/2 NSS @ 30 ml per hr	D_5 1/2 NSS @ 30 ml per hr
Pulmonary Respiratory rate 12 to 20 at rest, quiet, regular and nonlabored. Lungs clear and aerated equally in all lobes. No SOB at rest. No abnormal breath sounds. Mucous membranes pink.		✓	✓	✔
O_2 therapy				
Taught coughing, deep breathing, incentive spirometer		✓	✓	✓
Musculoskeletal Extremities pink, warm, and without edema; sensation and motion present. Normal joint ROM, no swelling or tenderness. Steady gait without aids. Pedal, radial pulses present. Rapid capillary refill.		✓	✓	✔
Activity (describe)		bed rest	OOB in chair	bed rest
Nurse's signature and title		Jane Snow, RN	Jane Snow, RN	Jane Snow, RN

Key: ✓ Meets assessment criteria

Face facts with FACT charting *(continued)*

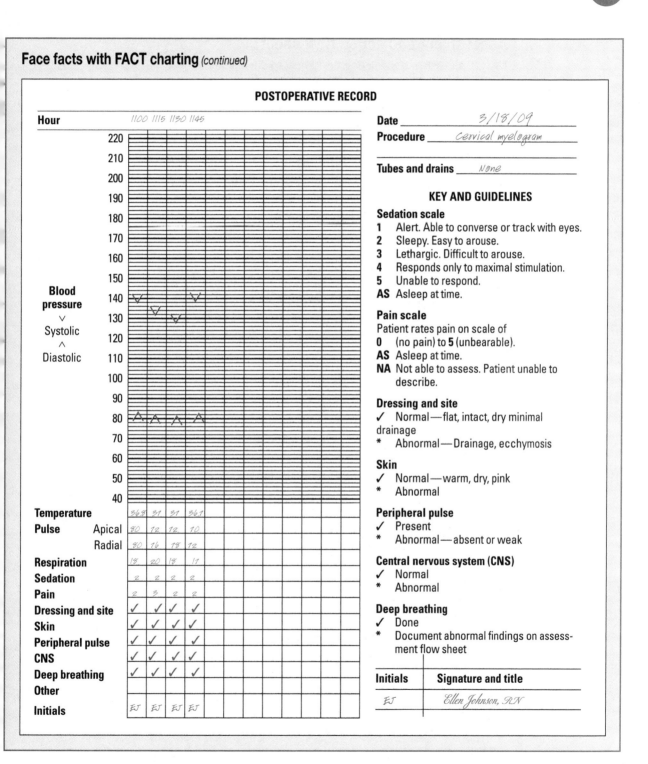

POSTOPERATIVE RECORD

Hour — 1100 1115 1130 1145

Date _3/18/09_

Procedure _Cervical myelogram_

Tubes and drains _None_

KEY AND GUIDELINES

Sedation scale
1. Alert. Able to converse or track with eyes.
2. Sleepy. Easy to arouse.
3. Lethargic. Difficult to arouse.
4. Responds only to maximal stimulation.
5. Unable to respond.
AS Asleep at time.

Pain scale
Patient rates pain on scale of
0 (no pain) to **5** (unbearable).
AS Asleep at time.
NA Not able to assess. Patient unable to describe.

Dressing and site
✓ Normal—flat, intact, dry minimal drainage
* Abnormal—Drainage, ecchymosis

Skin
✓ Normal—warm, dry, pink
* Abnormal

Peripheral pulse
✓ Present
* Abnormal—absent or weak

Central nervous system (CNS)
✓ Normal
* Abnormal

Deep breathing
✓ Done
* Document abnormal findings on assessment flow sheet

Blood pressure — ∨ Systolic, ∧ Diastolic

Blood pressure scale (mmHg): 220, 210, 200, 190, 180, 170, 160, 150, 140, 130, 120, 110, 100, 90, 80, 70, 60, 50, 40

	1100	1115	1130	1145
Temperature	36.8	37	37	36.7
Pulse Apical	80	72	72	70
Radial	80	76	78	72
Respiration	18	20	18	17
Sedation	2	2	2	2
Pain	2	3	2	2
Dressing and site	✓	✓	✓	✓
Skin	✓	✓	✓	✓
Peripheral pulse	✓	✓	✓	✓
CNS	✓	✓	✓	✓
Deep breathing	✓	✓	✓	✓
Other				
Initials	EJ	EJ	EJ	EJ

Initials	Signature and title
EJ	Ellen Johnson, RN

Assessment and action flow sheet

Use the assessment and action flow sheet to document ongoing assessments and interventions. Normal assessment parameters for each body system are printed on the form, along with the planned interventions. You may individualize the flow sheet according to the patient's needs.

Frequent assessment flow sheet

Use the frequent assessment flow sheet to chart vital signs and frequent assessments. On a surgical unit, for example, this form would include a postoperative assessment section.

Progress notes

The FACT system requires an integrated progress record. Use narrative notes to document the patient's progress and any significant incidents. As in FOCUS charting, write narrative notes using the data-action-response method. Update progress notes related to patient outcomes every 48 hours or according to facility policy.

Favorable FACTs

The FACT charting system has many good points. For example, this system:
• eliminates repetition and encourages consistent language and structure
• eliminates detailed charting of normal findings and incorporates each step of the nursing process
• is outcome oriented and communicates the patient's progress to all health care team members
• permits immediate recording of current data and is readily accessible at the patient's bedside
• eliminates the need for many different forms and reduces the time spent writing narrative notes
• is cost-effective.

Finding fault with FACT

However, FACT charting does have some problems:
• Development of standards and implementation of a facility-wide system requires a major time commitment.
• Narrative notes may be sketchy, and the nurse's perspective on the patient may be overlooked.
• The nursing process framework may be difficult to identify.

> The FACT system eliminates repetitive charting? Thank goodness!

Core charting system

The core system focuses on the nursing process, which is the core of documentation. It's most useful in acute care and long-term care facilities.

Core framework

This system requires you to assess and record a patient's functional and cognitive status within 8 hours of admission. It consists of:
- database
- care plan
- flow sheets
- progress notes
- discharge summary.

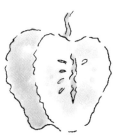

Database

The database (initial assessment form) focuses on the patient's body systems and activities of daily living. It includes a summary of his problems and appropriate nursing diagnoses. The nurse enters the completed database onto the patient's medical record card or Kardex.

Care plan

The completed care plan (like the database) goes on the patient's medical record card or Kardex.

Flow sheets

Use flow sheets to document the patient's activities and his response to nursing interventions, diagnostic procedures, and patient teaching.

Progress notes

On the progress notes sheet, record the DAE — that's data (D), action (A), and evaluation (E) or response — for each problem.

Discharge summary

The discharge summary includes information about the nursing diagnoses, patient teaching, and recommended follow-up care.

Core gets a high score

The core charting system with DAE has several things going for it:
• It incorporates the entire nursing process.
• The DAE component helps ensure complete documentation based on the nursing process.
• It encourages concise documentation with minimal repetition.
• It allows the daily recording of psychosocial information.

Core concerns

Oh no! Core with DAE has a worm (four worms, actually). They are:
• Staff members who are used to other documenting systems may need in-depth training.
• Development of forms may be costly and time-consuming.
• The DAE format doesn't always present information chronologically, making it difficult to quickly perceive the patient's progress.
• The progress notes may not always relate to the care plan, so you must monitor carefully to make sure the record shows high-quality care.

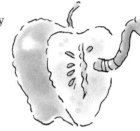

Choosing a charting system

Health care facilities are always striving for greater efficiency and quality of care. A top-notch charting system can help a facility reach these goals.

Remember, documentation is examined often to make sure a facility meets the profession's minimum acceptable level of care. If efficiency and quality levels are low, your charting system may need to be modified or replaced. (See *Does your charting system measure up?*)

Getting better and better

Continuous quality improvement programs are mandated by the state and The Joint Commission. Committees that set up these programs choose well-defined, objective, and easily measurable indicators that help them assess the structure, process, and outcome of patient care. They also use these indicators to monitor and evaluate the contents of a patient's medical record.

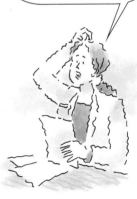

What charting system should I use? Let's see, I need to consider the type of care my facility provides.

Advice from the experts

Does your charting system measure up?

How useful is your current charting system? Is it incomplete, disorganized, or confusing? If so, it won't stand up to later scrutiny in case of a lawsuit or formal review. To evaluate your charting system, ask yourself the following questions. If you answer "no" to any of them, a closer evaluation of your system might be warranted.

Documenting interventions and patient progress

• Does your current system reflect the patient's progress and the interventions based on recorded evaluations? Look for records that describe the patient's progress, actual interventions, and evaluations of provided care.

• Does the record include evidence of the patient's response to nursing care? For example, does it report the effectiveness of analgesics or the patient's response to I.V. medications?

• Does it show that care was modified according to the patient's response to treatment? For example, does it show what action was taken if the patient tolerated only half of a prescribed tube feeding?

• Does the record note continuity of care, or do unexplained gaps appear? If gaps appear, are notes entered later that document previous happenings? If late entries appear in the nurses' notes on subsequent days, do you have to check the entire record to validate care?

• Are daily activities documented? For example, do the notes include evidence that the patient bathed himself or indicate that the patient could independently transfer himself to a wheelchair?

Documenting the health care team's actions

• Does the record portray the nursing process clearly? Look for actual nursing diagnoses, written assessments, interventions, and evaluation of the patient's responses to them.

• Does the current documentation system facilitate and show communication among health care team members? Check for evidence that calls were made, that doctors were paged and notified of changes in a patient's condition, and that actions reflected these communications.

• Is discharge planning clearly documented? Do the records show evidence of interdisciplinary coordination, team conferences, completed patient teaching, and discharge instructions?

• Does the record reflect current standards of care? Does it indicate that caregivers and administrators follow facility policies and procedures? If not, does the system provide for explanations of why a policy wasn't implemented or was implemented in a different way?

Checking for clarity and comprehensiveness

• Are all portions of the record complete? Are all flow sheets, checklists, and other forms completed according to facility policy? Are all necessary entries apparent on the medication forms? If not, does the record describe why a medication wasn't given as ordered and who was informed of the omission, if necessary?

• Does the documentation make sense? Can you track the patient's care and hospital course on this record alone?

Does your charting measure up?

Shorter hospital stays and the requirement to verify the need for supplies and equipment have placed greater emphasis on nursing documentation as a yardstick for measuring the quality of patient care and determining if it was required and provided.

To verify that treatment was required and provided or that medical tests and supplies were used, the insurers (also called *third-party payers*) review nursing documentation carefully. As a result, nurses now need to document more information than ever

Don't miss the review of charting systems on the next page.

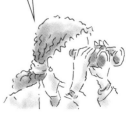

before, including every I.V. needle used to start an infusion, each use of an I.V. pump to deliver a specific volume of medication, and every test that the patient undergoes.

Are you committed? Serve on a committee...

When changes are called for, you may be asked to serve on a committee that decides whether your charting system needs a simple revision or total overhaul. Before committing to a totally new system, your committee should discuss the possibility of revising the current system. This, of course, is easier than switching to a new system and changing the way information is collected, entered, and retrieved. (See *To change or not to change.*)

When choosing a new charting system, consider the type of care that's provided at your facility. For example, some systems work better in acute care than in long-term care settings.

Cost is another important factor to consider. Although computer systems are used in almost every care setting, the cost of a new system can be astronomical.

If a new charting system is selected, staff will require plenty of training. The system may be initiated on one unit at a time to make the transition easier.

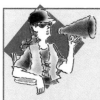

That's a wrap!

Review of charting systems

Traditional narrative
• Flexible, easy-to-learn system that keeps notes in chronological order, making them accessible, but may be time-consuming, repetitive, and difficult to read and understand
• Requires the nurse to be descriptive and specific about patient progress

POMR
• Problem-oriented medical record (POMR) system, which uses multidisciplinary progress notes and a five-part format (database, problem list, initial plan, progress notes, discharge summary)
• Works well in acute and long-term care settings

• Facilitates communication between disciplines, which results in continuity of care
• Organization by problem makes assessments and interventions difficult to follow and allows routine care to go undocumented

PIE
• Problem-intervention-evaluation (PIE) system that isn't multidisciplinary and uses daily assessment flow sheets and nursing-focused progress notes, eliminating the need for a separate care plan
• Ensures that notes have necessary information: problems, interventions, and evaluation of the patient's response
• Elimination of planning step makes tracking patient evaluation difficult

---

To change or not to change

Whether you're selecting a new charting system or modifying an existing one, ponder the following questions:

• What are the specific positive features of our current charting system?

• What are the specific problems or limitations of our current system? How can they be resolved?

• How much time will we need to develop a new system, educate the staff, and implement the changes?

• Will a new system be cost-effective?

• How will changing the charting system affect other members of the health care team, including the business office staff and medical staff?

• How will we handle resistance to the proposed changes?

Review of charting systems *(continued)*

FOCUS
• Adaptable system that typically uses a nursing diagnosis–based focus to organize information
• Use of three categories (data, action, response) guarantees complete documentation that's based on the nursing process
• Use of many flow sheets can cause inconsistent documentation and problems tracking patient complications

CBE
• Charting by exception (CBE) system that was designed to eliminate repetitive notes, poor organization, and other charting problems by requiring that only significant or abnormal findings be documented
• Requires the nurse to adhere to established guidelines and follow written standards of practice
• Includes a standardized care plan based on the nursing diagnosis and several types of flow sheets (nursing and medical order flow sheets, graphic form, patient-teaching record, patient discharge note)

FACT
• Computer-ready, outcome-oriented system that incorporates the CBE principles of documenting only significant or abnormal findings but attempts to reduce charting time and costs
• Eliminates repetition and detailed charting of normal findings
• Development and implementation may be difficult and time-consuming

Core
• Nursing process–focused system that uses a database, care plan, flow sheets, progress notes, and discharge summary
• Progress notes record the data, action, and evaluation (DAE)
• Incorporates the entire nursing process, which ensures complete documentation but isn't always presented chronologically, making evaluation difficult

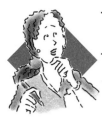

Quick quiz

1. The PIE charting format is useful in which setting?
    A.   Acute care
    B.   Long-term care
    C.   Home care
    D.   Ambulatory care

Answer: A. Acutely ill patients should be assessed at least every 8 hours, which the PIE system requires. However, such frequent assessment of patients in these other care settings would generate lengthy, repetitive notes.

2. A disadvantage of POMR documentation is its emphasis on:
    A.   priority of problems.
    B.   chronology of problems.
    C.   SOAP notes.
    D.   nursing process.

Answer: B. When the emphasis is put on chronology instead of priority, teammates may disagree about which problems to list.

3.   An advantage of narrative documentation is:
    A.   it clearly tracks trends and problems.
    B.   it's flexible in various clinical settings.
    C.   it uses flow charts.
    D.   it clearly identifies problems.

Answer: B. The most flexible of all charting systems, narrative charting suits any clinical setting and strongly conveys your nursing interventions and your patients' responses.

4.   When deciding which charting system to use, give the least consideration to:
    A.   your geographic area.
    B.   legal issues.
    C.   professional standards.
    D.   type of care provided at your facility.

Answer: A. Health care facilities also consider accrediting requirements when deciding which charting system would be the most effective.

Scoring

★★★   If you answered all four questions correctly, great job. Without exception, your knowledge of charting systems is FOCUSed.

★★   If you answered three questions correctly, three cheers! You've gotten to the core (with DAE) of charting systems.

★   If you answered fewer than three questions correctly, don't fret! You'll have plenty of opportunities to document your way to distinction, using narrative notes, POMR, the PIE system, FOCUS charting…

5

Computerized charting

Just the facts

In this chapter, you'll learn:

♦ advantages and disadvantages of computerized charting

♦ procedures to follow for computerized charting

♦ different types of computerized documentation systems.

A look at computerized charting

Whenever a patient enters a health care facility—whether it's a hospital, nursing home, or doctor's office—a lot of information about that patient is obtained, recorded, and processed. This information must be recorded so that it's easily retrievable as well as meaningful and useful to other health care providers. Computerized patient records are rapidly becoming the standard in most health care facilities.

Information station

Computerized charting systems consist of a complex, interconnected set of software applications that process and transport data that are input by the health care team. A computerized patient record categorizes the patient's data and stores the patient's health care history, including inpatient and outpatient records from various facilities. This information helps guide the health care team in providing care and identifying patient education needs.

Multitasker

In addition to helping with patient needs, computerized documentation can assist with:
• nurse-management reports
• staff scheduling

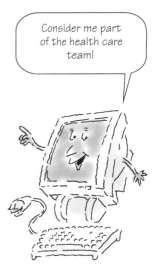

Consider me part of the health care team!

- staffing projections
- patient classification data
- federal and state licensure and accreditation surveys
- nursing research data.

Continuing ed advantage

Computerized documentation systems can also provide mandatory staff education modules, in which the nurse participates in interactive teaching modules and then takes a test. The computer system automatically records the score and keeps a log of the completed sessions. The nurse can then print out a certificate of completion for her continuing education record.

The upside

The advantages of computerized patient records include:
- improved standardized charting
- higher quality of clinical information within the medical record
- quick access to patient information across all departments
- reduction in redundant charting
- improved legibility of doctor's orders and progress notes.

The downside

Computerized patient records also have their disadvantages:
- Computer crashes or breakdowns can make patient information temporarily unavailable.
- Computer downtime for system updates makes information unavailable for a short period each day.
- Staff may be unfamiliar with the system.
- Breaches in patient confidentiality may occur.

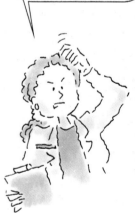

Can't make heads or tails of a doctor's written orders? A computerized patient record can help clear things up!

Using a computerized system

Most health care facilities have a mainframe computer as well as personal computers or terminals at workstations throughout the facility. These terminals provide quick access to vital information and allow staff to easily enter patient care orders. Some facilities have bedside terminals that make data even more accessible.

Mum's the word

Each team member accesses the record by entering an individual username and password. Don't share your password with anyone else. Your password is a legal electronic signature that's individual to you. Also, make sure to log off when leaving a computer terminal. Staying logged in allows someone else to record entries using your name. It also leaves the computer open for confidentiality breaches.

Starting the record

When a patient is admitted into the facility, a staff member logs into the computer system. The patient's name, account number, medical record number, and other demographic data are then entered into the computer system. This begins the patient's computerized record.

To each his own access

With computerized documentation, different members of the health care team can have access to different types of patient information. For example, a dietician who logs into the patient record with her username and password may see dietary orders but not physical therapy orders. When used correctly, this feature can help maintain a patient's privacy. (See *Maintaining patient confidentiality*.)

"Doctoring" the documentation

After the patient's computerized record is started, the doctor can log into the system and access the doctor's order screens. From

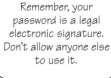

Remember, your password is a legal electronic signature. Don't allow anyone else to use it.

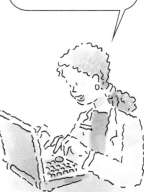

Maintaining patient confidentiality

The American Nurses Association and the American Records Association offer these guidelines for maintaining confidentiality of computerized medical records.

Never share
Never give your personal password or computer code to anyone — including another nurse in the unit, a nurse serving temporarily in the unit, or a doctor. Your health care facility can issue a short-term password that allows infrequent users to access certain records.

Log off
After you log on to a computer terminal, don't leave the terminal unattended. Although some computer systems have a timing device that automatically logs off the user after an idle period, you should get in the habit of logging off the system before leaving the terminal.

Don't display
Don't leave information about a patient displayed on a monitor where others can see it. Also, don't leave print versions or excerpts of the medical record unattended.

these screens, the doctor can choose the orders that are appropriate for the patient. Then the computer system transmits the orders to the patient's nursing department and other appropriate departments. For example, if the doctor orders medications for the patient, the order is transmitted to the patient's nursing department and the pharmacy.

Help for managing meds

Computerized documentation allows for direct order transmittal, which cuts down on medication errors by eliminating order transcription errors. It also alerts the doctor to patient allergies. Additionally, the system's medication order screens typically provide the doctor with choices of dosages and administration routes, which can help prevent dosing errors.

Ready, set, retrieve

After the doctor's orders are entered, you can log into the system to update the patient record as needed. To display the patient's electronic chart on screen, enter the patient's name or account number, or choose the patient's name from a patient census list. After retrieving the patient's information, you can enter new data into the care plan or progress notes, sign out medications that you've administered, or compare data on vital signs, laboratory test results, or intake and output.

Fast and functional

Typically, computerized documentation systems allow health care providers to retrieve information more quickly than traditional documentation systems do. Most systems allow you to print a patient Kardex each shift that contains information to guide your care. (See *Computer-generated Kardex*.)

Follow protocol

Be sure to follow your facility's protocol for correcting errors. Computer entries are part of the patient's permanent record and, as such, can't be deleted. Most systems have a special feature that allows you to correct a charting error. You simply access a screen that prompts you to make the correction. Then you enter the date and time the error was made, locate the error in the record, and correct it. Just as with traditional charting, the correction is shown along with the original error.

Back up

Make sure that stored records have backup files—an important safety feature. If you inadvertently delete part of the permanent

I can't find anything in this mess! Get me a computerized documentation system STAT!

(Text continues on page 101.)

Art of the chart

Computer-generated Kardex

The computer-generated Kardex contains vital information to help guide your nursing care throughout your shift. It may be necessary to print out a new Kardex at various times throughout your shift so new doctor's orders are reflected.

Medical ICU—4321 Patient Care Hospital   PAGE 01
03/14/09   07:00   **PATIENT KARDEX**

WILLIAMS, HENRY   68   MWMC
MR#: 5555555   DOB 10/26/40   MICU   302
FIN#: 1010101010   Admitted: 03/12/09
DR: Daniel Smith   Service: Internal Medicine

Summary: 03/14 07:00 to 15:00

ALLERGIES AND CODE STATUS:
  3/12/09   MED ALLERGY: NO KNOWN DRUG ALLERGY   NO INTUBATION

PATIENT INFORMATION:
  03/12/09   Admit Dx: TIA
  03/13/09   Final Dx: Stroke
  03/12/09   Patient condition: Fair
  03/13/09   Clinical guideline: Stroke
  03/12/09   Language: English
  03/12/09   PMH: No problems—respiratory, HTN, No problems—GI, No problems—GU, Type 2 diabetes, No
               problems—skin, No problems—blood, No problems—musculoskeletal, No problems—psych, No
               problems—hearing, glasses, cholecystectomy 1982, Tobacco use: denies, Alcohol use: current,
               1 beer a day, Illicit drug use: denies, Immunizations: Flu vaccine: 2008
  03/12/09   Living will: yes, on chart
  03/12/09   Durable power of attorney: yes, Name of DPOA: June Smith, Phone number 9875551234
  03/12/09   Organ donor: yes, card on chart
CONSULTS:
  03/12/09   Consult Westside Neurological Associates to see patient regarding flaccid left side and expressive aphasia
               Nurses, call consult now
ISF NOTES:
  03/12/09   Care plan: General care of the adult
  03/12/09   Nursing protocol: Falls prevention
  03/12/09   Nursing protocol: Skin breakdown (prevention)
  03/12/09   Goal: Patient will tolerate a progressive increase in activity level.   CONTINUED

(continued)

Computer-generated Kardex *(continued)*

03/14/09	07:00	**PATIENT KARDEX**

WILLIAMS, HENRY   68   MWMC
MR#: 5555555   DOB 10/26/40   MICU   302
FIN#: 1010101010   Admitted: 03/12/09
DR: Daniel Smith   Service: Internal Medicine

Summary: 03/14 07:00 to 15:00

NURSE COMMUNICATIONS:
   03/12/09   I.V. site — RA2, #20 inserted, restart on 03/15/09

ALL CURRENT MEDICAL ORDERS

Doctor to nurse orders:
   03/12/09   Blood cultures × 2 if temperature greater than 101° F, Nurse please enter as a secondary order, when necessary.
   03/12/09   Cardiology: ECG 12 lead Stat, prn chest pain, Nurse please enter as a secondary order, when necessary.
   03/12/09   Sequential Teds: Patient to wear continuously while in bed.
   03/12/09   Indwelling urinary catheter to urometer, measure output q 1 hour, notify MD if urine output less than 30 ml in one hour or greater than 300 ml in 2 hours.
   03/12/09   Notify MD for SBP greater than 180 mm Hg or less than 110 mm Hg
   03/12/09   Notify MD for change in mental status
   03/12/09   Accucheck q 6 hours

Vital sign orders:
   03/12/09   VS: q 1 hour with neurological checks

Diet:
   03/12/09   Diet: NPO

I&O orders:
   03/12/09   Per ICU routine

Activity:
   03/12/09   Activity: Bedrest with HOB elevated 30 degrees

IVS:
   03/12/09   I.V. line — Dextrose 5% & Sodium Chloride 0.45% 1000 ml, Rate: 80 ml per hour, 2 bags

Scheduled medications:
   03/12/09   Dexamethasone 4 mg, I.V., q 6 hours
   03/12/09   Metoprolol 5 mg, I.V., q 6 hours
   03/12/09   Heparin 5,000 units, subcutaneously, q 12 hours

Miscellaneous Medications:
   03/13/09   Furosemide 40 mg, I.V., Now

PRN Medications:
   03/12/09   Acetaminophen Supp 650 mg, #1, PR, q 4 hour prn pain or temperature greater than 101° F   CONTINUED

Computer-generated Kardex *(continued)*

PAGE 03

03/14/09   07:00   **PATIENT KARDEX**

WILLIAMS, HENRY   68   MWMC
MR#: 5555555   DOB 10/26/40   MICU   302
FIN#: 1010101010   Admitted: 03/12/09
DR: Daniel Smith   Service: Internal Medicine

Summary: 03/14 07:00 to 15:00

Laboratory:
    03/14/09   Basic metabolic panel tomorrow, collect at 05:00
    03/14/09   CBC/Diff/Plts tomorrow, collect at 05:00
    03/14/09   Cardiac troponin, tomorrow, collect at 05:00
Radiology:
    03/12/09   Computed tomography: CT scan of the head without contrast STAT
Ancillary:
    03/12/09   Respiratory care: Oxygen via nasal cannula at 2 L/minute
    03/12/09   Physical therapy: Patient evaluation and treatment   LAST PAGE

record (even though there are safeguards against this), type an explanation into the file along with the date, time, and your initials. Submit an explanation in writing to your nurse-manager, and keep a copy for your records.

Types of computerized documentation systems

Specialized nursing information systems can increase your efficiency in all phases of documentation. (See *Computerized charting and the nursing process*, page 102.)

Talk, touch, or click

Depending on which type of computer hardware and software your health care facility has, you may access information by using your voice, a keyboard, a light pen, a touch-sensitive screen, or a mouse.

Adding your personal touch

With some systems, you can use a menu of common phrases to quickly create a narrative note. You can also elaborate on a

Computerized charting and the nursing process

A computer information system can either stand alone or be a subsystem of a larger hospital system. Nursing information systems (NISs) can increase efficiency and accuracy in all phases of the nursing process—assessment, nursing diagnosis, planning, implementation, and evaluation—and can help nurses meet the standards established by the American Nurses Association and The Joint Commission. In addition, NISs can help nurses spend more time meeting patient needs. Consider these uses of computers in the nursing process.

Assessment

You can use the computer terminal to record admission information. As you collect data, enter additional information as prompted by the computer's software program. Enter data about the patient's health status, history, chief complaint, and other assessment factors.

Some software programs prompt you to ask specific questions and then offer pathways to gather further information. In some systems, the computer program flags assessment values that are outside the usual acceptable range to call attention to them.

Nursing diagnosis

Most current programs list standard diagnoses with associated signs and symptoms as references. However, you must still use clinical judgment to determine a nursing diagnosis for each patient. With this information, you can rapidly obtain diagnostic information. For example, the computer can generate a list of possible diagnoses for a patient with selected signs and symptoms, or it may enable you to retrieve and review the patient's records according to the nursing diagnosis.

Planning

To help nurses begin writing a care plan, some computer programs display recommended expected outcomes and interventions for the selected diagnosis. Computers can also track outcomes for large patient populations. You can use computers to compare large amounts of patient data, help identify outcomes the patient is likely to achieve based on individual problems and needs, and estimate the time frame for reaching outcome goals.

Implementation

You can also use the computer to record actual interventions and patient-processing information, such as transfer and discharge instructions, and to communicate this information to other departments. Computer-generated progress notes automatically sort and print out patient data—such as medication administration, treatments, and vital signs—making documentation more efficient and accurate.

Evaluation

During evaluation, you can use the computer to record and store observations, patient responses to nursing interventions, and your own evaluation statements. You may also use information from other members of the health care team to determine future actions and discharge planning. If a desired patient outcome has not been achieved, record new interventions taken to ensure desired outcomes. Then reevaluate the second set of interventions.

problem or clarify flow sheet documentation in the comment section of a computerized form by entering standardized phrases or typing in comments.

What's your type?

Types of computerized documentation systems include:
- specialized nursing information systems (NISs)
- nursing minimum data set (NMDS)
- nursing outcomes classification (NOC) system
- voice-activated systems.

Nursing information systems

Current NIS software programs allow nurses to record nursing actions in the patient's electronic record. These systems incorporate most or all of the components of the nursing process so they can meet the standards of the American Nurses Association and The Joint Commission. Furthermore, each NIS provides different features and can be customized to conform to a facility's documentation forms and formats. For example, some systems offer automated drug information, guidelines regarding facility policies and procedures, and intranet access. Other systems may provide the capability for online literature searches, which keeps the latest health care information at the nurse's fingertips.

From passive to interactive

NIS programs can manage information passively, actively, or interactively. Passive systems collect, transmit, organize, format, print, and display information that you can use to help make a decision, but they don't make that decision for you. Active systems suggest nursing diagnoses based on predefined assessment data that you enter. The most recent NIS programs take this functionality a step further, interacting with you based on the information you enter. (See *Computerized give-and-take.*)

Nursing minimum data set

The NMDS is a means of standardizing nursing information. It contains three categories of data:

🖐 nursing care, such as nursing diagnoses and interventions

✌ patient demographics, such as the patient's name, birth date, gender, race or ethnicity, and residence

✋ service elements, such as length of hospitalization.

Consistent and coded

The standardized format of the NMDS encourages consistent documentation. Data are coded, making documentation and information retrieval faster and easier. For example, NANDA-International assigns numerical codes to all nursing diagnoses so they can be used with the NMDS.

Nurse's little helper

The NMDS charting system helps you to:
• collect nursing diagnoses and intervention data, which can be used to plan patient care
• identify the nursing needs of various patient populations

Computerized give-and-take

Most nursing information systems interact with you, prompting you with questions and suggestions about the information you enter. Ultimately, this computerized, sequential decision-making format should lead to more effective nursing care and documentation.

An interactive system requires you to enter only a brief narrative. The questions and suggestions the computer program provides make your documentation thorough and quick. The program also allows you to add or change information so that your documentation is tailored to fit your patient.

- track patient outcomes
- describe nursing care received in different settings, including the patient's home
- establish accurate estimates for nursing service costs
- compare nursing trends locally, regionally, and nationally
- compare nursing data from various clinical settings, patient populations, and geographic areas
- obtain data about nursing care that may influence health care policy and decision making.

But it's always about the patient

Above all, the NMDS helps you provide better patient care. For example, examining the outcomes of various patient populations may help set realistic outcomes for an individual patient.

Nursing outcomes classification system

The NOC system provides the first comprehensive, standardized method of measuring nursing-sensitive patient outcomes. This system benefits the nursing profession by:
- allowing the comparison of patient outcomes with the outcomes of larger groups that share similar ages, diagnoses, or health care settings
- serving as an essential tool in ongoing nursing research
- including patient data-related outcomes, which in the past have been absent from computerized medical information databases.

Voice-activated systems

Some facilities have voice-activated nursing documentation systems. A voice-activated system combines a specialized knowledge base of words, phrases, and report forms with automated speech recognition technology. Voice-activated systems are most useful in departments that have a high volume of structured reports, such as operating rooms.

Look ma, no hands!

Voice-activated systems require little or no keyboard use—you simply speak into a telephone handset and the text appears on the computer screen. You can record complete nurses' notes by using your voice.

Report support and more

In addition to report forms, the computer program includes information on the nursing process, nursing

Can we talk?

theory, and nursing standards of practice. Trigger phrases spoken by the nurse cue the system to display passages of report text and allow word-for-word dictation and editing. You can use the text displayed to design an individualized care plan or to fill in standard facility forms.

Hanging on every word

Although voice-activated systems work most efficiently with trigger phrases, word-for-word dictation and editing are also possible.

Additional system features

Depending on the system type, a computerized documentation system may provide the ability to print out patient schedules. The system may also be equipped with bar code technology.

Patient schedules

Most systems have the ability to print out schedule lists for patients. For example, you can print out a schedule of patients who require fingerstick glucose level tests. If the situation requires you to delegate the task, the list may be given to ancillary staff members. The list lets them know exactly when they're supposed to obtain the fingerstick glucose level for each patient.

Bar code technology

Bar code technology allows you to scan a drug's bar code, scan the patient's identification bracelet, and then scan your own identification badge before administering a drug to the patient. The information immediately appears on a mobile computer screen, documenting the administration.

The Joint Commission and the Institute for Safe Medication Practices support use of medical bar code technology at the bedside. Additionally, the Food and Drug Administration's requirement that all drug makers use bar codes on medications commonly used in hospitals has led to widespread use of this system.

To be discontinued...

Bar code technology helps keep track of discontinued medications. The system connects to the order-entry system, so if a doctor discontinues a medication, it won't show up on the patient's listed medications when you scan the patient's wristband.

Sorry, wrong number

Scanning of medications also ensures that the nurse hasn't inadvertently picked the wrong medication out of the medication drawer or received the wrong medication from the pharmacy.

Streamlined service

Other advantages of bar code technology include saved time and streamlined documentation. If a patient refuses a medication, the nurse can document it immediately into the mobile computer. At the end of the shift, the nurse-manager can print a report to identify patients who didn't receive their medications.

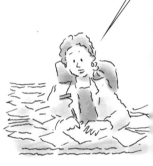

Technology is great, but it isn't perfect. You'll still need to be familiar with paper documentation in case the computer system fails.

When computers fail

Most nurses have good things to say about computerized charting. It makes storing and retrieving information fast and easy. But what happens when the computer system fails? Many facilities keep backup paperwork in case the computerized system fails. For this reason, you should familiarize yourself with the paper documentation forms that are available to you. Documentation must be thorough — even under extreme circumstances — so make sure that you're familiar with your facility's forms and that your documentation is complete.

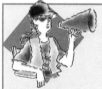

That's a wrap!

Computerized documentation review

Advantages
- Improved standardized charting
- Higher quality of the clinical information within the medical record
- Quick access to patient information across all departments
- Reduction in redundant charting
- Improved legibility of doctors' orders and progress notes

Disadvantages
- Computer crashes or breakdown make patient information temporarily unavailable.

- Computer downtime to update the system makes information unavailable for a short period of time each day.
- Staff may be unfamiliar with the system.
- Breaches in patient confidentiality can occur.

Using a computerized system
- The system includes a mainframe computer and personal computers or terminals at workstations throughout the facility.
- A username and password must be entered to access the patient's clinical record.

Computerized documentation review (continued)

• The patient's name, account number, medical record number, and other demographic data are entered on admission.

• The doctor enters orders into the system. The system transmits orders to the patient's nursing department and other appropriate departments.

• The nurse can enter new data on the care plan or progress notes, sign out medications that have been administered, or compare data on vital signs, laboratory test results, or intake and output.

Types of computerized documentation systems

Nursing information system
• Incorporates components of the nursing process
• Allows users to record nursing actions in the patient's electronic record
• Can be customized

Nursing minimum data set
• Standardizes nursing data
• Contains three categories of nursing data: nursing care, patient demographics, and service elements

Nursing outcomes classification system
• Standardizes method of measuring nursing-sensitive patient outcomes
• Essential tool in nursing research
• Includes patient data-related outcomes, which have been absent in the past

Voice-activated system
• Combines a specialized knowledge base of words, phrases, and report forms with automated speech recognition technology
• Requires little or no keyboard use

Additional system features

Patient schedules
• Provides ability to print patient schedules
• Useful if tasks need to be delegated

Bar code technology
• The drug's bar code, the patient's identification bracelet, and the nurse's identification badge are scanned.
• Scanned information appears on a mobile computer screen and documents the administration.

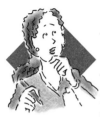

Quick quiz

1. Computerized systems cut down on medication errors because they eliminate:

    A.   administration errors.
    B.   transcription errors.
    C.   drug interactions.
    D.   allergic reactions.

Answer: B. Computerized systems provide direct order transmittal, which eliminates the possibility of transcription errors.

2. The NMDS organizes nursing information into which three categories of data?

    A.   Nursing care, patient demographics, and service elements

    B.   Nursing actions, nursing diagnoses, and patient outcomes

    C.   Nursing care plans, progress notes, and discharge summaries

    D.   Nursing care plans, patient demographics, and discharge summaries

Answer: A. The NMDS program attempts to standardize nursing information by dividing data into three categories: nursing care, patient demographics, and service elements.

3. Which action is acceptable practice when using a computerized documentation system?

    A.   Allowing a temporary staff member to use your computer username and password

    B.   Remaining logged in to a computer when you leave to administer a medication

    C.   Allowing the doctor covering your patient to quickly input an order using your computer password

    D.   Preventing others from seeing a display monitor that contains patient information

Answer: D. You should prevent others from seeing a display monitor that contains patient information. This ensures confidentiality of the computerized patient record.

4. A disadvantage of computerized charting is that:

    A.   charting isn't standardized.

    B.   access to patient information is slower than with standardized charting.

    C.   breaches in patient confidentiality can occur.

    D.   charting is often redundant.

Answer: C. A disadvantage of computerized charting is that breaches in patient confidentiality can occur.

Scoring

☆☆☆   If you answered all four questions correctly, right on! It didn't take long for you to process this information.

☆☆   If you answered three questions correctly, good work! You certainly took a "byte" out of the data in this chapter.

☆   If you answered fewer than three questions correctly, no need to crash. Take a moment to reboot your system before you continue.

6

Enhancing your charting

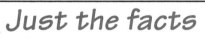

Just the facts

In this chapter, you'll learn:

♦ seven rules of clear charting and how to follow them

♦ different types of doctor's orders and how to clarify them

♦ the nurse's role in documenting doctor's orders.

A look at expert charting

Charting like a pro can be simple, but it requires adherence to seven fundamental rules:

1. Document care completely, concisely, and accurately.

2. Record observations objectively.

3. Document information promptly.

4. Write legibly.

5. Use approved abbreviations.

6. Use the proper technique to correct written errors.

7. Sign all documents as required.

Following these rules enhances communication between all members of the health care team and ensures reimbursement for your facility.

Charting completely, concisely, and accurately

Here are a few quick tips for expressing yourself as well as you possibly can:

• Write clear sentences that get right to the point.

• Use simple, precise language.

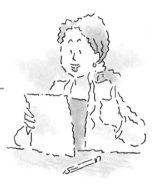

- Clearly identify the subject of each sentence.
- Don't be afraid to use the word *I*.

Say what?

If you don't use these tips, a rambling, vague, and ultimately meaningless note might be written such as *Communication with patient's home initiated today to delineate progression of disease process and describe course of action.* That's mind-boggling.

Instead, put the four tips to work for you, and your charting savvy will show. Here's how this note should be written: *I contacted Andrea Sovak's daughter by phone at 1300 hours; I explained that Mrs. Sovak's respiratory status had worsened and that she would be moved to the ICU for monitoring.* This note clearly differentiates your actions from those of the patient, the doctor, or another staff member. (See *Tell it like it is.*)

Don't be wishy-washy

Because we are taught that nurses don't make diagnoses, many of us qualify our observations with words like *appears* or *apparently*. However, using vague language in a patient's chart tells the reader

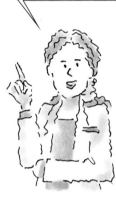

Don't be shy; say "I."

Art of the chart

Tell it like it is

In the examples below, the first is incomplete, leaving the reader wondering what really happened. The second is both complete and precise.

The wrong way

Not clear who this is

Date	Time	Sign entries	
1/20/09	0200	*Patient deceased at 0150. Next of kin notified.*	*Ann Pine, RN*

Vague wording

Concisely states what occurred

The right way

Date	Time	Sign entries	
1/20/09	0150	*Patient pronounced dead by Dr. Ted Burns.*	*Ann Pine, RN*
1/20/09	0155	*Dr. Ted Burns notified Mary Ritt, sister of patient, via telephone of patient's death.*	*Ann Pine, RN*

Clearly states who was notified and by whom

that you aren't sure what you're describing or doing. The right approach is to clearly and succinctly describe what occurred without sounding tentative.

Maintaining objectivity

Knowing what to chart is important, too. Record just the facts— exactly what you see, hear, and do—not your opinions or assumptions. Chart only relevant information relating to patient care and reflecting the nursing process.

Don't put words in other people's mouths

Avoid subjective statements such as *Patient's level of cooperation has deteriorated since yesterday.* Instead, use the patient's exact words to describe the facts that led you to this conclusion. You might write: *The patient stated, "I don't want to learn how to inject insulin. I tried yesterday, but I'm not going to do it today."* (See *Quotations are key,* page 112.)

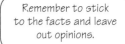
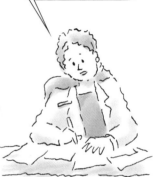

Remember to stick to the facts and leave out opinions.

You may also want to chart your subjective conclusion about the patient's condition. Doing so is okay, as long as you also record the objective assessment data that supports it. For example, *Pt sad and tearful with flat affect; states "I miss my family."*

Secondhand data

Document only data that you collect or observe yourself or data from a reliable source, such as the patient or another nurse. When you include data reported by someone else, always cite your source. For example, you may write, *Nurse Ray found pt attempting to climb OOB. Pt was assisted to the bathroom, then back to bedside chair.*

Ensuring timeliness

Timely charting includes these essentials:
- charting as soon as possible
- noting exact times
- charting chronologically
- handling late entries correctly.

Chart ASAP

Record information on the patient's chart as soon as possible after you make an observation or provide care. Information charted immediately is more likely to be accurate and complete. If you leave your charting until the end of the shift, you might forget important details.

Art of the chart

Quotations are key

Using the patient's exact words makes your charting accurate and objective. The notes below show how.

> Use the patient's own words as much as possible.

> Special instructions are documented precisely.

> Here's proof of patient teaching.

Date	Time	Sign entries
02/10/09	1300	Pt states she has been "voiding" drops of bloody urine every 5 to 10 minutes for the last hour. She states she feels "pressure" and a "burning-pain" with voiding. Pt states pain is a "7" on a scale of 1 to 10, in which 10 is the most severe. Dr. K. Jones was called. Dr. K. Jones's answering service responded. Dr. K. Jones will call back. ———— Tina Clark, RN
2/10/09	1310	Dr. K. Jones returned call; was informed of pt's symptoms. Order given for Bactrim DS, one, P.O. now and Pyridium 200 mg P.O. now. Dr. K. Jones will see pt this afternoon. —— Tina Clark, RN
2/10/09	1320	Bactrim DS, one P.O. and Pyridium 200 mg P.O. given. ———— Tina Clark, RN
2/10/09	1320	I gave pt instructions regarding medication uses and adverse effects; encouraged her to drink plenty of fluids. I explained that Pyridium may stain clothing and turn urine orange-red. Pt stated, "I understand" and had no further questions. ———— Tina Clark, RN
	1420	Pt states she has no pain with voiding and that "pressure is also gone." —— Tina Clark, RN

One way to chart on time is by keeping charting materials at the patient's bedside. However, this system can compromise confidentiality. (See *Keeping it confidential.*)

If your facility uses computerized charting, remember that most computerized programs record the date and time that entries are made. Therefore, it's important to specifically state in the body of your note the time that events occurred and the action taken.

Give them the time of day

Be specific about times in your charting, especially the exact time of sudden changes in the patient's condition, significant events, and nursing actions. Don't chart in blocks of time such as 0700 to

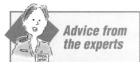

1500. This looks vague, implies inattention to the patient, and makes it hard to determine when specific events occurred. (See *Marking time.*)

Most facilities require nurses to chart in military time, which expresses time as 24 one-hour-long periods per day, rather than 2 sets of 12 one-hour periods. (See *Time marches on*, page 114.)

Put your chart in order

Most assessments and observations are useful only as parts of a whole picture. Isolated assessments reveal very little but, in chronological order, they tell the patient's story over time and reveal a pattern of improvement or deterioration.

Charting in chronological order is easy if you jot down your observations and assessments when they occur. Too often, however, nurses chart at the end of a shift, and then record groups of assessments that fail to accurately reflect variations in the patient's condition over time. (See *Correct and chronological*, page 115.)

Advice from the experts

Keeping it confidential

Bedside computers are the ultimate in easy charting, and bedside flow sheets or progress notes run a close second. However, facility policy must be followed to ensure compliance with confidentiality protocols and regulations.

One solution is to keep confidential records in a locked, fold-down desk outside the patient's room. Having a handy writing surface also makes it easier to chart promptly. If your facility doesn't use bed-side forms or computers, keep a worksheet or pad in your pocket for note keeping. Jot down key phrases and times, and then transcribe the information onto the chart later.

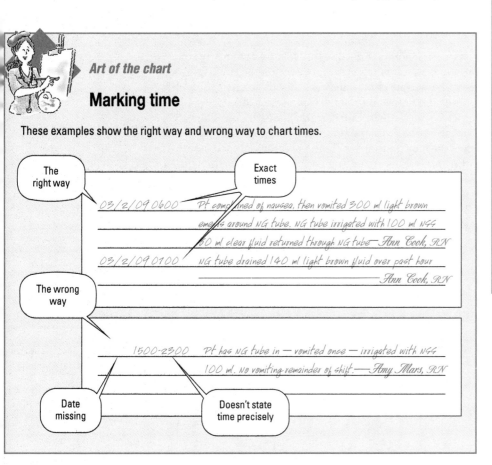

Art of the chart

Marking time

These examples show the right way and wrong way to chart times.

The right way

Exact times

03/2/09 0600 — Pt complained of nausea, then vomited 300 ml light brown emesis around NG tube. NG tube irrigated with 100 ml NSS 60 ml clear fluid returned through NG tube.— Ann Cook, RN
03/2/09 0700 — NG tube drained 140 ml light brown fluid over past hour
— Ann Cook, RN

The wrong way

1500-2300 — Pt has NG tube in — vomited once — irrigated with NSS 100 ml. No vomiting remainder of shift.— Amy Mars, RN

Date missing

Doesn't state time precisely

Time marches on

Many facilities use military time because it alleviates confusion over a.m. and p.m. entries. Here's how it works.

0100 hours = 1 a.m.	1300 hours = 1 p.m.
0200 hours = 2 a.m.	1400 hours = 2 p.m.
0300 hours = 3 a.m.	1500 hours = 3 p.m.
0400 hours = 4 a.m.	1600 hours = 4 p.m.
0500 hours = 5 a.m.	1700 hours = 5 p.m.
0600 hours = 6 a.m.	1800 hours = 6 p.m.
0700 hours = 7 a.m.	1900 hours = 7 p.m.
0800 hours = 8 a.m.	2000 hours = 8 p.m.
0900 hours = 9 a.m.	2100 hours = 9 p.m.
1000 hours = 10 a.m.	2200 hours = 10 p.m.
1100 hours = 11 a.m.	2300 hours = 11 p.m.
1200 hours = 12 noon	2400 hours = 12 midnight

If you're using computerized records, know that many software programs require nurses to answer predetermined questions or fields with multiple choice answers. Although this approach will capture core data and prompt responses to key issues, it will never replace a patient-specific narrative note. If possible, combine a narrative note with the prompted charting.

Review the charting entries for the previous 24 to 48 hours. If the charting is so generic that you can't identify the patient, then you'll need to incorporate narrative notes in your charting.

Better late than never

You may occasionally need to add a late entry in certain situations, such as:
- when the chart is unavailable at the time of the event
- if you forgot to document something
- if you need to add important information.

Bear in mind, however, that late entries can look suspicious during a malpractice trial. Find out if your facility has a protocol for late entries. If not, add the entry on the first available line and label it *late entry* to indicate that it's out of sequence. Then record the date and time of the entry as well as the date and time when the entry should have been made.

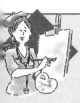

Art of the chart

Correct and chronological

Here's an example of charting that's done correctly in chronological order.

01/14/09	0800	Neuro: Pt AAO x 3, follows commands, moves all extremities, speech clear and appropriate. *Jane Klass, RN*
		CV: Afebrile; skin warm, dry and intact; palpable pulses; no edema. ———————— *Jane Klass, RN*
		Resp: Bilateral breath sounds, no shortness of breath, lungs clear, on room air. ———— *Jane Klass, RN*
01/14/09	0915	Pt complaining of sudden shortness of breath, O_2 2 L/ minute applied. Stat chest X-ray obtained, Dr. Kenneth
		Jones notified. ————————————————————————— *Jane Klass, RN*
01/14/09	0920	Lasix 40 mg I.V. provided to pt per Dr. Kenneth Jones's order. ——————— *Jane Klass, RN*
01/14/09	0930	Shortness of breath continues, pulse oximetry 87%. O_2 increased to 50% face mask. ——— *Jane Klass, RN*
01/14/09	0935	Pt transferred to ICU, report provided to Sally Brown, RN. Pt's family notified by Dr. Kenneth Jones. —
		——————————————————————————————————— *Jane Klass, RN*

Events are documented in correct time sequence.

Ensuring legibility

One of the main reasons to document your nursing care is to communicate with other members of the health care team. Trying to decipher sloppy handwriting wastes people's time and puts the patient in jeopardy if critical information is misinterpreted. (See *Neatness counts!* page 116.)

Use printing instead of cursive writing because it's usually easier to understand. If you don't have room to chart something legibly, leave the section blank, put a bracket around it, and write *See progress notes;* then record the information fully and legibly in the notes.

No pencils, please

Because it's a permanent document, the clinical record should be completed in ink or by computer. Use only black or blue ink. Don't use felt-tipped pens on forms with carbon copies because these pens usually don't hold up under the pressure needed to produce copies, and the ink is more likely to bleed through to another page or smear if the paper gets wet.

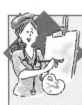

Art of the chart

Neatness counts!

Make sure your handwriting is as neat and clear as possible. Legible charting is vital in communications among colleagues. The flow sheet below shows legible and illegible charting.

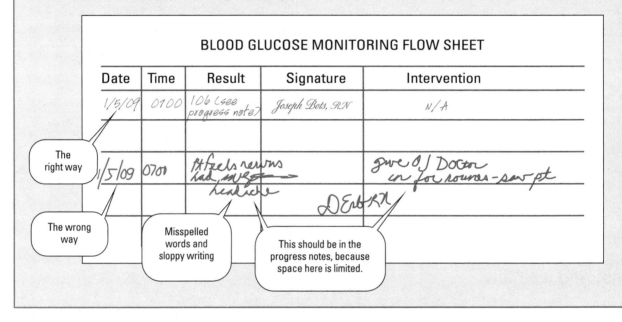

BLOOD GLUCOSE MONITORING FLOW SHEET

Date	Time	Result	Signature	Intervention
1/5/09	0100	106 (see progress note)	Joseph Bots, RN	N/A
1/5/09	0700	Pt feels nervous, had mild headache	D Eb RN	give OJ Doctor in for rounds - saw pt

The right way

The wrong way

Misspelled words and sloppy writing

This should be in the progress notes, because space here is limited.

Spelling counts

Notes filled with misspelled words and incorrect grammar create the same negative impression as illegible handwriting. Try hard to avoid these errors; information can be misrepresented or misconstrued if an error-filled medical record ends up in court. (See *Tips for improving spelling and grammar,* page 119.)

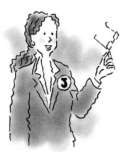

Using abbreviations appropriately

Standards set by The Joint Commission and many state regulations stipulate that health care facilities develop a list of approved abbreviations to use during charting. (See Avoid these abbreviations!*) Make sure you know and use your facility's approved abbreviations. When you have doubts about an abbreviation's meaning, spell it out.*

(Text continues on page 120.)

Avoid these abbreviations!

The Joint Commission requires every health care facility to develop a list of approved abbreviations for staff use. Certain abbreviations should be avoided because they're easily misunderstood, especially when handwritten. The Joint Commission has identified a minimum list of dangerous abbreviations, acronyms, and symbols. This do-not-use list includes the following items.

Abbreviation	Intended meaning	Misinterpretation	Correction
U or u	unit	Frequently misinterpreted as a "0" or a "4," causing a ten-fold or greater overdose	Write "unit."
IU	international unit	Frequently misinterpreted as I.V. or 10	Write "international unit."
q.d., q.o.d.	every day, every other day	Mistaken for each other. The period after the "q" has sometimes been misinterpreted as "i," the "o" can be mistaken for "i" and the drug has been given q.i.d. rather than daily.	Write "daily" or "every other day."
Trailing zero (X.0 mg) Lack of leading zero (.X mg)	10 mg, 0.1 mg	Frequently misinterpreted dosage	Never write a zero by itself after a decimal point (10.0 mg should be 10 mg) and always use a zero before a decimal point if no other number is present, such as 0.1 mg.
MS, MSO$_4$, MgSO$_4$	morphine sulfate magnesium sulfate	Confused with each other	Write "morphine sulfate" or "magnesium sulfate."

(continued)

Avoid these abbreviations! *(continued)*

In addition to the minimum required list, the following items should also be considered when expanding the do-not-use list.

Abbreviation	Intended meaning	Misinterpretation	Correction
℥	fluid ounce	Misinterpreted as "mcg"	Use the metric equivalents.
ʒ	fluid dram	Misinterpreted as "zinc"	Use the metric equivalents.
♏	minim	Misinterpreted as "molar"	Use the metric equivalents.
℈	scruple	Misinterpreted as "day"	Use the metric equivalents.
MTX	methotrexate	Misinterpreted as mustargen (mechlorethamine hydrochloride)	Write "methotrexate."
CPZ	Compazine (prochlorperazine)	Misinterpreted as chlorpromazine	Write "compazine."
HCl	hydrochloric acid	Misinterpreted as potassium chloride ("H" is misinterpreted as "K")	Write "hydrochloric acid."
DIG	digoxin	Misinterpreted as digitoxin	Write "digoxin."
MVI	multivitamins without fat-soluble vitamins	Misinterpreted as multivitamins with fat-soluble vitamins	Write "multivitamins."
HCTZ	hydrochlorothiazide	Misinterpreted as hydrocortisone (HCT)	Write "hydrochlorothiazide."
ara-A	vidarabine	Misinterpreted as cytarabine (ara-C)	Write "vidarabine."

Avoid these abbreviations! *(continued)*

Abbreviation	Intended meaning	Misinterpretation	Correction
au	*auris uterque* (each ear)	Frequently misinterpreted as "OU" (*oculus uterque*— each eye)	Write "each ear."
ʮg	microgram	Frequently misinterpreted as "mg"	Use "mcg."
cc	cubic centimeter	Frequently misinterpreted as U (units)	Write "ml" for milliliters.
A.S., A.D., and AU	Latin abbreviations for left ear, right ear, and both ears, respectively	Frequently misinterpreted as O.S., O.D., and OU	Write "left ear," "right ear," or "both ears."
OD	once daily	Frequently misinterpreted as "O.D." (*oculus dexter*— right eye)	Write "once daily."
OJ	orange juice	Frequently misinterpreted as "O.D." (*oculus dexter*— right eye) or "O.S." (*oculus sinister*— left eye). Medications that were meant to be diluted in orange juice and given orally have been given in a patient's right or left eye.	Write "orange juice."
Per os	orally	The "os" is frequently misinterpreted as "O.S." (*oculus sinister*— left eye).	Use "PO," "by mouth," or "orally."
qn.	nightly or at bedtime	Frequently misinterpreted as "q.h." (every hour)	Write out "nightly" or "at bedtime."

(continued)

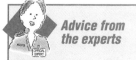

Advice from the experts

Tips for improving spelling and grammar

Want to look smart when you chart? Here are a few pointers:

• Keep both standard and medical dictionaries in charting areas, and refer to them as needed.

• Post a list of commonly misspelled or confusing words, especially terms and medications regularly used on the unit. Many medications have very similar names but extremely different actions.

• If your computer system includes a spelling or grammar check, use it. Understand, however, these are far from foolproof and don't replace careful proofreading.

Avoid these abbreviations! (continued)

Abbreviation	Intended meaning	Misinterpretation	Correction
S.C. SQ	subcutaneous	Mistaken as SL for sublingual or "5 every"	Use "Sub-Q," "subQ," or write out "subcutaneous."
D/C	discharge or discontinue	Frequently misinterpreted as each other	Write "discharge" or "discontinue."
h.s.	half-strength or at bedtime	Frequently misinterpreted as each other	Write out "half-strength" or "at bedtime."
T.I.W.	three times per week	Frequently misinterpreted as three times per day or twice weekly	Write "three times per week."

Using unapproved or ambiguous abbreviations can endanger a patient. For example, if you use *o.d.* for "once per day," another nurse might think you mean "oculus dexter" (right eye) and instill medication into the patient's eye instead of giving it orally. (See *Acceptable vs. unacceptable abbreviations.*)

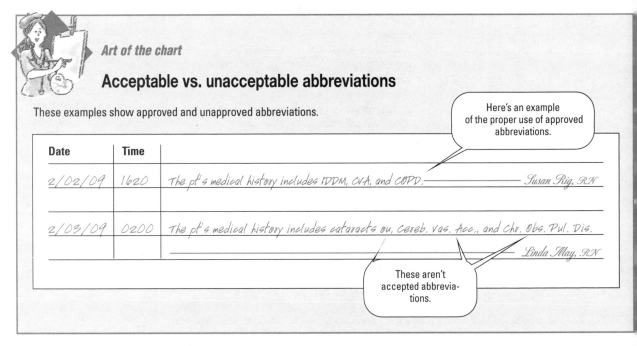

Art of the chart

Acceptable vs. unacceptable abbreviations

These examples show approved and unapproved abbreviations.

Here's an example of the proper use of approved abbreviations.

Date	Time	
2/02/09	1620	The pt's medical history includes IDDM, CVA, and COPD. — Susan Rig, RN
2/03/09	0200	The pt's medical history includes cataracts ou, Cereb. Vas. Acc., and Chr. Obs. Pul. Dis. — Linda May, RN

These aren't accepted abbreviations.

► *Art of the chart*

Correct correctly!

When you make a mistake on the clinical record, correct it by drawing a single line through the entry and writing the words *mistaken entry* above or beside it (don't use an abbreviation like *m.e.*, which could be someone's initials). Follow this with your initials and the date. If appropriate, briefly explain why the correction was necessary.

Make sure that the mistaken entry is still readable to indicate that you're only trying to correct a mistake, not cover something up.

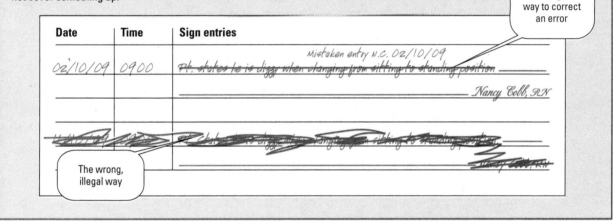

The right way to correct an error

Date	Time	Sign entries
02/10/09	0900	*Mistaken entry N.C. 02/10/09* ~~Pt. states he is dizzy when changing from sitting to standing position~~
		Nancy Cobb, RN

The wrong, illegal way

Correcting errors properly

When you make a mistake on a chart, correct it immediately by drawing a single line through the entry and writing *mistaken entry* above or beside it, along with the date and time. Then sign your name. Never erase a mistake, cover it with correction fluid, or completely cross it out because this looks as if you're trying to hide something. Also, writing *oops* or *sorry* or drawing a happy or sad face anywhere on a document is unprofessional and inappropriate. (See *Correct correctly!*)

Changing a record in any way is illegal and constitutes tampering. If the chart ends up in court, the plaintiff's lawyer will be looking for red flags that cast doubt on the chart's accuracy. (See *Altered records*, page 122.) So heed the following list of five don'ts:

✍ Don't add information at a later date without indicating that you did so.

✌ Don't date the entry so that it appears to have been written at an earlier time.

An important charting rule: Never erase a mistake.

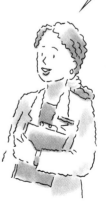

Case in point

Altered records

Cagnolatti v. Hightower (1996) is an example of the consequences of altering records. In this case, a 72-year-old female patient was admitted to the hospital after having a stroke. The night before discharge, the nurse assisted the doctor in administering I.V. edrophonium (Tensilon). Shortly after the drug's administration, the patient developed adverse reactions. The drug was discontinued. Most of the patient's symptoms disappeared within 15 minutes of stopping the drug. However, about 30 minutes after the drug was stopped, the patient went into cardiac arrest. The patient was resuscitated but remained comatose and died about 2 months later.

Record review
The patient's pulse after drug administration was documented as 88 beats/minute, but the nurse testified that this pulse was likely taken before the drug was given. Documentation also showed that the patient's pulse rate was 88 beats/minute 15 minutes after drug administration. However, a handwriting expert testified that the second pulse rate was originally entered as 58 beats/minute and had been altered. In addition, there was no documentation that a nursing assessment was performed during the 30-minute period after the drug was stopped.

The verdict
Any pulse rate below 60 beats/minute is bradycardic and requires intervention, especially after edrophonium administration. The pulse should have been brought to the attention of the treating doctor. Furthermore, the nurse should have monitored the patient more closely and documented the results of her assessment.

Don't add inaccurate information.

Don't omit information.

Don't destroy records.

If your facility uses computerized records, follow the protocols for the correction of entries made in the chart. Once notes are entered into the computer, they become the permanent record and shouldn't be deleted or edited at a later time without an explanation that's documented, signed, and dated.

Art of the chart

Charting do's and don'ts

The samples below illustrate some important rules about charting care.

> **Do draw a line** through the blank space to your signature. This discourages anyone from adding a note to yours.

> **Don't** skip lines or leave blank spaces.

> **Don't forget to provide** the caregiver's name.

> **Do make clear the** identity of key caregivers.

Date	Time	Sign entries
02/5/09	1200	I.V. of NSS absorbing at 125 ml per hr. Site of insertion observed. No adverse effects noted. ——————————— Tim Smith, RN
02/14/09	0600	Pt assisted to bathroom by nurse's aide.——————— Mary Rob, RN
02/14/09	0810	Loud noise heard in pt's room. Pt found lying on right side on floor near bathroom by Brian Sim, nurse technician. Pt awake, confused; one-inch laceration noted above right eyebrow. ——————————— James Born, RN

Signing documents

Sign each entry you make in your progress notes with your first name or initial, last name, and professional licensure, such as RN or LPN. Your employer may also require that you include your job title. If you find the last entry unsigned, immediately contact the nurse who made the entry and have her sign her name. If you can't locate her, simply write and sign your progress notes. The difference in charting times and handwriting should make it clear who the author was. (See *Charting do's and don'ts*.)

To be continued...

When charting continues from one page to the next, sign the bottom of the first page. At the top of the next page, write the date, the time, and *continued from previous page*. Make sure that each page is stamped or labeled with the patient's identifying information.

Never leave blank spaces on forms. Doing so could imply that you failed to give complete care or to assess the patient completely. If information listed on a form doesn't apply to your patient, write *N/A* (not applicable) in the space. If your charting doesn't fill the designated space, draw a line through the empty space until you reach your signature.

What you didn't see can hurt you

If you need to chart the actions of nursing assistants or technicians, write the caregiver's full name—not just his initials. Many nurses worry about countersigning care that they didn't actually see performed. If this is the case, you may refer to your facility's policy, contact your state board of nursing, or discuss the issue with your nurse-manager. Remember, your signature makes you responsible for everything in the notes.

If your facility uses computerized records, know that most software programs establish an electronic signature based on your personal user password. It's extremely important to guard your password and not share it with others. This is your legal signature! Always be sure to log off when leaving the computer station. Don't allow anyone else to use the computer with your password logged in. Any entries the other person makes will be stamped with your electronic signature.

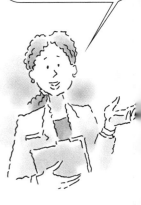

Write out the full names of nursing assistants or technicians when charting their actions.

Doctor's orders

Almost every treatment you give a patient requires a doctor's or a licensed independent practitioner's order, so accurate documentation of these orders is critical. Orders fall into four categories:

- written or electronic orders
- preprinted orders
- verbal orders
- telephone orders.

Written or electronic orders

No matter who transcribes an order—an RN, an LPN, or a unit secretary—a second person must double-check the transcription for accuracy. An effective method used by many facilities is the "chart check"—rechecking orders from the previous shift once per shift.

Checking for transcription errors at least once every 24 hours is also a good idea. These checks are usually done on the night shift. A line is placed across the order sheet to indicate that all orders above the line have been checked. Then the sheet is signed and dated to verify that the check was done.

Heading off mistakes

When checking a patient's order sheet, make sure that the orders were written for the right patient. An order sheet might be stamped with one patient's identification plate and then inadvertently placed in another patient's chart. Double-checking averts potential mistakes.

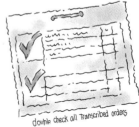

double check all transcribed orders

If an order is unclear, call the doctor who wrote the order for clarification. Don't ask other people for their interpretation; they'll only be guessing, too. If a doctor is notorious for his poor handwriting, ask him to read his orders to you before he leaves the unit.

If you use computerized charting, be aware that some programs allow you to select more than one patient at a time. Be sure to double-check the patient's name on the computer screen before charting.

Some facilities that use a computerized system require the doctors to enter all of their orders into the computer system. This system greatly reduces errors because it eliminates transcription. However, it's still important to check for accuracy and make sure orders are written for the right patient.

Preprinted orders

Many health care facilities use preprinted order forms for specific procedures, such as cardiac catheterization, or for admission to certain units such as the coronary care unit. As with other standardized documents, blank spaces are used for information that must be individualized according to the patient's needs.

If your facility uses these forms, don't assume that they're flawless just because they're preprinted. You may still need to clarify an order by discussing it with the doctor who gave it. (See *Preprinted orders*, page 126.)

Verbal orders

Verbal orders are easy to misinterpret. Errors in understanding or documenting such orders can cause mistakes in patient care and liability problems for you and your facility. Try to take verbal orders only in an emergency when the doctor can't immediately attend to the patient. As a rule, do-not-resuscitate and no-code orders should *not* be taken verbally.

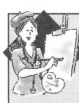

Art of the chart

Preprinted orders

The following is an example of a preprinted form for charting doctor's orders. This form specifies the treatment for a patient who's about to undergo cardiac catheterization.

DOCTOR'S ORDERS

Allergies: *None known*

Date/Time	PRECARDIAC CATHETERIZATION ORDERS:
2/1/09 0130	1. NPO after _midnight_ except for sips of water with medications.
	2. Shave and prep right and left groin areas.
	3. Premedications:
	Benadryl _25_ mg
	Xanax _0.5_ mg } P.O. on call to Cath lab
	4. Have ECG, PT, PTT, creatinine, Hgb, Hct, and platelet count on chart prior to sending the patient to the Cath lab.
	5. Have patient void before leaving for the Cath lab.
2/1/09 0200	*John Smith, MD* ———————
2/1/09 0200	*Mona Jones, RN* ———————

> Blanks are left for information that should be individualized according to the patient's needs.

From words to paper

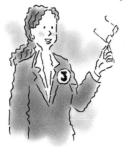

Carefully follow your facility's policy for documenting verbal orders, using a special form if one exists. Here's the usual procedure:
• Record the order verbatim on the doctor's order sheet, or enter it into a computer. Note the date and time.
• On the first line, write "verbal order." Then write the doctor's name and your name as the nurse who received the order.

Art of the chart

Charting verbal orders

This form shows the correct way to chart verbal orders. Make sure that the doctor countersigns the order.

Date/time	Sign entries
1/16/09 1500	Verbal order. Dr. J. Marks to Mary Jones, RN
	Lasix 40 mg I.V. now and daily starting in a.m. ——
	————————————— Mary Jones, RN

• *Read the order back, and receive confirmation from the person who gave the order. (This step is called "The Joint Commission read back requirement" and applies to all verbal and telephone orders.)*
• Sign your name.
• Draw lines through any space between the order and your verification of the order.
• When taking a medication order, include the type of drug, the dosage, the time you administered it, and any other information. (See *Charting verbal orders*.)
• Make sure the doctor countersigns the order within the time limits set by your facility. Without his countersignature, you may be held liable for practicing medicine without a license.

Telephone orders

Ideally, you should accept only written orders from a doctor. However, telephone orders are permissible when:
• the patient needs immediate treatment and the doctor isn't available to write an order
• you're providing care to the patient at home (If so, the orders must be signed by the doctor according to state nursing practice regulations. Under Medicare guidelines, verbal orders must be

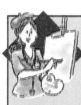

Art of the chart

Taking telephone orders

This form shows the correct way to chart telephone orders. Make sure that the doctor counter-signs the order.

Date/Time	Sign entries
2/4/09 0900	Telephone order. Dr. Bartholomew White to Cathy Phillips, RN
	Demerol 15 mg and Vistaril 50 mg I.M. now for pain.
	—————————————————— *Cathy Phillips, RN*

signed within 30 days. Other agencies impose their own, stricter rules. Failure to obtain a signed order could jeopardize reimbursement.)

• new information (laboratory data, for example) has become available and the telephone order will enable you to expedite care. (See *Taking telephone orders*.)

From phone to paper

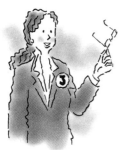

Telephone orders should be given directly to you; they should never go through a third party. Carefully follow your facility's policy for documenting these orders. Usually, you'll follow this procedure:

• Record the order verbatim on the doctor's order sheet or enter it into a computer. First, note the date and time. On the next line, write "telephone order." (Don't use *P.O.* for phone order—it could be mistaken for "by mouth.") Then write the doctor's name, and sign your name.

• *Read the order back and receive confirmation from the person who gave the order. (This step is called "The Joint Commission read back requirement" and applies to all verbal and telephone orders. The read back requirement also applies to critical test results reported verbally or by telephone.)*

• If you're having trouble understanding the doctor, ask another nurse to listen in as the doctor gives you the order. Then have her read it back and sign the order, too.

• Draw lines through any blank spaces in the order.

• Make sure that the doctor countersigns the order within the time limits set by your facility. Without his signature, you may be held liable for practicing medicine without a license.

• To save time and avoid errors (and if permitted by your facility's confidentiality policy), ask the doctor to fax you a copy of the order. Make sure that you wait at the fax machine for the transmission to protect the patient's right to confidentiality.

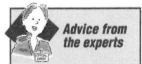

Advice from the experts

When in doubt, check it out

An order may be correct when issued but incorrect later because of changes in the patient's status. When this occurs, delay the treatment until you have contacted the doctor and clarified the situation.

Questioning doctor's orders

Although the unit secretary may transcribe orders, you're ultimately responsible for the transcription's accuracy.

Chart authority

Only you have the authority and the knowledge to question the validity of orders and to spot errors. This is why a chart check is so important.

Stop, question, and chart

What if an order seems vague or even wrong? Refuse to carry it out until you talk to the doctor. (See *When in doubt, check it out* and *Failure to question*, page 130.)

Your facility should have a written procedure for clarifying orders. If it doesn't, take these steps:

• Contact the prescribing doctor for clarification.

• Document that you made this contact.

• Document whether you carried out the order.

• If you refuse to carry out an order, document your refusal, including the reasons why you refused and your communications with the doctor. Inform your immediate supervisor.

• Ask your nursing administrator for a step-by-step policy to follow so you'll know what to do if the situation recurs.

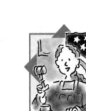

Case in point

Failure to question

In *Poor Sisters of Saint Francis Seraph of the Perpetual Adoration, et al. v. Catron (1982),* a hospital was sued for negligence because a nurse failed to question a doctor's order regarding an endotracheal tube.

The doctor ordered that the tube be left in place for 5 days instead of the standard 2 to 3 days. The nurse knew that 5 days was exceptionally long but, instead of clarifying the doctor's order and documenting her actions, she followed the order. As a result, the patient's larynx was irreparably damaged, and the court ruled the hospital negligent.

That's a wrap!

Expert charting review

Seven fundamental rules
- Chart completely, concisely, and accurately.
- Avoid using opinions; stick to the facts.
- Chart as soon as possible, making sure the information is in chronological order and noting exact times.
- Make sure your charting is legible. (Use printing instead of cursive, and use black or blue ink.)
- Use only accepted abbreviations.
- Follow protocols for correcting written errors and adding late entries.
- Sign your notes with your first name or initial, last name, and licensure.

Doctor's orders
- *Written or electronic*—Double-check all orders and clarify them, if necessary.
- *Preprinted*—Orders must be individualized according to the patient's needs; don't assume they're flawless; you may still need to clarify an order.
- *Verbal*—Take verbal orders only in an emergency, and make sure the doctor countersigns within the time limits set by your facility.
- *Telephone*—Take telephone orders only under certain circumstances, and make sure to take the order yourself.

Quick quiz

1. When documenting objectively, you should chart:
A. what you see, hear, and do.
B. the opinions of the health care team.
C. what you think the patient's response will be.
D. rambling, vague sentences.

Answer: A. Objective statements include facts, not opinions or assumptions.

2. When documenting events in a patient's chart, you should chart:
A. the period of time the shift covers (such as 0700 to 1500 hours).
B. the specific time of each event.
C. every hour on the hour.
D. every 2 hours.

Answer: B. Chart the exact time of all sudden changes in a patient's condition, significant events, and nursing actions.

3. Assessments and observations should be charted in chronological order because:
A. your facility requires it.
B. it's more convenient to chart this way.
C. The Joint Commission requires it.
D. they'll reveal a pattern of improvement or deterioration.

Answer: D. Usually, an isolated assessment tells very little about a patient.

4. If you make a mistake on a chart, correct it by immediately:
A. covering it with correction fluid.
B. crossing it out completely so it can't be read and adding the date, time, and your signature.
C. drawing a single line through the entry, writing *mistaken entry*, and adding the date, the time, and your signature.
D. highlighting the entry in yellow.

Answer: C. Incorrect entries shouldn't look as if you're trying to hide something. A single line through an incorrect entry is sufficient, along with a note stating "mistaken entry" and the date, the time, and your signature.

Scoring

☆☆☆ If you answered all four questions correctly, wow! Your charting is complete, concise, accurate, and all that good stuff. Turn to the next chapter, and keep mastering the art of the chart.

☆☆   If you answered three questions correctly, that's great! Your charting skills are definitely in order.

☆   If you answered fewer than three questions correctly, don't worry! In keeping with the tenets of good charting, we'll keep it confidential.

7

Avoiding legal pitfalls

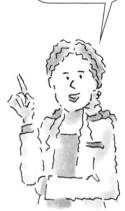

Just the facts

In this chapter, you'll learn:

♦ the legal significance of the medical record

♦ defensive charting

♦ the relationship between charting and risk management

♦ eight charting pitfalls and how to handle them.

A look at legal pitfalls in charting

As your professional responsibility grows, so does your legal accountability. Complete, accurate documentation proves that you're giving quality care and meeting the standards set by the nursing profession, state and federal regulatory agencies, accreditation organizations, your health care facility, and the law. It's your best protection if you're named in a malpractice lawsuit. (See *What sways the jury?* page 134.)

The aim is communication

Faulty charting is a pivotal issue in many malpractice cases. Medical records are reviewed by health care experts and can be presented in court case trials. Think of the medical record as a communication tool, and document accordingly. Focus on the facts, be objective, and document chronologically.

> Remember, charts are communication tools first and foremost.

Legal standards

What and how you chart on the medical record is controlled by:
• nurse practice acts
• American Nurses Association (ANA) credentialing committee certification requirements
• malpractice litigation
• your facility's policies and procedures.

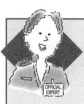

Advice from the experts

What sways the jury?

The outcome of every malpractice trial boils down to one question: Who will the jury believe? The answer depends on the credibility of the evidence. Jurors usually view the medical record as the best evidence of what really happened. It's commonly the hinge on which the verdict swings.

A general overview

In a nutshell, here's what happens in court: The plaintiff's (patient's) lawyer presents evidence showing that the patient was harmed because care provided by the defendant (in this case, the nurse) failed to meet accepted standards. The defendant's (nurse's) lawyer presents evidence showing that his client provided a standard of care that would be used by other nurses given the same circumstances.

If the nurse wasn't negligent, the medical record will provide evidence of quality care. However, if she *was* negligent or didn't document her care, the medical record is the plaintiff's best evidence. The jury will almost certainly rule in favor of the patient. Don't believe the myth that all cases settle out of court. Some do, but you don't want to be the exception.

Nurse practice acts

Nurse practice acts are state laws that designate what a nurse can do in that state. Today, nurses are considered managers of care as well as practitioners; states revise their laws and documentation requirements to keep up with changes like this in the nursing profession.

In a confused state? Read on...

The range of a nurse's legal responsibilities may vary from state to state—perhaps only to a small degree in certain cases. However, if licensed in more than one state, you must take care to follow precisely the specific guidelines of the state you're practicing in at the time. Always be familiar with your scope of practice. You'll be held liable if you're found practicing outside of your designated scope of practice.

ANA credentialing

What you write in a medical record shouldn't be dictated by the courts; it should be guided by the nursing profession's own standards. Charting that meets these standards describes the patient's status, medical treatment, and nursing care. The ANA sets standards for most nursing specialties. It says that documentation must be:

- systematic
- continuous and timely
- accessible and retrievable on a permanent basis
- communicated, accurate, and consistent
- recorded and able to be audited
- readily available to all members of the health care team.

The more things change, the more they stay the same

Although documentation goals haven't changed much over the years, documentation methods have. Nurses now use flow sheets, graphic records, and checklists in place of long narrative notes. In malpractice cases, the charting method used isn't important, as long as it's used consistently and provides comprehensive, factual information that's relevant to the patient's care.

Malpractice litigation

When charting, your main goal is to convey information. However, keep the legal implications in the back of your mind. If the care you provide and your charting are both top-notch, the records may be used to refute a plaintiff's accusation of nursing malpractice.

A malpractice verdict depends on three factors:

breach of duty

damage

causation.

Every relationship brings with it responsibility

The courts have ruled that it's your duty to provide an appropriate standard of care once a nurse-patient relationship is established— even if the relationship takes place over the phone. Breach of duty means that your care didn't meet that standard.

Proving that a nurse was guilty of breach of duty is difficult because her duties overlap with those of other health care providers. The court will ask, "How would a reasonable, prudent nurse with comparable training and experience have acted in the same or a similar circumstance?"

Once the plaintiff establishes a breach of duty, he must then prove that the breach caused the patient's injury (damage and causation).

Facility policies and procedures

How you chart is also controlled by the policies and procedures in your facility's employee and nursing manuals. Straying from

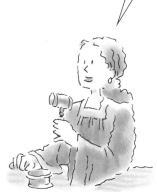

When you establish a relationship with a patient, you take on a legal responsibility.

these rules suggests that you failed to meet the facility's standards of care.

Although the courts have yet to decide whether these policies actually establish a legal standard of care, there are legal standards in place. In each nursing malpractice case, the courts compare a nurse's actions with regularly updated, national minimum standards established by professional organizations and accrediting bodies such as The Joint Commission.

The ties that bind

According to insurance company data, lawsuits naming nurses as defendants are increasing. Why? Two reasons are a nurse's expanding role and the breakdown of the nurse-patient relationship due to shorter hospital stays.

Developing a rapport with your patients, even on a short-term basis, can help decrease errors and foster a nurse-patient relationship—both of which help prevent lawsuits. Patients who feel their nurse attempted to do all in her power to provide care—usually despite short staffing—typically don't sue the nurse. However, they may sue the facility as the responsible party, which can still have legal ramifications for the nurse because the nurse may be called to testify.

> Establishing a strong nurse-patient relationship may help reduce legal risks.

Charting defensively

In the world of nursing and malpractice, a defensive attitude has become necessary—that is, chart factually but defensively as well. This involves knowing:

- how to chart
- what to chart
- when to chart
- who should chart.

How to chart

A skilled nurse charts with possible litigation in mind and knows that how she charts is just as important as what she charts.

Rule #1: Stick to the facts

Record only what you see, hear, smell, feel, measure, and count—not what you suppose, infer, conclude, or assume. For example, if a patient pulled out his I.V. line but you didn't witness it, write *Found pt, arm board, and bed linens covered with blood. I.V. line and venipuncture device were untaped and hanging free.* If the patient says he pulled out his I.V. line, record that.

Don't chart your opinions. If the chart is used as evidence in court, the plaintiff's lawyer might attack your credibility and the medical record's reliability.

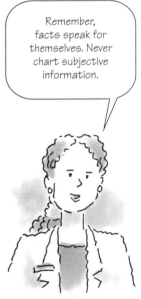

Remember, facts speak for themselves. Never chart subjective information.

Rule #2: Avoid labeling

Objectively describe the patient's behavior instead of subjectively labeling it. For example, write *Pt found pacing back and forth in his room, muttering phrases such as, "I'll take care of him my way" while punching one hand into the other.* Avoid using expressions such as *appears spaced out, flying high, exhibiting bizarre behavior,* or *using obscenities,* which can mean different things to different people. Ask yourself, could I define these terms in court? Objectivity in charting will increase your credibility with the jury.

Rule #3: Be specific

Your charting goal is to present the facts clearly and concisely. To do so, use only approved abbreviations and express your observations in quantifiable terms. (See *Specifics are terrific!* page 138.)

For example, writing *output adequate* isn't as helpful as writing *output 1,200 ml.* And *Pt appears to be in pain* is vague compared with *Pt requested pain medication after complaining of lower back pain radiating to his Ⓡ leg, which he rated 7 out of 10 on the visual analogue scale.* Also, avoid catch-all phrases such as *Pt comfortable.* Instead, describe how you know this. For instance, is the patient resting, reading, or sleeping?

Rule #4: Use neutral language

Don't use inappropriate comments or language in your notes. This is unprofessional and can cause legal problems.

In one case, an elderly patient developed pressure ulcers and his family complained that he wasn't receiving adequate care. The patient later died, probably of natural causes. Because family members were dissatisfied with the patient's care, they sued. The insurance company questioned the abbreviation *PBBB* in the chart, which the doctor had written under prognosis. After learning that this stood for "pine box by bedside," the family was awarded a significant sum.

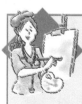

Art of the chart

Specifics are terrific!

The note below is clear and concise because it uses approved abbreviations and specific measurements.

5/16/09	1100	Complaining of pain at Ⓛ antecubital I.V. site at 1000. Pain rated on VAS
		3/10. Dressing removed. Redness 2 cm wide around I.V. insertion site. No
		drainage. Quarter-sized area of edema above insertion site, I.V. removed; site
		cleaned with chlorhexidine and sterile dressing applied. Warm compress applied
		to site × 20 min. Dr. John Smith notified. Acetaminophen 650 mg given P.O. at
		1015. Pt now reports pain 0/10 on VAS. ———————— Margaret Doherty, RN

Rule #5: Eliminate bias

Don't use language that suggests a negative attitude toward the patient. Examples include *obstinate*, *drunk*, *obnoxious*, *bizarre*, or *abusive*. The same goes for what you say out loud and then document. Disparaging remarks, accusations, arguments, or name calling could lead to a defamation of character or libel suit. In court, the plaintiff's lawyer might say, "This nurse called my client 'rude, difficult, and uncooperative.' It's right here in her own handwriting! No wonder she didn't take good care of him—she didn't like him." Remember, the patient has a legal right to see his chart. If he spots a derogatory reference, he'll be hurt, angry, and more likely to sue.

If a patient is difficult or uncooperative, document the behavior objectively and let the jurors draw their own conclusions. (See *Polite and to the point.*)

Rule #6: Keep the record intact

Be sure to keep the patient's chart complete. Let's say that you spill coffee on a page and blur several entries. Don't discard the original! Keep it on the chart. Discarding pages, even for innocent reasons, raises doubt in a lawyer's mind. (See *Missing records*, page 140.)

Always keep the original pages in a patient's chart.

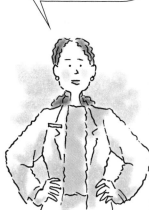

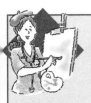

Art of the chart

Polite and to the point

The note below describes a difficult situation dispassionately, while still getting the point across.

3/11/09	1300	I attempted to perform the daily abdominal dressing change, but pt stated,
		"This doesn't need to be done every day. It doesn't hurt and I don't want you
		to touch it. Leave me alone." I explained the importance of monitoring and clean-
		ing the incision and offered an analgesic to be given 20 min before dressing
		would be changed. Pt became agitated and still refused. Dr. B. Humbert
		notified that incisional site was not assessed nor was dressing changed and
		that pt is agitated. ———————————————— Mary Marley, R.N.

What to chart

Caring for patients seems more important than documenting every detail, doesn't it? However, legally speaking, an incomplete chart reflects incomplete nursing care. Neglecting to record every detail is such a serious and common charting error that malpractice lawyers have coined the expression "Not charted, not done."

This doesn't mean that you have to document everything. Some information, such as staffing shortages and staff conflicts, is definitely off limits. (See *Charting don'ts*, page 141.)

Rule #1: Chart significant situations

Learn to recognize legally dangerous situations as you give patient care. Assess each critical or out-of-the-ordinary situation, and decide whether your actions might be significant in court. If they could be, chart them as well as every other detail of the situation in the progress notes. (See *Understanding negligence*, page 142, and *Out of the ordinary*, page 142.)

Rule #2: Chart complete assessment data

Failing to perform and document a complete physical assessment is a key factor in many malpractice suits. During your initial assess-

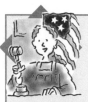

Case in point

Missing records

The case of *Keene v. Brigham and Women's Hospital* (2003) shows how missing records can raise doubt about whether proper care was given to a patient. In this situation, a neonate developed respiratory distress and cyanosis within hours of birth. He was transferred to the neonatal intensive care unit. Blood tests, including a complete blood count and a blood culture, were performed. The patient was then transferred back to the regular nursery for "routine care" with instructions for staff to watch for signs and symptoms of sepsis and to withhold antibiotic therapy pending the results of the complete blood count. About 20 hours after the transfer, the neonate went into septic shock and started having seizures. Antibiotics were given at this time.

Record skips

Subsequent testing revealed that the neonate had neonatal sepsis and meningitis and tested positive for group B beta-hemolytic streptococci. However, no one could determine whether anyone was notified about the patient's condition or if appropriate actions were taken because about 18 hours worth of hospital records relating to the patient couldn't be found.

The verdict

The court held that a party who has negligently or intentionally lost or destroyed evidence known to be relevant for an upcoming legal proceeding should be held accountable for any unfair prejudice that results. Therefore, the court inferred that without evidence to the contrary, the missing records would have likely contained proof that the antibiotics should have been administered sooner and that the defendant's failure to do so caused the neonate's injuries.

---

ment, focus on the patient's reason for seeking care, and then follow up on all other problems he mentions. Be sure to chart everything you do as well as why. (See *The trouble with charting by exception*, page 143.)

After completing the initial assessment, write a well-constructed care plan. Doing so gives you a clear approach to the patient's problems and helps defend your care if you're sued.

Phrase each problem statement clearly, and modify them as you gather new assessment data. State the care plan for solving each problem; then identify the actions you intend to take.

Rule #3: Document discharge instructions

Because of insurance constraints, facilities are now discharging patients earlier than they once did. This change means that patients and family members are changing dressings, assessing wounds, and tackling other tasks that nurses have traditionally performed. Patient and family teaching is your responsibility. If a

> Family teaching is part of your professional responsibility.

Advice from the experts

Charting don'ts

Negative language and inappropriate information don't belong in a medical record and can return to haunt you in a lawsuit. The charting mistakes below are legal land mines. Avoid them.

1. Don't record staffing problems
True, staff shortages may affect patient care or contribute to an incident. However, you shouldn't mention this in a patient's chart because it can be used as legal ammunition against you if the chart lands in court. Instead, write a confidential memo to your nurse-manager, and review your facility's policy and procedure manuals to see how you're expected to handle this situation.

2. Don't record staff conflicts
Don't chart:
• disputes with other nurses (including criticisms of their care)
• questions about a doctor's treatment
• a colleague's rude or abusive behavior.

Personality clashes aren't legitimate patient care concerns. In the event of a lawsuit, the plaintiff's lawyer will exploit conflicts among codefendants.

Instead of charting these problems, talk with your nurse-manager, or consult with the doctor directly if an order puzzles you. If another nurse writes personal accusations or charges of incompetence in a chart, talk to her about the implications of doing this. Remember, you're responsible for your actions.

3. Don't mention incident reports
Incident reports are confidential and filed separately from the patient's chart. Document only the facts of an incident in the chart, and never write *incident report* or indicate that you filed one.

For example, write: *Found pt lying on the floor at 1250 hours. Vital signs BP 110/70, P 82, R 20, T 98.6° F. No visible bleeding or trauma. AA Ox3, PERLA, + ROM to all extremities. Pt returned to bed with all side rails up and bed in low position. Pt. stated, "I must have been sleepwalking." Notified Dr. Gary Dietrich at 1253 hours, and he saw pt at 1300 hours.*

4. Don't use words associated with errors
Terms like *by mistake, accidentally, somehow, unintentionally, miscalculated,* and *confusing* are bonus words to the plaintiff's attorney. Steer clear of words that suggest an error was made or a patient's safety was jeopardized. Let the facts speak for themselves.

For example, suppose you gave a patient 100 mg of Demerol instead of 50 mg. Here's how to chart this without calling undue attention to it: *Pt was given Demerol 100 mg I.M. at 1300 hours for abdominal pain VAS 7/10. Dr. Smith was notified but gave no orders. Pt's vital signs remained stable.*

5. Don't name a second patient
Naming a second patient in a patient's chart violates confidentiality. Instead, write *roommate*, the patient's initials, or his room and bed number.

6. Don't chart casual conversations with colleagues
Telling your nurse-manager in the elevator or restroom about a patient's deteriorating condition doesn't qualify as informing her. She's likely to forget the details or may not even realize you expect her to intervene. Before notifying someone, clearly state why you're notifying the person so she can focus on the facts and take appropriate action. Otherwise, you can't chart that you informed her.

patient receives inadequate or incorrect instructions and an injury results, you could be held liable.

Many facilities give patients printed instruction sheets that describe treatments and home care procedures. (Make sure your patient can read English before giving printed instruction sheets.) In court, these materials may be used as evidence that instruction took place. To support testimony, they should be tailored to each

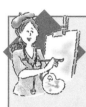

Art of the chart

Out of the ordinary

This note shows the right way to chart atypical information.

2/18/09	1900	Furosemide 40 mg P.O. not given because of
		impending upper GI series. Dr. T. Wenger
		notified that furosemide was not given. Dr. T.
		Wenger gave order for furosemide 20 mg I.V.
		Administered at 0915.—— Charles Cashman, RN

patient's specific needs and contain any verbal or written instructions you provided. Documentation of referrals to home health care agencies or other community providers is another essential component of discharge planning.

When to chart

Finding time to chart can be hard during a busy shift. However, the timeliness of entries is a major issue in malpractice suits.

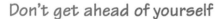

Don't get ahead of yourself

Document nursing care when you perform it or shortly afterward. Never document ahead of time — your notes will be inaccurate, and you'll leave out information about the patient's response to treatment. Even if you did what you charted, a lawyer might ask, "Do you occasionally chart something before doing it?" If you answer "yes," the jury won't see the chart as a reliable indica-

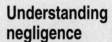

Document ahead of time? Never! My credibility is at stake.

Understanding negligence

Inadequate observation of patients that leads to misdiagnosis or injury is a common cause of lawsuits involving nurses. Most of these lawsuits involve issues of negligence — the failure to exercise the degree of care that a person of ordinary prudence would exercise under the same circumstances. A claim of negligence requires that there be a duty owed by one person to another, that the duty be breached, and that injury resulted.

Malpractice is a more restricted, specialized type of negligence, defined as a violation of professional duty to act with reasonable care and in good faith. Several states have begun to recognize nursing negligence as a form of malpractice.

Avoid negligence cases by documenting any and all unusual patient events.

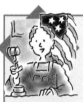

Case in point

The trouble with charting by exception

The case of *Lama v. Borras* (1994) shows the importance of thoroughly documenting assessment findings.

"Back"ground
The patient underwent disc surgery for which prophylactic antibiotics weren't ordered. Postoperatively, the patient started to show signs of infection, including "very bloody" dressings and pain at the incision site. Ultimately, the patient was diagnosed with discitis (an infection of the space in-between discs) and was given antibiotics. The patient was hospitalized for several months while undergoing treatment for the infection.

Exception = incomplete
Details regarding the patient's infection symptoms weren't known because the hospital's nurses were instructed to "chart by exception," a system in which nurses don't record qualitative observations at each shift; rather, they record such observations only when it's deemed necessary to document important changes in the patient's condition. It was alleged that the nurses' failure to report the patient's symptoms during each nursing shift caused the late detection of the patient's infection.

The verdict
The court stated there was evidence to suggest that charting by exception didn't regularly record information important to an infection diagnosis, such as the changing characteristics of the surgical wound and the patient's complaints of postoperative pain. One of the attending nurses conceded that under the charting by exception policy, she wouldn't report a patient's pain if she didn't administer medicine or if she gave the patient only an aspirin-type medication. The court also concluded that the intermittent charting of possible signs of infection failed to record the sort of continuous danger signals that would most likely spur early intervention by a doctor.

tor of what you actually did, which wrecks your credibility. (See *Charting ahead*, page 144.)

Who should chart

State nurse practice acts have strict rules about who can chart. Breaking these rules can cause you to have your nursing license suspended.

Finish what you started

No matter how busy you are, never ask another nurse to complete your charting (and never complete another nurse's charting). Doing so is a dangerous practice that may be specifically prohibited by your state's nurse practice act. If the other nurse makes an error

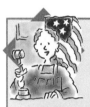

Case in point

Charting ahead

In the case of *Beene v. St. Vincent Mercy Medical Center* (2000), a court upheld a hospital's disciplinary suspension of a nurse after the death of a patient under her care. The patient had a heart attack, but no audible alarm was sounded when the patient went into arrest because the alarms on his cardiac monitor were disengaged. During the subsequent investigation, it was discovered that the nurse noted on the patient's medical chart that the alarms were active at 4:00 p.m., 5:00 p.m., and 6:00 p.m.; however, the patient was already dead at these times. The nurse admitted that to save time she had made all entries regarding the alarms at the beginning of her shift rather than at hourly intervals as suggested on the medical chart. The nurse attempted to establish that it was common practice for nurses to "chart ahead," or mark hourly intervals 3 or 4 hours before treatment is administered. The court found that charting ahead was a violation of hospital policy and, in the circumstances of the case, the action amounted to falsifying medical records.

or misinterprets information, the patient can be harmed. Then if the patient sues you for negligence, both you and your facility will be held accountable because delegated documentation doesn't meet nursing standards.

Delegating charting has another consequence: It destroys the credibility and value of the medical record both in the facility and in court. Judges give little, if any, weight to medical records containing secondhand observations or hearsay evidence.

Risk management and documentation

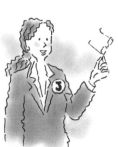

A health care facility's reputation for safe, reliable, and effective service is its main defense against liability claims. Well-coordinated risk management and performance improvement programs show the public that the facility is being managed in a legally responsible manner. If complaints arise, a good program ensures that they're handled promptly to contain the damage and minimize liability claims. (See *Understanding risk management and performance improvement.*)

In addition, The Joint Commission requires health care facilities to identify and manage sentinel events. A sentinel event is an unexpected occurrence involving death or serious physical or psychological injury. When an organization suspects an undesirable event, it's required to initiate an intense analysis of the situation.

Understanding risk management and performance improvement

Do the terms *risk management* and *performance improvement* confuse you? Here's how to tell them apart: Risk management focuses on the patient's and family members' perceptions of the care provided; performance improvement focuses on the role of the health care provider.

Two for one

Many facilities combine these two programs in their educational efforts. They place a high priority on teaching new medical residents and nurses about malpractice claims, staff members' reporting obligations, proper informational and reporting channels, and principles of risk management and performance improvement.

This analysis should lead to performance improvement concerns and then to changes as necessary. Analysis should start when a sentinel event or one of the following situations has occurred:

- confirmed transfusion reaction
- significant adverse drug reaction
- significant medication error.

Mining the records for potential risk

Sometimes, documentation reveals potential problems within a health care facility. For example, documentation might reveal that a certain procedure repeatedly leads to patient injury or another type of accident. Risk management programs help reduce injuries and accidents, minimize financial loss, and meet the guidelines of The Joint Commission and other regulatory agencies.

In the past, the focuses of risk management and performance improvement programs were to maintain and improve facilities and equipment and ensure employee, visitor, and patient safety. Today, the focus is on identifying, evaluating, and reducing patient injury in specialty units that have the greatest malpractice risks.

Preventing adverse events

Risk management has three main goals:

decreasing the number of claims by promptly identifying and following up on adverse events (early warning systems)

reducing the frequency of preventable injuries and accidents leading to lawsuits by maintaining or improving the quality of care

controlling costs related to claims by pinpointing trouble spots early and working with the patient and his family.

Early warning systems

Early warning systems can pinpoint much useful information. However, to be effective they need:

- a strong organizational structure
- cooperation between risk management and performance improvement departments
- the commitment of all staff members to report adverse events to the appropriate clinical chairperson, so he can study the medical records more closely or talk to the staff member involved and recommend remedial education, monitoring, or restricted privileges
- the commitment of key staff members — such as nurses, doctors, administrators, and chiefs of high-risk services — to analyze the information

• the commitment of all staff members to be compliant with policies and procedures in order to maintain and maximize quality patient care.

The most commonly used early warning systems are *incident reporting* and *occurrence screening.*

Reporting the out of the ordinary

An incident report refers to the documentation of events that are inconsistent with a health care facility's ordinary routine, regardless of whether injury occurs. Doctors, nurses, or other staff are responsible for reporting such events when they're observed or shortly afterward. Examples include the unplanned return of a patient to the operating room or a medication error.

Let's review

Occurrence screening involves reviewing medical records to find adverse events. Both general indicators of adverse events (such as a nosocomial infection or medication error) and more specific indicators (such as an incorrect sponge count during surgery) are considered.

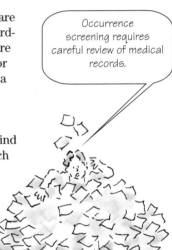

Occurrence screening requires careful review of medical records.

Reducing injuries and accidents

Many health care facilities coordinate educational efforts to help prevent injuries and accidents that may lead to lawsuits.

Making sure everyone is on the same page

The facility may reach out to a specific employee, such as a nurse or doctor, who has been identified as having a particular problem, or to a larger population, such as new nurses or residents, that may face the same types of problems. Required teaching topics for new employees include malpractice claims, reporting obligations, proper informational and reporting channels, and principles of risk management and performance improvement.

Cost control

Systematic, well-coordinated risk management and performance improvement programs demonstrate to the public that the facility is managed in a legally responsible way. When complaints do arise, risk managers handle them promptly to contain the damage and minimize liability claims.

Managing incidents

Despite risk management programs, adverse events still occur. Health care facilities rely on the following sources to identify dangerous situations or trends:

• *Incident reports*, also called *quality tracking forms*, are a primary source of information for lawyers. Lawyers use the reports when researching potential lawsuits and in court as evidence.

• *Nurses* are usually the first ones to recognize potential problems because they spend so much time with patients and families. They know which patients are dissatisfied with their care and which ones have complications that may lead to injuries.

• *Patient-representatives* keep files of patient complaints, identify litigious patients, and maintain contact with the patient and his family after an incident has occurred.

• *The business office and medical records department* may be alerted to potential lawsuits when a patient threatens to sue after he receives his bill or when a patient or a lawyer requests a copy of the medical record.

• *Other sources* can also help. For example, the engineering department has information on the safety of the hospital environment; purchasing, biomedical engineering, and the pharmacy can report on the safety and adequacy of products and equipment; and social workers, hospital clergy, volunteers, and patient escorts commonly know about highly dissatisfied patients. *Remember:* Whenever you get a report from one of these sources, document it thoroughly on the patient's medical record and fill out an incident report.

Other members of the health care team can provide information to help manage incidents.

The claim chain reaction

Once the risk manager learns of a potential or actual lawsuit, he notifies the medical records department and the facility's insurance company. The medical records department makes copies of the patient's chart and files the original in a safe place to prevent tampering.

A claim notice should also trigger a performance improvement peer review of the medical record. This review measures the health care provider's conduct against the professional standards of conduct for the particular situation. This information is used by the risk manager and the facility's attorney to investigate the claim's merit, the facility's responsibility, and areas where changes are needed. The standard required for a successful defense isn't always as high as the facility's optimal standard.

Eight legal hazards

Every day, you face patient care situations that could land you in court. Your challenge is to watch out for potential pitfalls and know how to chart them defensively when they arise. This section describes eight volatile legal situations.

Hazard #1: Incident reports

Whenever you witness an adverse event, file an incident report. Some things to report are injuries from restraints, burns, or other causes; falls (even if the patient wasn't injured); and a patient's insistence on being discharged against medical advice. If an incident report form doesn't leave enough space to fully describe an incident, attach an additional page of comments. (See *Completing an incident report.*)

Following the guidelines here will reduce your legal risks.

The form's function

An incident report isn't part of the patient's chart, but it may be used later in litigation. A report has two functions:

☞ It informs the administration of the incident so the risk management staff can work on preventing similar incidents.

✌ It alerts the administration and the facility's insurance company to a potential claim and the need for further investigation.

It's an eyewitness report

Only people who witnessed an incident should fill out and sign an incident report, and each witness should file a separate report. After the report is filed, it may be reviewed by the nursing supervisor, the doctor who examined the patient after the incident, various department heads and administrators, the facility's attorney, and the insurance company.

Because incident reports will be read by many people and may even turn up in court, you must follow strict guidelines when completing them. (See *Tips for reporting incidents*, page 150.)

Facilities are continually revising their incident report forms; some have begun to use computerized forms. Incident reports are also processed by computer, which permits classifying and counting incidents to indicate trends.

Charting incidents in progress notes

When documenting an incident in the medical record, follow these guidelines:

Art of the chart

Completing an incident report

When you witness a reportable event, you must fill out an incident report. Forms vary, but most include the following information.

INCIDENT REPORT

Name _Greta Manning_
Address _1 Worth Way, Boston, MA_
Phone _(617) 555-1122_

9. DATE OF INCIDENT	10. TIME OF INCIDENT
3-14-09	1442

11. EXACT LOCATION OF INCIDENT (Bldg., Floor, Room No., Area)
4-Main, Rm. 441

Addressograph if patient

12. TYPE OF INCIDENT (CHECK ONE ONLY)   ☐ PATIENT   ☐ EMPLOYEE   ☑ VISITOR   ☐ VOLUNTEER   ☐ OTHER   (Specify)

13. DESCRIPTION OF THE INCIDENT (WHO, WHAT, WHEN, WHERE, HOW, WHY) (Use Back of Form if Necessary)

Wife of pt found on floor next to left side of bed. States "I was trying to put the siderail of the bed down to sit on my husband's bed and I fell down."

State only what you saw or heard.

Describe relevant conditions.

14. FLOOR CONDITIONS   ☑ CLEAN & SMOOTH   ☐ OTHER ____   ☐ SLIPPERY (WET) | FRAME OF BED   ☑ LOW   ☐ HIGH | NIGHT LIGHT

15. WERE BED RAILS PRESENT?   ☐ NO   ☐ 1 UP   ☐ 2 UP   ☐ 3 UP   ☑ 4 UP | 17. OTHER RESTRAINTS (TYPE & EXTENT)   N/A

18. AMBULATION PRIVILEGE   ☐ UNLIMITED   ☐ LIMITED WITH ASSISTANCE   ☐ COMPLETE BEDREST   ☐ OTHER ____

19. WAS NARCOTICS, ANALGESICS, HYPNOTICS, SEDATIVES, DIURETICS, ANTIHYPERTENSIVES OR ANTICONVULSANTS GIVEN DURING LAST 4 HOURS?   ☐ YES   ☑ NO

| DRUG | AMOUNT | TIME |

PATIENT INCIDENTS

20. PHYSICIAN NOTIFIED   NAME OF PHYSICIAN   J. Reynolds, MD | DATE   3-14-09 | TIME | COMPLETE IF APPLICABLE   1445

EMPLOYEE INCIDENTS

21. DEPARTMENT | 22. JOB TITLE | 23. SOCIAL SECURITY #

24. MARITAL STATUS

ALL INCIDENTS

27. SUPERVISOR NOTIFIED   NAME OF SUPERVISOR   C. Jones, RN   DATE   3-14-09   TIME   1500 | 28. LOCATION (WHERE TREATMENT WAS RENDERED)

29. NAME, ADDRESS AND TELEPHONE NUMBER OF WITNESS(ES) OR PERSONS FAMILIAR WITH INCIDENT - WITNESS OR NOT
Connie Smith, RN   (617) 555-0912   1 Main St., Boston, MA

List the name, telephone number, and address of anyone involved.

SIGNATURE OF PERSON PREPARING REPORT   Connie Smith | TITLE   RN | 31. DATE OF REPORT   3-14-09

- To be completed for all cases involving injury or illness   (DO NOT USE ABBREVIATIONS) (Use back of Form if necessary)

Pt in Emergency Department after reported fall in husband's room. 12 cm x 12 cm ecchymotic area noted on right hip. X-rays negative for fracture. Good range of motion. no c/o pain. VAS 0/10. Ice pack applied. ____ — J. Reynolds, MD

33. DISPOSITION   sent home, written instructions provided to pt and wife; pt and wife verbalized understanding of instructions.

| 34. PERSON NOTIFIED OTHER THAN HOSPITAL PERSONNEL NAME AND ADDRESS   R. Manning (daughter) address same as pt | 35. DATE 3-14-09 | 36. TIME 1500 |

| 37. PHYSICIAN'S SIGNATURE   J. Reynolds, MD | 38. DATE 3-14-09 |

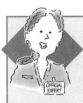

Advice from the experts

Tips for reporting incidents

In the past, a plaintiff's lawyer wasn't allowed to see incident reports. Today, however, many states allow lawyers access to incident reports if they make their requests through proper channels. So, when writing an incident report, keep in mind who may read it and follow these guidelines:

• Include essential information, such as the identity of the person involved in the incident, the exact time and place of the incident, and the name of the doctor you notified.

• Document any unusual occurrences that you witnessed.

• Record the events and the consequences for the patient in enough detail that administrators can decide whether or not to investigate further.

• Write objectively, avoiding opinions, judgments, conclusions, or assumptions about who or what caused the incident. Tell your opinions to your supervisor or the risk manager later.

• Describe only what you saw and heard and the actions you took to provide care at the scene. Unless you saw a patient fall, write *Found pt lying on the floor.*

• Don't admit that you're at fault or blame someone else. Steer clear of statements such as *Better staffing would have prevented this incident.*

• Don't offer suggestions about how to prevent the incident from happening again.

• Don't include detailed statements from witnesses and descriptions of remedial action; these are normally part of an investigative follow-up.

• Don't put the report in the medical record. Send it to the person designated to review it according to your facility's policy.

• Write a factual account of the incident, including treatment and follow-up care as well as the patient's response. This account shows that the patient was closely monitored after the incident. Make sure the descriptions in the chart match those in the incident report.

• Don't write *incident report completed* after charting the event. This destroys the confidential nature of the report and may result in a lawsuit. For the same reason, the doctor shouldn't write an order for an incident report in the chart.

• In charting the incident, include everything the patient or family member says about the patient's role in the incident. For example, you might write *Pt stated, "The nurse told me to ask for help before I went to the bathroom, but I decided to go on my own."* In a negligence lawsuit, this information may help the defense lawyer show that the incident was entirely or partially the patient's fault.

The information I document in the incident report...

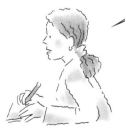

...has to match the information in the medical record.

If the jury finds that the patient was partially at fault, the concept of *contributory negligence* may be used to reduce or even eliminate the patient's recovery of damages.

Hazard #2: Informed consent

A patient must sign a consent form before most treatments and procedures. Informed consent means that he understands the proposed therapy and its risks and agrees to undergo it. The doctor performing the procedure is legally responsible for explaining the procedure and its risks and for obtaining consent. However, he may ask you to witness the patient's signature. Some facilities may specifically require the person who informs the patient of the treatment or procedure to be the one to obtain the consent. Check with your facility's legal counsel if you have any questions. (See *Sign here: Witnessing a consent form.*)

Advice from the experts

Sign here: Witnessing a consent form

After the doctor informs the patient about a medical procedure, he may ask you to obtain the patient's signature on the consent form and then sign as a witness. Before doing so, review this checklist:

• Make sure that the patient is competent, awake, alert, and aware of what he's doing. He should not be under the influence of alcohol, illicit drugs, or prescribed medications that impair his understanding or judgment.

• Ask the patient whether the doctor explained the diagnosis, proposed treatment, and expected outcome to his satisfaction. Also ask whether he understands all that was said.

• Ask the patient whether he has been told about the risks of the treatment or procedure, the possible consequences of refusing it, and alternative treatments or procedures.

• Ask the patient whether he has any concerns or questions about his condition or the treatment. If he does, help him get answers from the doctor or other appropriate sources.

• Tell the patient that he can refuse the treatment without having other care or support withdrawn and that he can withdraw his consent after giving it.

• Notify your nurse-manager and the doctor immediately if you suspect that the patient has doubts about his condition or the procedure, hasn't been properly informed, or has been coerced into giving consent. Performing a procedure without voluntary consent may be considered battery.

• Objectively document your assessment of the patient's understanding in the chart, noting the situation, his responses, and the actions you took.

• When you're satisfied that the patient is well informed, have him sign the consent form including the date and time, and then sign your name as a witness.

• Remember that you're responsible for obtaining oral informed consent for any procedures that you'll be performing, such as inserting an I.V. catheter or a urinary catheter, even though a general treatment consent was signed upon admission.

Art of the chart

Informed consent

A patient's signature on a consent form implies that he understands the risks of a procedure and agrees to undergo it. Here's a typical form.

CONSENT FOR OPERATION AND RENDERING OF OTHER MEDICAL SERVICES

1. I hereby authorize Dr. ___Wesley___ to perform upon ___Joseph Smith___ (Patient name), the following surgical and/or medical procedures: (State specific nature of the procedures to be performed) ___Exploratory laparotomy___

2. I understand that the procedure(s) will be performed at Valley Medical Center by or under the supervision of Dr. ___Wesley___, who is authorized to utilize the services of other doctors, or members of the house staff as he or she deems necessary or advisable.

> The form should state the specific procedure under consideration.

3. ___ned to me that during the course of the operation, unforeseen conditions may be revealed that necessitate an ex-___nal procedure(s) or different procedure(s) than those set forth in Paragraph 1, I therefore authorize and request ___ed doctor, and his or her associates or assistants, perform such medical surgical procedures as are necessary ___e exercise of professional judgment.

4. ___nature and purpose of the procedure(s), possible alternative methods of dia___ed, the possibility of complications, and the consequences of the procedure(s). I acknowledge ___een made as to the results that may be obtained.

> The patient acknowledges that he understands therapy and its risks and agrees to undergo it.

5. I authorize the above named doctor to administer local or regional anesthesia (for all other ___on-sent must be signed by the patient or patient's authorized representative).

6. I understand that if it is necessary for me to receive a blood transfusion during this procedure or this hospitalization, the blood will be supplied by sources available to the hospital and tested in accordance with national and regional regulations. I understand that there are risks in transfusion, including but not limited to allergic, febrile, and hemolytic transfusion reactions, and the transmission of infectious diseases, such as hepatitis and AIDS (Acquired Immune Deficiency Syndrome). I hereby consent to blood transfusion(s) and blood derivative(s).

7. I hereby authorize representatives from Valley Medical Center to photograph or videotape me for the purpose of research or medical education. It is understood and agreed that patient confidentiality shall be preserved.

8. I authorize the doctor named above and his or her associates and assistants and Valley Medical Center to preserve for scientific purposes or to dispose of any tissue, organs, or other body parts removed during surgery or other diagnostic procedures in accordance with customary medical practice.

9. I certify that I have read and fully understand the above consent statement. In addition, I have been afforded an opportunity to ask whatever questions I might have regarding the procedure(s) to be performed and they have been answered to my satisfaction.

___Joseph Smith___   ___03/15/09___   ___C. Gurney, RN___
Legal Patient or Authorized Representative   Date   Witness
(State Relationship to Patient)

If the patient is unable to consent on his or her own behalf, complete the following:

Patient _____ is unable to consent because _____

> Signing indicates only that you're witnessing the patient's signature.

_____

Legally Responsible Person _____ Doctor Obtaining Consent ___M. Wesley, MD___

Waive it good-bye

The legal requirement for obtaining informed consent can be waived only if:

• a mentally competent patient says that he doesn't want to know the details of a treatment or procedure

• an urgent medical or surgical situation occurs (many facilities specify how you should document such an emergency).

Most facilities use a standard consent form that lists the legal requirements for consent. If the patient doesn't understand the doctor's explanation or asks for more information, answer all questions that fall within the scope of your practice. Be sure to document your interaction with the patient. (See *Informed consent*.)

Hazard #3: Advance directives

The Patient Self-Determination Act requires health care facilities to provide information about the patient's right to choose and refuse treatment. Facilities must also ask patients whether they have advance directives, which are documents that state a patient's wishes regarding life-sustaining medical care in case the patient is no longer able to indicate his own wishes. Your job is to document that the patient received the required information and whether he brought an advance directive with him. (See *Tips for dealing with advance directives*, page 154.) Facility policies and state laws vary, so make sure you know what's required in your state and facility.

A change may be in order

When a patient's advance directive is given to the doctor, the nurse's orders may change, depending on the patient's wishes. For example, if the patient's family submits an advance directive that includes the information that the patient doesn't want to be resuscitated, a do-not-resuscitate (DNR) order may be written.

Don't forget this

DNR orders are instructions not to attempt to resuscitate a patient who has suffered cardiac or respiratory failure. A DNR order may be appropriate if the patient has a terminal illness, is permanently unconscious, or won't respond to cardiopulmonary resuscitation (CPR). A terminally ill patient may ask not to be resuscitated if he experiences sudden cardiac arrest, or he may write this request into his advance directive.

A DNR order should be reviewed periodically or whenever a significant change occurs in the patient's clinical status. (See *Charting last wishes*, page 155.)

Advice from the experts

Tips for dealing with advance directives

Many patients wait until they're hospitalized to consider an advance directive or to make significant legal decisions. So, be prepared to offer information and advice and to record the patient's wishes in a legally appropriate manner. Here are some important points to remember.

Legal competence

Only a competent adult can execute a legally binding document. To prevent a patient's relatives from raising questions about his competence later, discuss his mental status with the doctor and, possibly, a psychiatrist. Be sure to document his mental status assessment in the chart before he signs any legal document.

Living will and durable power of attorney

If a patient has a living will or durable power of attorney for health care, a copy should be in his chart. Also, you should know how to contact the person with decision-making power. If the patient doesn't have the document with him, ask a family member to bring it to the health care facility. As your patient's advocate, you must ensure that his wishes are properly executed. If conflicts arise, discuss them with your nurse-manager as well as with a risk manager.

If a patient wants to execute a living will during his hospital stay, you aren't required, or even allowed in some states, to sign as a witness. Many facilities have the social service or risk management department oversee this process. Find out who is responsible in your facility. The person who acts as witness can be held accountable for the patient's competence. Place the signed and witnessed document in the chart.

Last will and testament

In some facilities, dictating a patient's last will and testament is so commonplace that special forms have been designed for it. If this situation occurs often in your facility, discuss creating a form with your manager.

If no form exists in your facility, and a patient wants to dictate his last will and testament to you, document his request and what has been done to facilitate it—for example, who has been contacted and when.

If an administrator isn't available, two nurses should be present during dictation of the will. One should record the information in the chart, and both should sign it. In most instances, the patient's family will obtain their own legal representatives to process the recording of the will.

Who else can give a DNR order?

If the patient doesn't ask for a DNR order, or if no policies exist, the doctor may write the order if it's medically appropriate and the patient understands the impact of the DNR order. If the patient is incompetent, an appropriate surrogate must give consent for the doctor to write the DNR order.

A patient's right

The patient has the right to change advance directives at any time. Because the patient's requests may differ from what the family or doctor wants, document discrepancies carefully. Use social services or the legal department for advice on how to proceed. (See *Check this out: Advance directive checklist*, page 156.)

Two common types of advance directives are living will and durable power of attorney for health care.

> When the patient's wishes about life-sustaining care clash with the doctor's or family members', document the discrepancy.

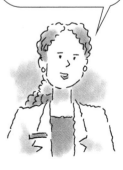

Advice from the experts

Charting last wishes

Because do-not-resuscitate (DNR) orders are legally recognized, you won't incur liability if you don't try to resuscitate a patient with a DNR order and that patient later dies. You may, however, incur liability if you initiate resuscitation on a patient who has a DNR order. Every patient with a DNR order should have a written order on file. But if a patient doesn't have a DNR order, you're obligated to call a code if the situation warrants it.

How should you proceed?
If a terminally ill patient without a DNR order tells you that he doesn't want to be resuscitated in a crisis, document the patient's wishes and chart his degree of awareness and orientation. Then contact his doctor and your nurse-manager, and ask for assistance from administration, legal services, or social services. Don't place yourself in the middle. Let the doctor and the patient's family make the decisions.

If the doctor knows about the patient's wishes but still refuses to write a DNR order, document this information in your notes. Like you, the doctor must abide by the patient's wishes and may be found liable if he doesn't. If the patient has prepared an advance directive, make sure the doctor has seen it.

Living will

In making a living will, a legally competent person declares what medical care he wants or doesn't want if he develops a terminal illness. Living wills may apply only to treatment decisions made after a terminally ill patient becomes comatose and has no reasonable chance of recovery. They usually authorize the doctor to withhold or discontinue lifesaving measures.

State-ments

Most states recognize living wills as valid legal documents. Although the legal requirements vary from state to state, most states specify:
• circumstances under which a living will applies
• who is authorized to make a living will (usually only competent adults)
• limitations or restrictions on care that can be refused (for example, some states don't allow refusal of food and water)
• elements the will must contain to be considered a legal document, including witnessing requirements

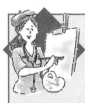

▶ *Art of the chart*

Check this out: Advance directive checklist

The Joint Commission requires that information on advance directives be charted on the admission assessment form. However, many facilities also use a checklist like the one below.

ADVANCE DIRECTIVE CHECKLIST

(Check appropriate boxes.)

I. DISTRIBUTION OF ADVANCE DIRECTIVE INFORMATION

    A. Advance directive information was presented to the patient: .... ☑

       1. At the time of preadmission testing .... ☑

       2. Upon inpatient admission .... ☐

       3. Interpretive services contacted .... ☐

       4. Information was read to the patient .... ☐

    B. Advance directive information was presented to the next of kin as
       the patient is incapacitated. .... ☐

    C. Advance directive information was not distributed as the patient is
       incapacitated and no relative or next of kin was available. .... ☐

                    Mary Barren, RN   03/15/09
                      RN   **DATE**

	Upon admission		Upon transfer to Critical Care Unit	
	YES	**NO**	**YES**	**NO**
II. ASSESSMENT OF ADVANCE DIRECTIVE UPON ADMISSION				
A. Does the patient have an advance directive?	☐	☑	☐	☐
If yes, was the attending physician notified?	☐		☐	
B. If no advance directive, does the patient want to execute an advance directive?	☑	☐	☐	☐
If yes, was the attending physician notified?	☑		☐	
Was the patient referred to resources?	☑		☐	

(Sign and date.)

       Mary Barren, RN
       RN   **RN**
          03/15/09
       DATE   **DATE**

III. RECEIPT OF AN ADVANCE DIRECTIVE AFTER ADMISSION

    A. The patient has presented an advance directive after admission,
       and the attending physician has been notified.

(Sign here if the patient brought an advance directive and presented it after admission.)

       RN   **DATE**

- who is immune from liability for following a living will's directions
- procedure for rescinding a living will.

Durable power of attorney

A durable power of attorney for health care enables a person to state what type of care he does or doesn't want. However, it also names another person to make health care choices if the patient becomes legally incompetent. This person is usually a family member or friend or, in rare instances, the doctor.

Hazard #4: Patients who refuse treatment

You're also responsible for helping patients make informed decisions about continuing treatment. When treatment is refused, important patient care, safety, and documentation issues come into play.

Refusing treatment

Any mentally competent adult can legally refuse treatment if he has been fully informed about his medical condition and the likely consequences of his refusal. Thus, he can refuse mechanical ventilation, tube feedings, antibiotics, fluids, and other treatments that are needed to keep him alive.

The patient who says "no"

When your patient refuses treatment, chart his exact words. Inform him of the risks involved in refusing treatment, preferably in writing. If he still refuses treatment, chart that you didn't provide the prescribed treatment, and then notify the doctor. The doctor will explain the risks to the patient again. If he continues to refuse treatment, the doctor will ask him to sign a refusal-of-treatment release form, which you may need to sign as a witness. (See *Witnessing refusal of treatment*, page 158.)

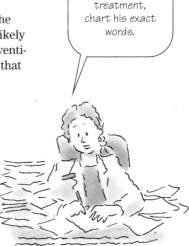

When a patient refuses treatment, chart his exact words.

If the patient won't sign this form, document this, too. For extra protection, your facility may require you to have the patient's spouse or closest relative sign another refusal-of-treatment release form.

Get to them early

More and more facilities are informing patients soon after admission about their future treatment options. Discuss the patient's wishes at your first opportunity, and document the discussion in case he becomes incompetent later. It may be helpful to use a

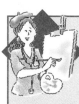

Art of the chart

Witnessing refusal of treatment

To prevent misunderstandings and lawsuits if a patient refuses treatment, the doctor must explain the risks involved in making this choice. If the patient still refuses treatment, the doctor will ask him to sign a refusal-of-treatment release form, such as the one below, which you may need to witness.

REFUSAL-OF-TREATMENT RELEASE FORM

I, ___*Joseph Arden*___, refuse to allow anyone to ___*administer parenteral nutrition*___
    (patient's name)   (insert treatment)

The risks attendant to my refusal have been fully explained to me, and I fully understand the benefits of this treatment. I also understand that my refusal of treatment seriously reduces my chances for regaining normal health and may endanger my life.

I hereby release ___*Memorial General*___ , its nurses and employees, together with all doctors in any way
                        (name of facility)
connected with me as a patient, from liability for respecting and following my express wishes and direction.

___*Donna Burns, RN*___   ___*Joseph Arden*___
(Witness's signature)   (Patient's or legal guardian's signature)

___*2/11/09*___   ___*16*___
(Date)   (Patient's age)

> The patient acknowledges that he understands the risks of refusing treatment.

chaplain or someone from social services to speak with the patient to verify his wishes.

Legal guidelines

Failure to respond appropriately to a patient's refusal to accept treatment may have serious legal consequences. To prevent problems, take these steps:

• Confirm the patient's condition and prognosis with the doctor, and record them in the medical record.

• Make sure that the doctor documented the patient's understanding of the consequences of his refusal, such as pain or decreased life expectancy or quality of life.

- Search the medical record for a living will, a durable power of attorney for health care, or letters from people who heard the patient express his wishes.
- Search the medical record for documentation of conversations between the patient and health care providers, including the conversation about the patient's final decision to withhold treatment. Documentation should include the dates of conversations, the full names of people involved, the circumstances, and what treatments and medical conditions were discussed.
- DNR orders should be reviewed every 48 to 72 hours, or according to your facility's policy.
- DNR orders must be written and signed by the doctor; they can't be provided as verbal orders or telephone orders.
- Refuse written or spoken orders for "slow codes," such as calling the doctor before resuscitating a patient, doing CPR but withholding drugs, giving oxygen but withholding CPR, or not putting a patient on a ventilator. These orders are unethical and illegal.
- Suggest that your facility set up an ethics committee to resolve problems about withholding treatment.

Hazard #5: Documenting for unlicensed personnel

Anyone reading your notes assumes these notes are a firsthand account of care provided—unless you chart otherwise. In some settings, nursing assistants and technicians aren't allowed to make formal chart entries. In such cases, determine what care was provided, assess the patient and the task performed (for example, a dressing change), and document your findings. Be sure to record the full names and titles of unlicensed personnel who provided care. Don't just record their initials.

Countersign-language

If your facility allows unlicensed personnel to chart, you may have to countersign their notes. If your facility's policy states that the unlicensed person must provide care in your presence, don't countersign unless you actually witness her actions. If the policy says that you don't have to be there, your countersigning indicates that the notes describe care that other people had the authority and competence to perform and that you verified that the procedures were performed. You can specifically document that you reviewed the notes and consulted with the technician on certain aspects of care. Of course, you must document any follow-up care you provide.

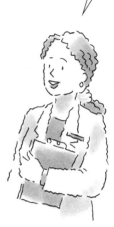

If you're charting care provided by unlicensed personnel, assess the patient and the task performed and document your findings.

Hazard #6: Using restraints

When physical restraints are ordered for a patient, you have several responsibilities, including:

• monitoring the patient frequently for problems associated with the restraints

• performing range-of-motion exercises on all extremities

• making sure the patient has access to the call signal

• assessing the patient's vital signs, circulation status, hydration and elimination needs, level of distress and agitation, mental status, cognitive functioning, and skin integrity

• documenting your care.

Most facilities have a policy outlining the proper procedure for using restraints that conforms to The Joint Commission standards and the Centers for Medicare and Medicaid Services (CMS) regulations. Make sure you know your facility's policy well.

The law recognizes the legitimate use of restraints for acute medical and surgical care as a measure to prevent patient injury. It also recognizes the use of restraints or seclusion to manage violent or self-destructive behavior that jeopardizes the immediate physical safety of the patient, a staff member, or others.

The laws, they are a-changing...

New state and federal regulations combine the standards for the use of restraints in acute medical and surgical care and seclusion for behavior management into a single standard. This new standard focuses on protecting patients from harmful behaviors, regardless of the patient's location. All health care facilities governed by the CMS must adhere to these regulations.

Putting restraints on abusing restraints

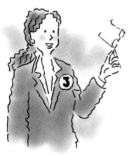

The law also states that a patient must be informed of his rights upon admission to a health care facility. Specifically, a patient has the right to be free from restraints or seclusion of any form imposed by staff members as a means of coercion, discipline, convenience, or retaliation. Restraints and seclusion may only be imposed to ensure the immediate physical safety of the patient, staff members, or others and must be discontinued at the earliest possible time.

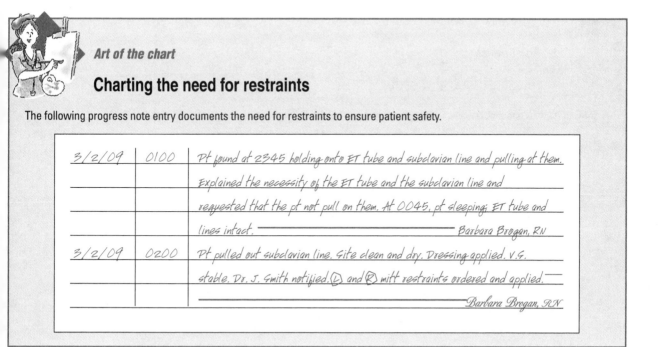

Art of the chart

Charting the need for restraints

The following progress note entry documents the need for restraints to ensure patient safety.

3/2/09	0100	Pt found at 2345 holding onto ET tube and subclavian line and pulling at them.
		Explained the necessity of the ET tube and the subclavian line and
		requested that the pt not pull on them. At 0045, pt sleeping; ET tube and
		lines intact. ———————————————————— Barbara Brogan, RN
3/2/09	0200	Pt pulled out subclavian line. Site clean and dry. Dressing applied. V.S.
		stable. Dr. J. Smith notified. (L) and (R) mitt restraints ordered and applied.—
		————————————————————————— Barbara Brogan, RN

Ordering restraints

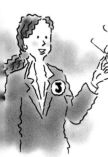

A doctor or other licensed independent practitioner (LIP) who is responsible for the care of the patient and who is authorized to order restraints or seclusion by hospital policy in accordance with state law is allowed to order restraints for a patient. You may recommend to the doctor that he order physical restraints for a patient and chart your observations in the progress notes. (See *Charting the need for restraints.*)

However, new regulations dictate that restraints or seclusion can be used only when less restrictive interventions have been determined to be ineffective to protect the patient or others from harm. Also, the least restrictive type or technique of restraint or seclusion must be used that will effectively protect the patient or others from harm.

Types of restraints

A *physical restraint* is any manual method or physical or mechanical device, material, or equipment attached or adjacent to the patient's body that the patient can't easily remove and that restricts

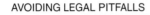

Art of the chart

Physical restraint order

A form such as the one below must be in the patient's chart before physical restraints are applied.

Date: _____3/5/09_____   Time: ___0315_____

Reason for restraint use (circle all that apply):
To prevent:
  (1.) Risk for self-harm
  2. Risk for harm to others
  (3.) High potential for removing tubes, equipment, or invasive lines
     Ⓡ *subclavian CV line*_____
  4. Risk for causing significant disruption of the treatment environment
  5. Other _____

Duration of restraint (Not to exceed 24 hr): _____24_____

Type of restraint (circle all that apply):
  Vest
  (Left mitt)   (Right mitt)
  Left wrist   Right wrist
  Left ankle   Right ankle
  Other _____

Doctor's signature _____ *J. Donnelly, MD* _____

---

his freedom of movement or normal access to his body. A *pharmaceutical restraint* is a medication used as a restriction to manage the patient's behavior or restrict the patient's freedom of movement that isn't part of standard treatment for the patient's condition.

The earlier, the better

When restraints are used for to ensure the safety of a nonviolent, nonself-destructive patient, the order may be renewed as authorized by the facility's policy. However, regardless of the length of the order, restraints and seclusion must be discontinued at the earliest possible time. (See *Physical restraint order.*)

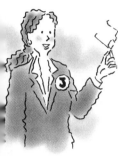

Violent and self-destructive patients

When restraints or seclusion are used to manage violent or self-destructive behavior that jeopardizes the immediate physical safety of the patient, a staff member, or others, the patient must be seen and evaluated face-to-face within 1 hour after initiating the restraint. A trained registered nurse or physician's assistant may perform this assessment, but the doctor or other LIP treating that patient must be consulted as soon as possible to further evaluate the patient's immediate status, his response to the use of restraints, his medical and behavioral history, and the need to continue or stop the restraint or seclusion.

One day at a time—no more

The restraint or seclusion order may be renewed up to a total of 24 hours, with different durations depending on age. The order may be renewed every 4 hours for adults 18 years and older, every 2 hours for children and adolescents between the ages of 9 and 17, and every hour for children younger than 9 years of age. After 24 hours, the doctor or LIP must see and assess the patient before a new order is written.

Getting into training

New regulations call for staff members who work with patients requiring restraints or seclusion to receive orientation training and periodic staff retraining, according to facility policy. Staff members must demonstrate competency in applying restraints and implementing seclusion as well as monitoring, assessing, and providing care for a patient in restraints or seclusion. If a competent patient refuses physical restraints, he may be required to sign a release absolving everyone involved of liability if he's injured as a result.

Hazard #7: Patients who request to see their charts

A patient has a legal right to read his medical record. He may ask to see it because he's confused about the care he's receiving. First, ask him whether he has questions about his treatment and try to clear up any confusion.

If he still wants to see the record, check your facility's policy to see whether he has to read it in your presence. Document questions the patient asks about the record or statements he makes about it as well as what you say to him.

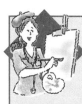

Art of the chart

The patient's progress

When a patient leaves against medical advice, document it in the progress notes as shown below.

| 3/5/09 | 1300 | Pt found in room dressed in own clothes with coat on. When asked why he was dressed, he stated, "They still don't know why I keep getting dizzy, and nothing is turning up in any of the tests. I don't want any more tests and I'm going home." Dr. J. McCarthy notified and came to speak with pt and his son. Pt willing to sign AMA form. AMA form signed. Pt told of the possible risks of his leaving the hospital with dizziness and hypertension. Pt verbalized his understanding of the risks of leaving AMA. Pt agrees to see Dr. C. McCarthy in office tomorrow. Discussed appointment with pt and son Tom Reynolds. Pt going to son's home after discharge. Accompanied pt in wheelchair to main lobby with son. Pt left at 1245. ——————————————————————————————— Lola Caudullo, RN |

Don't just hand it over

Never release medical records to unauthorized people, including family members and police officers. Refer all requests from insurance companies to the appropriate administrator, and refer other requests to your nurse-manager. Be sure to notify your nurse-manager if you have any doubts about the validity of a request — she may want to notify the facility's administrator.

Hazard #8: Patients who leave against medical advice

The law says that a mentally competent patient can leave a facility at any time. Having the patient sign an against medical advice (AMA) form protects you, the doctors, and the facility if problems arise from his unapproved discharge.

That's a wrap!

Legal pitfalls review

Basics
- Complete, accurate documentation proves that you're providing quality care and meeting standards.
- Faulty charting is a pivotal issue in many malpractice cases.

Legal standards
- Nurse practice acts — state laws that designate nursing scope of practice
- ANA requirements — standards set by the nursing profession
- Malpractice litigation — previous rulings, which are influenced by breach of duty, damage, and causation
- Facility policies and procedures — rules that are developed by each facility to identify standards of care

Defensive charting
How to chart
- Stick to facts.
- Avoid labeling.
- Be specific.
- Use neutral language.
- Eliminate bias.
- Keep the chart intact.

What to chart
- Significant situations
- Complete assessment data and care plan
- Discharge instructions

Other charting tips
- Always document care when it's performed or shortly after.
- Never delegate your charting.

Risk management goals
- Decreasing claims
- Reducing preventable accidents
- Controlling costs related to claims

Eight legal hazards
- Incident reports
- Informed consent
- Advance directives
- Patients who refuse treatment
- Documentation for unlicensed personnel
- Restraints
- Patients who request to see their charts
- Patients who leave against medical advice

Taking aim at the AMA form

The AMA form should clearly document that the patient knows he's leaving against medical advice, that he has been advised of and understands the risks of leaving, and that he knows he can come back. Use his own words to describe his refusal.

Here's what to include on the AMA form:
- names of relatives or friends notified of the patient's decision and the dates and times of the notifications
- explanation of the risks and consequences of the AMA discharge, as told to the patient, and the name of the person who provided the explanation

- other places the patient can go for follow-up care
- names of people accompanying the patient at discharge and the instructions given to them
- patient's destination after discharge.

If the patient leaves without anyone's knowledge or if he refuses to sign the AMA form, check your facility's policy; you most likely will need to fill out an incident report in either situation.

Relate the patient's state

In the progress notes, document statements and actions that reflect the patient's mental state at the time he left your facility. Doing so helps protect you, the doctor, security personnel, and the facility against a charge of negligence if the patient later claims that he was mentally incompetent at the time of discharge and was improperly supervised while in that state. (See *The patient's progress*, page 164.)

The case of the missing patient

Suppose a patient never says anything about leaving but, on rounds, you discover he's missing? If you can't find him in the facility, notify your nurse-manager, facility security, and the doctor; then try to contact the patient's home. If he isn't there, call the police if you think the patient might hurt himself or others, especially if he left the hospital with any medical devices.

Chart the time you discovered the patient missing, your attempts to find him, the people you notified, and other pertinent information.

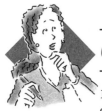

Quick quiz

1.   Failure to provide patient care and follow appropriate standards is called:
    A.   breach of duty.
    B.   breach of promise.
    C.   negligent duty.
    D.   faulty duty.

Answer: A. When investigating breach of duty, the courts ask, "How would a reasonable, prudent nurse with comparable training and experience have acted in the same or similar circumstances?"

2. Professional standards for most nursing specialties are set by:
   A.   the court system.
   B.   ANA.
   C.   The Joint Commission.
   D.   CMS.

Answer: B. The ANA sets standards for most nursing specialties.

3. If you spill something on a page of the medical record, you should:
   A.   throw the old page away after copying it.
   B.   copy it and leave both pages in the chart.
   C.   leave the stained page in the chart.
   D.   get staff to rewrite the page and throw the old page away.

Answer: C. Discarding pages from the medical record, even for innocent reasons, will raise doubt in the jury's mind if the chart ends up in court.

4. If your facility uses flow sheets, checklists, and graphic forms, you still must chart in the progress notes if:
   A.   you filled out an incident report.
   B.   there's any out-of-the-ordinary information.
   C.   there are staff conflicts.
   D.   you want the doctor to see it.

Answer: B. Anticipate litigation, and include in the progress notes anything that needs further explanation or clarification.

5. One way to expedite the charting process is to:
   A.   ask another nurse to help with some of your charting.
   B.   chart before you perform care.
   C.   chart all your care at the end of the shift.
   D.   chart your care as close to the time of the event as possible.

Answer: D. If you chart care right away, you'll be able to record it faster because events will be fresh in your mind.

Scoring

☆☆☆ If you answered all five questions correctly, way to go! Document your achievement and move on to the next chapter.

☆☆ If you answered four questions correctly, terrific! Document your score on a DNR — definitely nice results — form.

☆ If you answered fewer than four questions correctly, don't worry. Draw a line through your test score, initial it, and try again.

Part II   Charting procedures and special situations

8

Charting procedures

Just the facts

In this chapter, you'll learn:

♦ charting requirements for several common nursing procedures

♦ guidelines for charting medication administration and I.V. therapy

♦ charting guidelines for assisted and miscellaneous procedures.

Guidelines for charting procedures

Your notes about routine nursing procedures usually appear in the patient's chart, on flow sheets, or on graphic forms. Whatever your health care facility's requirements are, you must include this information in your documentation:
• what procedure was performed
• when it was performed
• who performed it
• how it was performed
• how well the patient tolerated it
• adverse reactions to the procedure, if any.
     The sections that follow outline information that must be documented for several nursing procedures.

Medication administration

A medication administration record (MAR) is part of most charting systems. It may be included in the medication Kardex, or it may be on a separate sheet. In either case, it's the central record of medication orders and their execution and is part of the patient's permanent record.

> Take the time to document accurately, objectively, thoroughly, consistently, and legibly — in routine and exceptional situations.

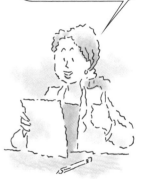

You chart MARvelously

When charting on the MAR, follow these guidelines:
• Follow your facility's policies and procedures for recording drug orders and administration.
• Record the patient's full name, medical record number, and allergy information on each MAR.
• Immediately document the drug's name, dose, route of administration, frequency, the number of doses ordered or the stop date (if applicable), and the administration time for doses given.
• Write legibly.
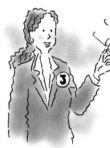
• *Use only standard abbreviations. Remember that The Joint Commission prohibits the use of certain abbreviations (those that appear on the "do not use" list).* When in doubt, write out the word or phrase.
• After administering the first dose, sign your full name, licensure status, and initials in the appropriate space.
• Record drug administration immediately after each dose is administered so that another nurse doesn't inadvertently repeat the dose.
• If you chart by computer, do so right after giving each drug — especially if you don't use printouts as a backup. Doing so gives all team members access to the latest drug administration data.
• If a specific assessment parameter must be monitored during administration of a drug, document this requirement on the MAR. For example, when digoxin is administered, the patient's pulse rate must be monitored and charted on the MAR.
• If you didn't give a drug, circle the time and document the reason for the omission.
• If you suspect that a patient's illness, injury, or death was drug-related, report this to the pharmacy department, who will relay the information to the Food and Drug Administration.

p.r.n. medications

Chart all p.r.n. (as needed) drugs when administered, including the reason for giving the drug and the patient's response. For specific drugs given p.r.n., follow these guidelines:
• For eye, ear, or nose drops, chart the number used as well as the administration route.
• For suppositories, chart the type (rectal, vaginal, or urethral) and how the patient tolerated it.
• For dermal drugs, chart the size and location of the area where you applied the drug and the condition of the skin or wound.
• For dermal patches, chart the location of the patch.
• For I.V., I.M., or subcutaneous medications, chart the dose given and the location of administration.

No room for exceptions

If you administer p.r.n. drugs according to accepted standards, you don't need to chart more specific information. However, if your MAR doesn't have space to document — for example, a patient's response to a drug or refusal to take a drug — document that information in the progress notes.

Drug abuse or refusal

If the patient refuses or abuses medications, describe the event in his chart. Here are some situations that require careful documentation:
• You discover nonprescribed drugs at the patient's bedside. Document the type of medication (pill or powder), the amount of medication, and its color and shape. (You may wish to send the drug to the pharmacy for identification.) Follow your facility's policy regarding the completion of the appropriate report.
• You find a supply of prescribed drugs in the patient's bedside table, indicating that he isn't taking each dose. Record the type and amount of medication.
• You notice a sudden change in the patient's behavior after he has visitors, and you suspect them of giving him opioids or other drugs. Document how the patient appeared before the visitors came and afterward. Notify the doctor immediately and follow your facility's policy.
• You offer prescribed medications and the patient refuses to take them. Document the refusal, the reason for it (if he tells you), and the medication. This prevents the refusal from being misinterpreted as an omission or a medication error on your part. Note the example below.

2/15/09	1100	Pt refused K-Dur tabs, stating that they were too big and made her feel like she was choking when she tried to swallow one. Dr. J. Boyle notified. K-Dur tabs order discontinued. KCl elixir ordered and given. ———— Kathy Collins, RN

Paging the doctor...

Report any medication abuse or refusal to the doctor. When you do so, document the name of the doctor, his response, and the date and time of notification.

Opioid administration

Whenever you give an opioid, you must document it according to federal, state, and facility regulations. These regulations require you to:
- sign out the drug on the appropriate form
- verify the amount of drug in the container before giving it
- have another nurse document your activity and observe you if you must waste or discard part of an opioid dose
- count opioids after each shift.

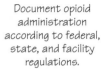

Document opioid administration according to federal, state, and facility regulations.

Double team

Depending on your facility's policy, two nurses should be present to count opioid drugs — preferably the oncoming and offgoing nurse. If you discover a discrepancy in the opioid count, report it, following your facility's policy. Also, file an incident report. An investigation will follow.

I.V. therapy

More than 80% of hospitalized patients receive some form of I.V. therapy, such as fluid or electrolyte replacement, total parenteral nutrition (TPN), drugs, and blood products. Document all facets of I.V. therapy carefully, including subsequent complications. Your facility may have you document in the progress notes, on a special I.V. therapy sheet, in a flowchart, or in another format.

Basic charting

After establishing an I.V. route, document:
- date, time, and venipuncture site
- equipment used such as the type and gauge of the catheter
- number of venipuncture attempts made, the type of assistance required (if applicable), and the patient's response.

Once per shift (or according to your facility policy), document:
- type, amount, and flow rate of I.V. fluid
- condition of the I.V. site
- that you flushed the I.V. catheter and what medication you used.

Update your records each time you change the insertion site, venipuncture device, or I.V. tubing. Also, document the reason you changed the I.V. site, such as extravasation, phlebitis, occlusion, patient removal, or a routine change.

Getting complicated

Document complications precisely. For example, record if extravasation occurs and what interventions you took, such as stopping the I.V. infusion, assessing the amount of fluid infiltrated, and notifying the doctor.

If a chemotherapeutic drug extravasates, stop the I.V. infusion immediately and follow the procedure specified by your health care facility. Document the appearance of the I.V. site, the treatment you gave (especially antidotes), and the kind of dressing you applied. Document the amount of any discarded medication.

If the patient has an allergic reaction during I.V. therapy, stop the infusion and notify the doctor immediately. Then document all pertinent information about the reaction as well as your interventions and the patient's response.

Don't forget the family

Record patient and family teaching, such as explaining the purpose of I.V. therapy, describing the procedure itself, and discussing possible complications.

Total parenteral nutrition

If a patient is receiving TPN, document:
- type and location of the central venous access device
- condition of the insertion site and type of dressing as well as when it was last changed
- that two nurses confirmed the doctor's order
- volume and rate of the solution infused.

We interrupt this service...

When you discontinue a central or peripheral I.V. catheter for TPN, record:
- date and time
- type of dressing applied
- appearance of the administration site
- why it was discontinued — for example, a doctor's order, infiltration, or phlebitis.

Blood transfusions

Whenever you administer blood or blood components — such as packed cells, plasma, platelets, or cryoprecipitates — use proper identification and crossmatching procedures.
- patient's name
- patient's medical record number
- patient's blood group or type
- patient's and donor's Rh factor
- crossmatch data
- blood bank identification number
- expiration date of the product

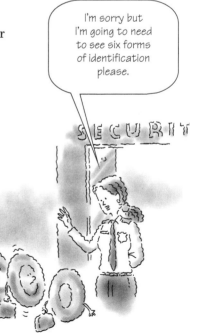

I'm sorry but I'm going to need to see six forms of identification please.

SECURIT

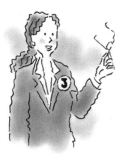

In addition, according to The Joint Commission's National Patient Safety Goals, the blood or blood component must be identified by two licensed health care professionals, both of whom sign the slip that comes with the blood and verify that the information is correct.

After you determine that the information on the blood bag label is correct, you may administer the transfusion. On the transfusion record, document:
- dates and times the transfusion was started and completed
- name of the health care professional who verified the information
- type and gauge of the I.V. catheter
- total amount of the transfusion and normal saline solution infused
- patient's vital signs before the transfusion, 15 minutes after the transfusion is started, and after the transfusion is completed, according to your facility's policy
- infusion device used, if any, and its flow rate
- blood warming unit used, if any
- patient's response to the transfusion.

Accounting for autotransfusions

If the patient receives his own blood, document the amount retrieved and reinfused in the intake and output records. Document laboratory tests during and after the autotransfusion, paying special attention to the coagulation profile, hematocrit, and arterial blood gas (ABG), hemoglobin, and calcium levels. Also chart the patient's pretransfusion, midtransfusion, and posttransfusion vital signs.

Reacting to a transfusion reaction

If the patient develops a transfusion reaction, stop the transfusion immediately, hang new tubing with normal saline solution running, and notify the doctor. On a transfusion reaction form or in the progress notes, document:
- time and date of the reaction
- type and amount of infused blood or blood products
- times you started and stopped the transfusion
- clinical signs in the order of occurrence
- patient's vital signs per facility protocol
- urine specimens and blood samples sent to the laboratory for analysis
- treatment you gave and the patient's response to it.

You may need to send the noninfused blood and tubing back to the blood bank. Follow your facility's policy. An example of a note documenting a reaction is shown on the next page.

1/16/09	1130	Pt reports nausea and chills. Transfusion started at 1030 hr. Cyanosis of the
		lips noted at 1100 hr with first unit of PRBCs transfusing. Stopped infusion.
		Approximately 100 ml infused. Tubing changed. I.V. of 1,000 ml NSS infusing at
		40 ml per hr in left hand. Dr. J. Dunn notified. BP 170/90; P 110; R 28; T
		99.4° F. Blood sample taken from PRBCs and sent to lab. Remaining blood
		discarded. Two red-top tubes of blood drawn from pt and sent to lab. Urine
		specimen obtained and sent to lab for UA. Pt given diphenhydramine 50 mg I.M.
		Two blankets placed on pt ———————————— Anne Grasso, RN
	1145	Pt reports he's getting warmer and less nauseated. BP 164/86; P 100;
		R 24; T 99.2° F. ———————————— Anne Grasso, RN
	1200	Pt without chills or nausea. I.V. 1,000 ml NSS infusing at 80 ml per hr in left
		hand. BP 156/82; P 92; R 22; T 98.9° F. ———————————— Anne Grasso, RN

Surgical incision care

When a patient returns from surgery, document his vital signs according to facility policy and level of consciousness (LOC) and carefully record information about his surgical incision, drains, and the care you provide. An example of a progress note documenting surgical incision care is shown below.

1/17/09	1030	Dressing removed from 4-cm right mastectomy incision; 1-cm sized area of serous
		sanguineous drainage on dressing. Incision well-approximated with staples intact.
		Site cleaned with sterile NSS. 4" x 4" sterile dressing applied. Teaching given
		to pt regarding dressing change and signs and symptoms of infection. See teach-
		ing flow sheet for more details. ———————————— Deborah Liu, RN

Records that get around

Study the records that travel with the patient from the post-anesthesia care unit. (See *Roaming records*, page 178.)

Who's up first?

Look for a doctor's order stating whether you or he will perform the first dressing change. If you'll be performing it, document:
• type of wound care performed (sterile or clean technique)
• wound's appearance (size, color, condition of margins, and presence of necrotic tissue); odor, if any; location of drains;

Advice from the experts

Roaming records

When your patient recovers from anesthesia, he'll be transferred from the postanesthesia care unit (PACU) to his assigned unit for ongoing recovery and care. As his nurse, you're responsible for the four-part document that travels with the patient. Make sure that the PACU report is complete by checking for the information below.

Part 1: History
This history section of the report should describe the patient's pertinent medical and surgical history, including drug allergies, medication history, chronic illnesses, significant surgical history, hospitalizations, and smoking history.

Part 2: Operation
This operation section describes the surgery itself and should include:
• the procedure performed
• the type and dosage of anesthetics
• how long the patient was anesthetized
• the patient's vital signs throughout surgery
• the volume of fluid lost and replaced
• drugs administered
• surgical complications
• tourniquet time
• drains, tubes, implants, or dressings used during surgery and removed or still in place.

Part 3: Postanesthesia period
The postanesthesia part of the record includes information about:
• pain medications and pain control devices the patient received and how he responded to them
• interventions that should continue on the unit, such as frequent circulatory, motor, and neuro-logic checks if the patient underwent leg surgery and had a tourniquet on for a long time
• a flow sheet showing the patient's postanesthesia recovery scores on arrival and discharge in the areas of activity level, respiration, circulation, and level of consciousness (LOC)
• unusual events or complications that occurred in the PACU; for example, nausea or vomiting, shivering, hypothermia, arrhythmias, central anticholinergic syndrome, sore throat, back or neck pain, corneal abrasion, tooth loss during intubation, swollen lips or tongue, pharyngeal or laryngeal abrasion, and postspinal headache.

Part 4: Current status
The current status section should describe the patient's status at the time of transfer back to the unit. Information should include his vital signs, LOC, sensorium, and the condition of the surgical site.

and drainage characteristics (type, color, consistency, and amount)
- condition of skin around drain or wound
- type and amount of dressing
- additional wound care procedures, such as drain management, irrigation, packing, or application of a topical medication
- how the patient tolerated the dressing change
- teaching provided to the patient (or family, if applicable).

Detailed care and discharge data

Document special or detailed wound care instructions and pain management measures on the nursing care plan. Also, chart the color and amount of measurable drainage on the intake and output form.

If the patient needs wound care after discharge, provide patient teaching and document it. Chart that you explained aseptic technique, described how to examine the wound for infection or other complications, demonstrated how to change the dressing, and gave written instructions for home care. Include the patient's understanding of the instructions, and chart if he can perform wound care measures or if further teaching is needed.

Pacemaker care

If the patient has a temporary pacemaker inserted, record:
- date and time of placement
- reason for placement
- pacemaker settings and type
- patient's response to the procedure
- patient's LOC and vital signs, including which arm you used to obtain the blood pressure reading
- complications, such as chest pain and signs of infection
- interventions such as X-rays to verify correct electrode placement
- medications that may have been given before or during the procedure.

Make sure that the rhythm strip includes the patient's name and the date and time of placement. An example of a progress note documenting pacemaker care is shown on the next page.

If the patient has a transcutaneous pacemaker, document the reason for this kind of pacing, the time pacing started, and the locations of the electrodes.

2/1/09	1315	Pt with temporary transvenous pacemaker in right subclavian vein. Heart rate
		60. Monitor showing 100% ventricular paced rhythm. ECG obtained. Pacemaker
		sensing and capturing correctly. Site without redness or swelling. Dressing dry
		and intact. ———————————————————————— Anne Salata, RN

Get a rhythm going

Document the information obtained from a 12-lead electrocardiogram (ECG). Put rhythm strips in the medical record before, during, and after pacemaker placement; any time pacemaker settings change; and any time the patient receives treatment for a pacemaker complication.

As ECG monitoring continues, record capture, sensing rate, intrinsic beats, and competition of paced and intrinsic rhythms.

Peritoneal dialysis

If your patient is receiving peritoneal dialysis, monitor and document his response to treatment during and after the procedure. Be sure to chart:
• patient's vital signs per facility protocol
• abrupt changes in the patient's condition and that you notified the doctor
• amount and type of dialysate infused and drained and medications added (Complete a dialysis flowchart every shift.)
• effluent's characteristics (color, clarity, and odor) and the assessed negative or positive fluid balance at the end of each infusion-dwell-drain cycle
• patient's daily weight (immediately after the drain phase) and abdominal girth when the treatment ends; note the time of day and variations in the weighing and measuring technique
• physical assessment findings
• fluid status
• equipment problems, such as kinked tubing or mechanical malfunction, and your interventions
• condition of the patient's skin at the dialysis catheter site
• patient's reports of unusual discomfort or pain and your interventions
• any break in aseptic technique and that you notified the doctor
• whether the patient or family member performs the peritoneal dialysis procedure.

An example of a progress note documenting peritoneal dialysis is shown at the top of the next page.

2/20/09	0300	Pt received peritoneal exchanges q2h of 1,500 ml 4.25 dialysate with 500
		units heparin and 2 mEq, KCl; infused over 15 min. Dwell time 15 min. Drain time
		30 min. Drainage clear, pale yellow fluid. Pt tolerated procedures without com-
		plications or discomfort. LLQ catheter site with no redness or drainage. Site
		cleaned and dressed per protocol. Pt weight after drain phase 205 lb.
		Abdominal girth 45 ½". ——————————————— Amanda Taylor, RN

Peritoneal lavage

For the patient recovering from peritoneal lavage, document:
• patient's vital signs and symptoms of shock, such as tachycardia, decreased blood pressure, diaphoresis, dyspnea, and vertigo
• condition of the incision site
• type and size of the peritoneal dialysis catheter used
• type and amount of solution instilled into the peritoneal cavity
• amount and color of the fluid withdrawn from the peritoneal cavity and whether it flowed freely in and out
• what specimens were obtained and sent to the laboratory for analysis
• complications that occurred and your interventions.

An example of a progress note documenting peritoneal lavage is shown below.

2/21/09	0400	#16 Fr. Foley catheter inserted without incident. NG tube inserted via right
		nostril to low intermittent suction. Placement confirmed with X-ray. Dr. T. Byrne
		inserted # 15 Fr. peritoneal catheter below umbilicus via trocar; 20 ml clear
		fluid withdrawn. 150 ml warm NSS instilled as ordered and clamped. Pt turned
		from side to side. NSS dwell time 10 min, then drained freely from abdomen. Fluid
		samples sent to lab as ordered. Peritoneal catheter removed and incision
		closed by Dr. T. Byrne. 4" x 4" gauze pad with povidone-iodine ointment applied
		to site. Pt tolerated procedure well and is in no distress. ——Lois Testa, RN

Thoracic drainage

If your patient has thoracic drainage, initially record:
• date and time the drainage began
• type of system used
• amount of suction applied (if any) to the pleural cavity

- presence or absence of bubbling or fluctuation in the water-seal chamber
- amount and type of drainage
- patient's respiratory status, including breath sounds.
    At the end of each shift, record:
- how frequently you inspected the drainage system
- presence or absence of bubbling or fluctuation in the water-seal chamber
- patient's respiratory status, including pulse oximetry readings
- condition of the chest dressings
- type, amount, and route of pain medication you gave
- complications and subsequent interventions and results.

The charting goes on and on

Ongoing documentation should include:

- amount of suction applied, if any
- color, consistency, and amount of thoracic drainage in the collection chamber as well as the time and date of each observation
- patient-teaching sessions and activities you taught the patient to perform, such as coughing and deep breathing exercises, sitting upright, and splinting the insertion site to minimize pain
- rate and quality of the patient's respirations and your auscultation findings
- complications, such as cyanosis, rapid or shallow breathing, crepitus, chest pain, or excessive bleeding, and the time and date you notified the doctor
- dressing changes and the patient's skin condition at the chest tube site.

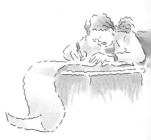

    An example of a progress note documenting thoracic drainage is shown below.

2/22/09	0100	Right anterior chest tube intact to 20 cm of H₂0 in Pleur-evac suction control
		chamber. 100 ml bright red bloody drainage noted in collection chamber since
		0300. No air leak noted. Positive water chamber fluctuation. Chest tube site
		dressing dry and intact; no crepitus palpated. Resp. assessment unchanged as
		per flow sheet. ———————————————— *Nancy Sigfried, RN*

Cardiac monitoring

For the patient receiving cardiac monitoring, include in your notes:

- date and time the monitoring began
- monitoring leads used

- rhythm strip readings every shift or with any rhythm change, labeled with the patient's name and room number and the date and time
- patient's response to rhythm changes.

An example of a progress note documenting cardiac monitoring is shown below.

2/24/09	1315	At 1245 monitor showing ST (HR 150s) with multifocal PVCs. Pt complaining of
		shortness of breath and palpitations. O₂ 2 L via nasal cannula placed. BP 178/96.
		ECG done. Dr. T. Corcoran notified and he administered Lopressor 5 mg I.V. at
		1250. Blood drawn for serum electrolytes and sent to lab. Monitor presently
		showing NSR with occasional multifocal PVCs. Pt denies shortness of breath,
		chest pain, or palpitations at present. ———————— Nancy Shwan, RN

Keep on chartin'

If the patient is to continue cardiac monitoring after discharge, document:

- which caregivers can interpret dangerous rhythms and perform cardiopulmonary resuscitation (CPR)
- patient and family teaching about monitor care, event recording, and equipment malfunction
- referrals to equipment suppliers, home health agencies, and other community resources.

Chest physiotherapy

Whenever you perform chest physiotherapy, document:

- date and time of your interventions
- patient's positions for secretion drainage and how long he remains in each
- chest segments you percussed or vibrated
- characteristics of the secretion expelled, including color, amount, odor, viscosity, and the presence of blood
- patient's tolerance of the chest physiotherapy
- breath sounds before and after treatment
- complications and your interventions.

An example of a progress note documenting chest physiotherapy is shown on the next page.

2/28/09	1130	Auscultated rhonchi in Ⓛ upper lobe. Pt placed on right side in Trendelenburg
		position. Chest physiotherapy and postural drainage performed for 10 min, from
		lower to middle then upper lobes as ordered. Productive cough produced large
		amount yellow tenacious sputum. Pt tolerated procedure without difficulty; lungs
		clear to auscultation. ————————————— Harry Moppert, RN

Mechanical ventilation

For patients receiving mechanical ventilation, initially chart:
• date and time the mechanical ventilation began
• type of ventilator used and its settings
• patient's responses to mechanical ventilation, including his vital signs, breath sounds, use of accessory muscles, secretions, intake and output, weight, and arterial oxygen saturation readings.

Take a deep breath — then chart!

Throughout mechanical ventilation, chart:
• complications and subsequent interventions
• pertinent laboratory data, including results of ABG analyses and oxygen saturation findings
• duration of spontaneous breathing and the ability to maintain the weaning schedule for patients receiving pressure support ventilation or those using a T-piece or tracheostomy collar
• rate of controlled breaths, the time of each breath rate reduction, and the rate of spontaneous respirations for patients receiving intermittent mandatory ventilation, with or without pressure support ventilation
• level of positive end-expiratory pressure or pressure support
• adjustments made in ventilator settings as a result of ABG levels
• adjustments of ventilator components, such as draining condensate into a collection trap and changing, cleaning, or discarding the tubing
• interventions to increase mobility, protect skin integrity, or enhance ventilation; for example, active or passive range-of-motion exercises, turning, or positioning the patient upright for lung expansion
• presence and characteristics of secretions
• type and frequency of oral care provided
• assessment findings related to LOC, peripheral circulation, urine output, decreased cardiac output, fluid volume excess, or dehydration
• patient's sleep and wake periods, noting significant trends
• patient and family teaching in preparation for the patient's discharge, especially that associated with ventilator care and set-

Don't forget to document the patient's responses to mechanical ventilation.

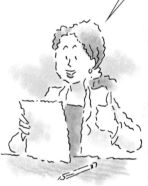

tings, artificial airway care, communication, nutrition, and therapeutic exercise
• teaching discussions and demonstrations related to signs and symptoms of infection and equipment functioning
• referrals to equipment vendors, home health agencies, and other community resources.

An example of a progress note documenting mechanical ventilation is shown below.

2/28/09	1100	ventilator wean started, placed 40% T-piece from 0930 to 1030. O₂ sat. remained above 90% during the entire weaning period (see flow sheet). Resp. assessment unchanged from flow sheet; pt in no distress at present. ———————————————————— John Devine, RN

Nasogastric tube insertion and removal

After you insert a nasogastric (NG) tube, record:
• type and size of the NG tube
• date, time, insertion route, and reason for insertion
• type and amount of suction
• amount, color, consistency, and odor of the drainage
• how the patient tolerated the insertion procedure
• signs and symptoms of complications, such as nausea, vomiting, and abdominal distention
• method of placement verification (for example, testing the pH of the gastric aspirate or X-ray)
• subsequent irrigation procedures and problems occurring afterward, if any.

Record information about irrigations on an input and output sheet. An example of a progress note documenting NG tube replacement is shown below.

1/30/09	2100	#12 Fr. NG tube placed in right nostril. Placement verified by X-ray and tube attached to low intermittent suction, as ordered. Drainage dark brown; heme positive. Dr. J. Cohen notified. Hypoactive bowel sounds in all four quadrants. Pt tolerated procedure well. ———————————————— Diane Harris, RN

The tube is removed — so chart some more!

After you remove an NG tube, record:
• date and time of removal
• how the patient tolerated the procedure
• unusual events accompanying tube removal, such as nausea, vomiting, abdominal distention, and food intolerance
• bowel sounds.

Seizure management

If your patient has a seizure while hospitalized, document:
• what seizure precautions you took
• date and time the seizure began and its duration
• precipitating factors, including auralike sensations reported by the patient
• involuntary behavior occurring before the seizure, such as lip smacking, chewing movements, or hand and eye movements
• incontinence, vomiting, or salivation during the seizure
• patient's vital signs (response to the seizure)
• what medications you gave, any complications, and your interventions
• your assessment of the patient's postseizure mental and physical status
• what and when you reported to the doctor.

An example of a progress note documenting seizure management is shown below.

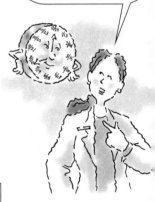

Document the date and time the patient's seizure began and its duration.

1/30/09	1615	At 1545 pt observed with generalized tonic-clonic seizure activity lasting 3
		min. Awake at time of onset and stated, "Here it comes!" Pt. had urinary
		incontinence during seizure. Siderail pads in place prior to seizure. Placed on
		left side, airway patent. Dr. G. Defabio notified of seizure. Diazepam 10 mg given
		I.V. as ordered. Pt sleeping at present. Vital signs stable (see graphic form).
		No further seizure activity noted. ———————— Barbara Chao, RN

Suture and staple removal

If the doctor writes an order for you to remove sutures or staples, document:
• date and time the sutures were removed and the patient's response
• appearance of the suture line

• appearance of the wound site, including the presence of purulent drainage
• if and when you notified the doctor
• if and when you collected a specimen and sent it to the laboratory for analysis.

Tube feedings

When documenting your care of a patient receiving tube feedings, write down:
• patient's tolerance of the feeding, including complications and your interventions
• assessment of bowel sounds
• kind of tube feeding the patient is receiving (such as duodenal or jejunal feedings or a continuous drip or bolus)
• amount, rate, route, and method of feeding (with continuous feedings, document the rate hourly)
• dilution strength if you need to dilute the formula (for example, half-strength or three-quarters strength)
• time you flushed the tube and the type and amount of solution used, if applicable
• time you replaced the tube and how the patient tolerated the procedure, if applicable
• amount of gastric residual, if applicable
• description of the patient's gastric function, including prescribed medications or treatments to relieve constipation or diarrhea
• urine and serum glucose, serum electrolyte, and blood urea nitrogen levels as well as serum osmolality values
• feeding complications, such as hyperglycemia, glycosuria, and diarrhea, and the time you notified the doctor
• patient and family teaching if the patient will continue receiving tube feedings after discharge
• referrals to suppliers or support agencies.

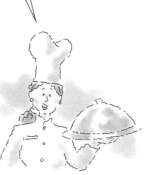

When giving tube feedings, be sure to document the patient's tolerance of the feeding formula.

Obtaining an arterial blood sample

When you obtain blood for ABG analysis, record:
• patient's vital signs and temperature
• arterial puncture site
• results of Allen's test
• indications of circulatory impairment, such as swelling, discoloration, pain, numbness, or tingling in the bandaged arm or leg, and bleeding at the puncture site
• time you drew the blood sample
• how long you applied pressure to the site to control bleeding
• type and amount of oxygen therapy that the patient was receiving (if applicable).

An example of a progress note documenting obtainment of an arterial blood sample is shown below.

1/31/09	0930	Blood drawn at 0800 from left radial artery after positive Allen's test, brisk
		capillary refill. Pressure applied to site for 5 min and pressure dressing
		applied. No swelling, bleeding, or hematoma noted. Hand pink and warm, with brisk
		capillary refill. Dr. G. Smith notified of ABG results; O₂ increased to 40%
		nonrebreather mask at 0845. Pt in no resp. distress. —Karen Andrews, RN

Need an ABG analysis? That's another form!

When filling out a laboratory request form for ABG analysis, include:
- patient's current temperature and respiratory rate
- his most recent hemoglobin level
- fraction of inspired oxygen and tidal volume if he's receiving mechanical ventilation.

Charting assisted procedures

When you assist a doctor during a procedure, you have the added responsibilities of providing patient support and teaching, evaluating the patient's response, and carefully documenting the procedure.

Procedures may change, but the charting remains the same

Regardless of the procedure, you must always document:
- date, time, and name of the procedure
- doctor who performed it and assistants who helped
- how it was performed
- how the patient tolerated it
- adverse reactions to the procedure, if any
- any teaching provided to the patient.

The section that follows describes documentation for several procedures during which you may assist the doctor.

Bone marrow aspiration

After assisting the doctor with bone marrow aspiration, document:
- date and time of the procedure
- name of the doctor performing the procedure

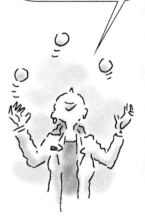

While assisting a doctor during a procedure, I have another important job to do — document the procedure. That's a lot of responsibilities to juggle!

- how the patient responded to the procedure
- location and appearance of the aspiration site, including bleeding and drainage
- patient's vital signs before and after the procedure
- teaching provided to the patient.

    An example of a progress note documenting assistance during bone marrow aspiration is shown below.

2/3/09	1015	Bone marrow aspiration explained to pt with questions answered. Refer to pt.
		education sheet for specific instruction and pt. responses. Bone marrow
		aspiration on left iliac crest performed by Dr. K. Wallace at 0945. No bleeding
		at site. Specimens sent to lab as ordered. Maintaining bed rest. Vital signs
		stable. Pt tolerated procedure well. Pt. denies any discomfort.
		—Pamela Clark, RN

Esophageal tube insertion and removal

After assisting with esophageal tube insertion or removal, document:
- date and time that you assisted in the insertion or removal
- name of the doctor who performed the procedure
- intragastric balloon pressure, amount of air injected into the gastric balloon port, amount of fluid used for gastric irrigation, and color, consistency, and amount of gastric return before and after lavage (if applicable)
- baseline intraesophageal balloon pressure, which varies with respirations and esophageal contractions
- patient's tolerance of the insertion and removal procedures
- patient's vital signs before, during, and after the procedure.

    An example of a progress note documenting esophageal tube insertion is shown below.

1/4/09	1320	Sengstaken-Blakemore tube placed by Dr. T. Weathers via left nostril. 50 cc air
		injected into gastric balloon, then 500 cc air injected into gastric balloon after
		abdominal X-ray confirmed placement. Tube secured to football helmet traction.
		Large amount of bright red blood drainage noted. Tube irrigated with 1,800 ml
		of iced NSS until clear. Esophageal balloon inflated to 30 mm Hg and clamped.
		Vital signs stable. Equal breath sounds bilat. Pt tolerated procedure well.
		Emotional support given. —James Carr, RN

Arterial line insertion and removal

When assisting a doctor who's inserting an arterial line, record:
- date and time
- doctor's name
- insertion site
- type, gauge, and length of the catheter
- patient's response to the procedure, including circulation status to the involved extremity.

An example of a progress note documenting insertion of an arterial line is shown below.

1/5/09	0820	20G 2½" arterial catheter placed in left radial artery and sutured in place by
		Dr. T. Watson after positive Allen's test. Transducer leveled and zeroed. Read-
		ings accurate to cuff pressures. Site without redness, swelling, or ecchymosis.
		Dressed per protocol. Line flushes easily. Arterial waveform visible on monitor.
		Hand warm and pink with brisk capillary refill. ————— Harry Nguen, RN

The arterial line's work may be done, but not yours...

After removing the arterial line, record:
- date and time
- doctor's name
- length of the catheter
- condition of the insertion site
- specimens that were obtained from the catheter for culture
- patient's response to the procedure
- amount of time pressure was held at site.

Central venous access device insertion and removal

When you help the doctor insert a central venous (CV) access device, you need to document:
- time and date of insertion
- doctor's name
- length and location of the access device
- solution infused
- patient's response to the procedure
- time that X-rays were done to confirm correct placement, the results, and when you notified the doctor of them. Also document if more than one attempt was made to insert the access device.

An example of a progress note documenting insertion of a CV access device is shown on the next page.

1/6/09	1030	Procedure explained to pt and consent obtained by Dr. E. Rafferty. Triple-lumen
		catheter placed by Dr. E. Rafferty on 2nd attempt in left subclavian. Catheter
		sutured in place and dressing applied as per protocol. All lines flushed with
		5 ml NSS. Portable chest X-ray obtained to confirm placement. Pt tolerated
		procedure well. Vital signs stable. ——————————— Eva Ryan, RN

Out with the access device, in with the documenting...

After assisting with removal of a CV access device, record:
- time and date of removal and the patient's response
- type of dressing applied
- condition of the insertion site
- catheter specimens you collected for culture or other analysis.

Lumbar puncture

During a lumbar puncture, observe the patient closely for signs of complications, such as a change in LOC, dizziness, or changes in vital signs. Report these to the doctor immediately and document them carefully.

Also document:
- color and clarity of the fluid obtained
- number of test tubes sent to the laboratory for analysis
- how the patient tolerated the procedure
- your interventions and care after the procedure, including keeping the patient in a supine position for 6 to 12 hours, encouraging fluid intake, and assessing for headache and leaking cerebrospinal fluid around the puncture site.

When documenting lumbar puncture, record how many test tubes were sent for analysis.

Paracentesis

When caring for a patient during and after paracentesis, document:
- date and time of the procedure
- puncture site
- whether the site was sutured
- amount, color, viscosity, and odor of the initially aspirated fluid (also, record this in the intake and output record).

With responsibility comes more charting

If you're responsible for ongoing patient care, document:
- running record of the patient's vital signs
- frequency of drainage checks per facility protocol

- patient's response to the paracentesis
- characteristics of the drainage, including color, amount, odor, and viscosity
- patient's daily weight and abdominal girth measurements (taken at about the same time every day)
- what fluid specimens were sent to the laboratory for analysis
- peritoneal fluid leakage, if any. (Be sure to notify the doctor and chart the time and date.)

An example of a progress note documenting paracentesis is shown below.

3/15/09	1300	Procedure explained to pt and consent obtained by Dr. T. Wolf. Dr. T. Wolf
		performed paracentesis in LLQ as per protocol. 1,800 ml of straw-colored fluid
		drained and sent to lab as ordered. Site sutured with two 3-0 silk sutures.
		Sterile 4" x 4" gauze pad applied. No leakage noted at site. Abdominal girth
		48" preprocedure and 45 ¼" postprocedure. Weight 210 lb preprocedure and
		205 lb postprocedure. Before the procedure, pt. stated "I'm afraid of this pro-
		cedure." Reinforced teaching as per teaching flow sheet and offered support.
		After procedure, pt. stated "that wasn't as bad as I thought it would be." ———
		——————————————————————— Owen Starr, RN

Thoracentesis

When assisting with thoracentesis, you need to document:
- date and time of the procedure
- name of the doctor who performed it
- amount and characteristics of fluid aspirated
- patient's response to the procedure
- if the patient had sudden or unusual pain, faintness, dizziness, or changes in vital signs and when you reported these problems to the doctor
- symptoms of pneumothorax, hemothorax, subcutaneous emphysema, or infection as well as when you reported them to the doctor along with your interventions
- when you sent a fluid specimen to the laboratory for analysis.

An example of a progress note documenting thoracentesis is shown at the top of the next page.

3/2/09	1100	Procedure explained to pt and consent obtained by Dr. F. McCall. Pt positioned
		over secured bedside table. RLL thoracentesis performed by Dr. F. McCall without
		incident. Sterile 4" x 4" gauze dressing applied to site; site without redness,
		edema, or drainage. 900 ml straw-colored fluid aspirated and specimens sent to
		lab as ordered. Vital signs stable. Lungs clear to auscultation. Patient reports
		pain at site as 1 on a 0-to-10 scale. ———————— Donna Taylor, RN

Charting miscellaneous procedures

Documentation isn't limited to procedures you perform or help the doctor perform. You'll also chart in other situations, including the ones described here.

Diagnostic tests

Before receiving a diagnosis, the patient usually undergoes testing, which can be as simple as a blood test or as complicated as magnetic resonance imaging. Record in the medical record all tests and how the patient tolerated them.

Chart your first impressions

Start your documentation by recording preliminary assessments you made of the patient's condition. For example, chart if she's pregnant or has allergies because these conditions might affect the way a test is performed or the test's result. If the patient's age, illness, or disability requires special preparation for a test, record this information as well.

Also chart what you taught the patient about the test and follow-up care, the administration or withholding of drugs and preparations, special diets, food or fluid restrictions, enemas, and specimen collection.

An example of a progress note documenting a diagnostic test is shown below.

> When charting a diagnostic test, begin by recording your preliminary assessment findings.

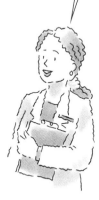

3/14/09	0600	24-hr test for urine protein started. Pt instructed on purpose of test and how
		to collect urine. Demonstrated correct technique. Sign placed on pt's door and
		in bathroom. Specimen containers placed on ice in bathroom. — Mary Brady, RN

Pain control

In your quest to eliminate or minimize your patient's pain, you may use a number of assessment tools to determine the degree of pain. When you use these tools, always document the results. (See *Chart pain three ways.*)

When charting pain levels and characteristics, determine whether the pain is internal, external, localized, or diffuse and whether it interferes with the patient's sleep or other activities of daily living. Describe the pain in the chart using the patient's own words.

Translating body language

Be aware of the patient's body language and behaviors associated with pain. Does he wince or grimace? Does he move or squirm in bed? What positions seem to relieve or worsen the pain? What other measures — such as heat, cold, massage, or drugs — relieve or heighten the pain? Also, note if the pain appears to worsen or improve when visitors are present. Document all of this information as well as your interventions and how the patient responded.

An example of a progress note documenting care for a patient with pain is shown below.

3/2/09	0800	Pt admitted with osteosarcoma and severe lower back pain. Pt. rates pain as 8
		on scale of 0-10. Has been taking ibuprofen 800 mg q, 6h at home without
		relief. Dr. S. Kobb notified. Morphine 2 mg ordered and given I.V. at 0715. vital
		signs stable. Pt states pain now a 2 on a 0-to-10 scale. ——Sarah Bane, RN

Intake and output

Many patients, including surgical and burn patients, those receiving I.V. therapy, and those with fluid and electrolyte imbalances, hemorrhage, or edema need 24-hour intake and output monitoring. To expedite documentation, you'll probably keep intake and output sheets at the bedside or by the bathroom door. If the patient is incontinent, document this as well as tube drainage and irrigation volumes.

Taking the intake charting challenge

Keeping track of foods and fluids that are premeasured is easy. You can list the volumes of specific containers for quick reference and use infusion devices to more accurately record enteral and I.V. intake.

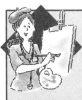

Art of the chart

Chart pain three ways

Some facilities use standardized questionnaires, such as the McGill-Melzack Pain Questionnaire or the Initial Pain Assessment Tool. Other facilities have devised their own pain measurement tools, such as the flow sheet and rating scales shown below. Whichever pain assessment tool you choose, remember to document its use and put the graphic form in your patient's chart.

Pain flow sheet

Flow sheets are convenient tools for pain assessment because they allow you to reevaluate the patient's pain at regular intervals. They're also useful when patients and families feel too overwhelmed to answer a long, detailed questionnaire.

Try to incorporate pain assessment into the flow sheet you're already using. The easier it is to use the flow sheet, the more likely you and your patient will be able to use it.

> Record the patient's pain rating before medication administration here.

> Record the patient's pain rating after medication administration here.

PAIN FLOW SHEET

Date and time	Pain rating (0 to 10)	Patient behaviors	Vital signs	Pain rating after intervention	Interventions
1/20/09 1100	7	Wincing, holding head	BP 186/88 HR 98- RR 22	5	Dilaudid 2 mg I.M. given
1/20/09 1200	3	Relaxing, reading	BP 160/80 HR 84 - RR 18	2	

Visual analog pain scale

In a visual analog pain scale, the patient marks a linear scale at the point that corresponds to his perceived degree of pain. The typical scale shown below uses the phrases "no pain" at one end and "pain as bad as it could be" at the other end.

VISUAL ANALOG SCALE

No pain ———————————————————✱——————————— Pain as bad as it could be

Graphic rating scales

Graphic rating scales are similar to visual analog scales, but they show more degrees of pain intensity. Have the patient mark the spot on the continuum that best describes his pain.

> The patient fills out these forms.

GRAPHIC RATING SCALE

No pain ——— Mild ——— Moderate ——— Severe ——— Pain as bad as it could be

Keeping track of intake that isn't premeasured is more difficult. For example, measuring and recording a food such as gelatin that's fluid at room temperature requires the cooperation of the patient and other caregivers. You'll also need to teach family members and friends to record or report to you all snacks and soft drinks they bring the patient and all meals they help him eat.

Don't forget these types of intake

Don't forget to document as intake I.V. piggyback infusions, drugs given by I.V. push, patient-controlled analgesics, and irrigation solutions that aren't withdrawn. Also, chart oral or I.V. fluids that the patient receives when he isn't on your unit. Doing so requires the cooperation of the patient and staff members in other departments. In addition, remind the ambulatory patient to use a urinal or commode.

Fluid loss through the GI tract is normally 100 ml or less daily. However, if the patient's stools become excessive or watery, you must document them as output. Vomiting, drainage from suction devices and wound drains, and bleeding are other measurable sources of fluid loss that require documentation.

> Keeping track of intake is a group effort! It requires the cooperation of the patient, his family and friends, and your colleagues.

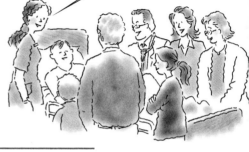

Transferring a patient to a specialty unit

If your patient's condition deteriorates and he requires transfer to a specialty unit, be sure to record:
• date and time of the transfer as well as the name of the unit receiving the patient
• that you received transfer orders
• patient's condition at the time of transfer, including his vital signs, descriptions of incisions and wounds, and locations of tubes or medical devices still in place as well as significant events during the hospital stay, noting whether the patient has advanced directives and special factors, such as allergies, a special diet, sensory deficits, and language or cultural issues
• medications, treatments, and teaching needs, noting which goals were and weren't met
• time that you gave a report to the receiving unit, including the name of the nurse who received the report
• how the patient was transported to the specialty unit along with who accompanied him
• any patient teaching related to the transfer such as the reason for transfer. (Some facilities use a transfer form to record this information.)

An example of a progress note documenting a patient transfer is shown on the next page.

3/24/09	1430	Pt is a 63 y.o. white English-speaking female with early Alzheimer's disease
		being transferred from medical unit to MICU by stretcher, accompanied by
		daughter and medical resident, Paul Reed. Report given to Sue Riff, RN. Advance
		directives in chart. Pt unresponsive to verbal stimuli, opens eyes to painful stim-
		uli. Prior to this episode, daughter reports pt. was alert and oriented to name
		but not always to place and time. Daughter states that pt's forgetfulness and
		confusion has recently gotten worse. Found alone in her apartment 2 days ago,
		unresponsive, no food eaten or dishes used since last groceries purchased for pt
		5 days ago. Pt is severely dehydrated despite 2,000 ml I.V. fluids given over
		last 24 hrs. Currently NPO. I.v. with #18 catheter in Ⓡ antecubital with
		0.45% NSS at 15 ml per hr. HR 124 irregular, BP 84/palp, R 28, rectal T
		100°F, weight 78 lb, height 64". Allergies to molds, pollen, and mildew. Lungs
		clear; normal heart sounds. Skin intact, pale and cool; poor skin turgor. Radial
		pulses weak; pedal pulses not palpable. Foley catheter in place draining approxi-
		mately 30 ml per hr. Dr's orders written. Medical record, MAR, and nursing
		Kardex transferred with pt. —————————————————— Diana Starr, RN

Termination of life support

According to the right-to-die laws of most states, a patient has the right to refuse extraordinary life-supporting measures if he has no hope of recovery. If the patient can't make the decision, the patient's next of kin is usually permitted to decide if life support should continue. A written statement of the patient's wishes is always preferable.

Advanced warning

Because of the Patient Self-Determination Act, each health care facility is required to ask the patient upon admission if he has an advance directive. An advance directive is a statement of the patient's wishes if he can't make decisions for himself. An advance directive may include a living will, which goes into effect when the patient can't make decisions for himself, as well as a durable power of attorney, which names a designated person to make these decisions when the patient can't. The act also states that the patient must receive written information concerning his right to make decisions about his medical care.

Match the patient's wishes to the situation

If life support is to be terminated, read the patient's advance directive to ensure that the present situation matches the patient's

> The Patient Self-Determination Act requires that the patient be asked upon admission if he has an advance directive.

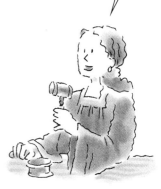

wishes and verify that the risk manager has reviewed the document. Check that the appropriate consent forms have been signed. Ask the family whether they would like to see the chaplain and if they would like to be with the patient before, during, and after life-support termination.

Charting directions for directives

If your patient has an advance directive, you need to record:
• if the patient's advance directive matches his present situation and life support wishes
• that your facility's risk manager has reviewed the advance directive
• that a consent form has been signed to terminate life support, according to facility policy
• the names of persons who were notified of the decision to terminate life support and their responses
• types of physical care for the patient before and after life-support termination
• whether the family was with the patient before, during, and after termination of life support as well as whether a chaplain was present
• time of termination, name of the doctor who turned off equipment, and names of people present
• patient's vital signs after extubation, the time the patient stopped breathing, the time he was pronounced dead, and who made the pronouncement
• family's response, your interventions for them, and after-care for the patient.

An example of a progress note documenting the terminating of life support is shown below.

2/02/09	1800	Advance directive provided by pt's wife. Document reviewed by risk manager, who verified that it matched the pt's present situation. Wife signed consent form to terminate life support. Wife spent approximately 10 min alone with pt before termination of life support. Declined to have anyone with her during this time. Mechanical ventilation terminated at 1730 by Dr. J. Brown, with myself, Chaplain Greene, and pt's wife present. VS after extubation: P 50, BP 50/20, no respiratory effort noted. Pronounced dead at 1731. Pt's wife tearful. Chaplain Greene and myself stayed with her, listening to her talk about her 35 years with her husband. Pt bathed and dressed in pajamas for family visitation. ———————————————————— Lucy Danios, RN

Charting CPR

A completed code record like the one below should be included in your patient's chart.

CODE RECORD

Pg. 1 of 1

Arrest Date: 1/9/09
Arrest Time: 0631
Rm/Location: 431-2
Discovered by:
C. Brown
☑ RN ☐ MD
☐ Other

Methods of alert:
☐ Witnessed, monitored: rhythm
☐ Witnessed, unmonitored
☑ Unwitnessed, unmonitored
☐ Unwitnessed, monitored; rhythm
Diagnosis: Post anterior wall MI

Condition when found:
☑ Unresponsive
☐ Apneic
☐ Pulseless
☐ Hemorrhage
☐ Seizure

Ventilation management:
Time: 0635
Method:
oral ET tube
Precordial thump:
CPR initiated at: 0631

Previous airway:
☐ ET tube
☐ Trach
☑ Natural

Addressograph

CPR PROGRESS NOTES

	VITAL SIGNS						I.V. PUSH		INFUSIONS	ACTIONS/PATIENT RESPONSE
Time	Pulse CPR	Resp. rate Spont; bag	Blood pressure	Rhythm	Defib (joules)		Atropine	Epinephrine	Amiodarone	Responses to therapy, procedures, labs drawn/results
0631	No pulse CPR	Bag	0	V fib	200					No change.
0632		Bag	0	V fib	300					No change
0633	No pulse CPR	Bag	0	Asystole	360			1 mg		No change
0635	40	Bag	60 palp	SB PVCs						Oral intubation by Dr. David Hart
0645	60	Bag	80/40	SB PVCs						ABGs drawn. @ fem pressure applied.

Time Spec Sent	ABGs & Lab Data						
	pH	PCO	Po₂	HCO₃⁻	Sat%	Fio₂	Other
0653	7.1	76	43	14	80%		

Resucitation outcome
☑ Successful ☑ Transferred to CCU at 0700
☐ Unsuccessful — Expired at
Pronounced by: _____ MD
Family notified by: S. Quinn, RN
Time: 0645
Attending notified by: S. Quinn, RN   Time 0645
Code Recorder S. Quinn, RN
Code Team Nurse B. Mullen, RN
Anesthesia Rep. J. Hanna, RN
Other Personnel Dr. Hart
B. Russo, RT
Signature Connie Brown, R N   Recorder

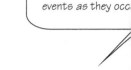

During CPR, a designated recorder should document events as they occur

Codes

Guidelines established by the American Heart Association direct you to keep a written, chronological account of a patient's condition throughout CPR. If you're the designated recorder, document therapeutic interventions and the patient's responses *as* they occur. Don't rely on your memory later.

Getting up to code

The form used to chart a code is the *code record*. It incorporates detailed information about your observations and interventions as well as drugs given to the patient. (See *Charting CPR*, page 199.)

A helpful critique

Some facilities use a *resuscitation critique* form to identify actual or potential problems with the resuscitation process. This form tracks personnel responses and response times as well as the availability of appropriate drugs and functioning equipment. Make sure that a copy of the completed critique form is submitted to the performance improvement department for analysis.

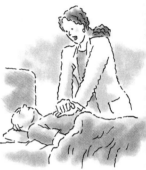

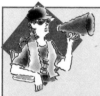

That's a wrap!

Charting procedures review

Charting nursing procedures
Include the following information when documenting nursing procedures:
• what procedure was performed
• when it was performed
• who performed it
• how it was performed
• how well the patient tolerated it
• adverse reactions to the procedure, if any.

Charting assisted procedures
Include the following information when documenting assisted procedures, such as bone marrow aspiration, esophageal tube insertion and removal, arterial line insertion and removal, central venous line insertion and removal, lumbar puncture, paracentesis, and thoracentesis:

• date, time, and name of the procedure
• doctor who performed it and the assistants who helped
• how it was performed
• how the patient tolerated it
• adverse reactions to the procedure, if any
• any teaching provided to the patient.

Charting miscellaneous procedures
• Document all diagnostic tests a patient receives and how they were tolerated.
• Use an assessment tool to determine the degree of pain your patient is experiencing.
• Document intake and output on an intake and output sheet, including enteral and I.V. intake, foods and fluids, and all output, including incontinence.

Charting procedures review *(continued)*

• Document transferring your patient to a specialty unit if his condition deteriorates.

• Document termination of life support if the patient refuses life support measures.

• Document codes using guidelines established by the American Heart Association. Use a code record, which allows you to keep a chronological account of a patient's condition throughout CPR.

Quick quiz

1. When using an MAR, you need to:
   A. use abbreviations that only people on your unit understand.
   B. squeeze in as much information as possible.
   C. record drugs immediately after you give them.
   D. record the patient's last name only.

   Answer: C. Recording a drug immediately after you give it prevents other nurses from inadvertently giving the drug again.

2. After you establish an I.V. route, document:
   A. each time you check the I.V. setup.
   B. the condition of the patient's veins.
   C. the number of venipuncture attempts if more than one is made.
   D. the number of I.V. start kits you used.

   Answer: C. Chart the number of attempts you made and the type of assistance required.

3. In charting about mechanical ventilation, include:
   A. only the ventilator adjustments you make.
   B. your assessment findings.
   C. only the patient's objective responses.
   D. family teaching only if the patient can't be taught.

   Answer: B. Document assessment findings related to peripheral circulation, urine output, decreased cardiac output, fluid volume excess, or dehydration.

4. When assisting a doctor with a procedure, document:
   A. only what you did.
   B. why you think the patient is having the procedure done.
   C. what you think the doctor should have done.
   D. the doctor's name and the patient's response.

Answer: D. Also, record the date and time of the procedure, pertinent information about the procedure, and your patient teaching.

5.   Before giving a blood transfusion:
    A.   ask another health care professional to identify and document the blood or blood component.
    B.   ask the patient if he'd rather receive his own blood.
    C.   try to figure out if he'll develop a reaction.
    D.   identify the patient by his last name only.

Answer: A. You also need to match the patient's name, medical record number, blood group or type, Rh factor (patient's and donor's), crossmatch data, and blood bank identification number with the label on the blood bag — and then document that you did so.

6.   Which of the following tools is used for documenting pain?
    A.   French scale
    B.   Graphic rating scale
    C.   Analogous graphic sheet
    D.   Thomas scale

Answer: B. The graphic rating scale allows the patient to chart his degree of pain on a linear scale.

Scoring

☆☆☆   If you answered all six questions correctly, gadzooks! You're able to complete tall stacks of medical records in a single round.

☆☆   If you answered four or five questions correctly, leaping lizards! You've performed your purpose: polishing off a plethora of paperwork.

☆   If you answered fewer than four questions correctly, don't worry! You can go back and review this chapter, take this book to work, and feel confident knowing you have a reference that makes charting incredibly easy.

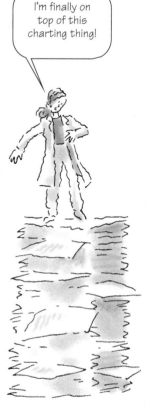

I'm finally on top of this charting thing!

Charting special situations

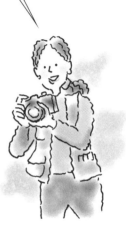

Just the facts

In this chapter, you'll learn:

♦ special situations related to patient rights and safety and the way a nurse should respond to them

♦ special situations that affect personal safety and the way a nurse should respond to them

♦ the proper way to document each of these special situations.

A look at special situations

Although proper charting is essential in all areas of health care, it plays a key role in protecting patient rights and ensuring patient safety in special situations. Thorough and objective documentation can also be effective in situations that affect the nurse's safety and well-being in the workplace.

> Don't take off that lens cap unless you have permission from the patient to take the photograph.

Situations related to patient rights and safety

Depending on your area of practice, you may need to:
• request permission to photograph a patient
• request permission for information to be released to the media
• search for contraband
• document instances of equipment tampering.

You'll need to document each of these special situations accordingly, while protecting patient rights and ensuring patient safety.

Photographing a patient

Photographs are commonly taken of child abuse, rape, or accident victims to document the severity of the injury and to serve as proof that the injury occurred. Occasionally, a doctor may want to document the severity or treatment of another type of injury, such as a wound, with photographs as well. Photographs provide important information about the progress of wound healing.

Get the old John Hancock

Most facilities require signed consent before taking photographs of the patient. It's the responsibility of the doctor or nursing personnel to obtain the patient's permission. (See *Permission to photograph.*) Keep in mind, however, that a health care facility has the right to refuse to take photographs, even if the patient has given permission, if the process interferes with delivering care to the patient.

Alas, you may bypass

Depending on the jurisdiction, permission to photograph may not be necessary in cases of suspected child abuse. For example, Section 2207 of the Pennsylvania statute concerning child abuse states that officials required to report cases of suspected child abuse may take photographs of visible trauma and obtain X-rays as needed. These photographs and X-rays must then be sent to child protective services along with a written report. When taking photographs of a suspected child abuse patient, make sure that the child's identity and the date are clearly visible.

Memento for those in mourning

In the case of a stillborn fetus of 16 weeks' gestation or older, photographs are taken as mementos for the bereaving parents. Permission is not required to take these photos. In many cases, the family is included in these photographs. Documentation involves noting on the fetus's chart that the photographs were taken. No other information is required. Photographs are provided to the parents at their request.

No signature required

Signed consent isn't required for photographs of personal or family situations that don't involve the health care facility. Examples include taking pictures of a new baby or a birthday celebration.

Permanent fixture

Photographs that do require permission to be taken become a permanent part of the patient's medical record. After signed consent is obtained, no further nursing documentation is required.

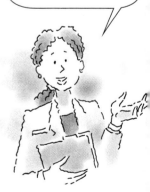

Photos relating to the patient's care become part of his medical record.

Permission to photograph

Depending on your facility's protocol, you may use a form similar to this one to obtain permission to photograph a patient.

Permission to photograph and release of photograph

Date _3/25/09_

I hereby give my permission for a photograph to be taken of _wound_

This photograph is being taken for the following purpose(s): _to monitor wound_ _healing progression_

I intend to be legally bound hereby.

Angela Steiner   Signed _Barry Arnold_
(Witness)

Address _771 Holly Drive_
Philadelphia, PA

If the patient is unable to sign or is a minor, complete the following:

Patient is a Minor who is _____ years of age and whose date of birth is
_____ , or the patient is unable to sign because:
(month, day, and year)

_____   _____
(Witness)   (Closest Relative or Guardian)

Releasing information to the media

Patient confidentiality continues to be a priority of health care workers and patients. When a patient seeks health care services, he trusts that the information shared with a health care provider will remain confidential. Those who come in contact with a patient in a health care setting have a legal and ethical obligation to maintain confidentiality and adhere to the guidelines of the Health Insurance Portability and Accountability Act. This obligation includes situations involving releasing information to the media.

Permission policy

Information regarding a patient's care or treatment—even if the patient is well-known—can't be disclosed without the patient's permission. Each health care facility has a policy for handling media requests for information. If permission to release information is granted, only people designated and trained to disclose information to the media are allowed to do so.

In the spotlight

If the situation involves a well-known patient (someone who is in the public eye or is newsworthy because of the nature of his condition), releasing information to the media on a regular basis may be in the patient's best interest. Without a formal statement, the media may distort the condition of the patient.

The doctor and the patient should agree on what information is included in the statement, thus ensuring an accurate release of information. This information is then released to the media by a designated facility spokesperson.

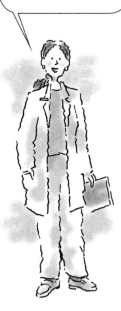

Releasing formal statements to the media about a patient's condition ensures that the information is accurate.

Documenting duties

Before a patient's information may be released to the media, the patient and the attending doctor must give their permission. This permission need not be written, but the permission is documented in the patient's chart. If the attending doctor's name is also to be released, the doctor's permission to do so must also be documented in the patient's chart.

Documentation in the nurses' notes should reflect consent from the patient and doctor to release information to the media. If the nurse assists the facility spokesperson in obtaining information or consent, this should also be documented in the nurses' notes. Remember to include the date, time, and name of the facility spokesperson in the note. (See *Permission to release information to the media.*)

For the (public) record

Information is releasable without the patient's consent if the case is on public record or if the case is reportable to civil authorities, as in police or coroner cases and situations involving accidents, fires, or disasters. Generally, patients involved in these situations are treated in the emergency department. Information released to the media would include the condition of the patient and whether

> **Art of the chart**
>
> ## Permission to release information to the media
>
> This example illustrates how to document whether a patient has given permission to release information to the media.
>
> | | | |
> |---|---|---|
> | 4/1/09 | 1300 | Pt. granted permission to Dr. W. Jones, attending physician, and Anita Robinson, public relations, to release a statement |
> | | | to the media regarding her condition. States, "All inquiries and/or calls are to be handled by Anita Robinson and her |
> | | | staff." Assured pt. her wishes would be honored and respected. ————————— J. Brown, RN |
> | 4/1/09 | 1315 | Dr. W. Jones placed order in chart reflecting his permission for Anita Robinson, public relations, to release his name to |
> | | | the media. ————————————————————— J. Brown, RN |

the patient was treated and released or transferred to another facility.

Terms used to describe a patient's condition under these circumstances include:

- good — patient is stable; indicators are excellent
- fair — patient is stable; indicators are favorable
- serious — patient may be unstable; indicators are questionable
- critical — patient is unstable; indicators are unfavorable.

Dealing with death

If a death occurs, the facility may release that information to the media after the patient's family and next of kin have been notified. The cause of death may be released with permission from the attending doctor. If the death is suspicious in nature, all inquires must be forwarded to the appropriate coroner. (See *Nonreleasable patient information.*)

Searching for contraband

Contraband is defined as any item that's prohibited from being in the patient's possession while he's in the facility. Examples include:

- controlled substances
- drug paraphernalia
- alcohol
- weapons (such as firearms, knives, explosive agents, or chemical agents).

Nonreleasable patient information

Patient information regarding these topics isn't releasable to the media even with consent from the patient:
- personal health information
- drug or alcohol intoxication
- circumstances surrounding a possible poisoning
- rape
- suicide or attempted suicide
- child abuse
- communicable or rare diseases
- abortions
- death that occurred during surgery.

Probable cause?

Searching a patient's possessions for contraband is appropriate only when there's clear evidence that a patient may possess a substance or object that may harm the patient or others. If you suspect that a patient has a dangerous substance or object, notify your nurse-manager and the security department immediately. You may be directed to ask the patient to disclose the possession of the contraband. If he doesn't disclose possession of the items, you need his permission to search his belongings.

Request denied

If a patient denies the request for a search, and you still suspect that the patient has dangerous contraband, notify the proper authorities so they can evaluate whether a search is necessary. This usually includes the attending doctor, the risk management officer, and an administrator of the health care facility. (See *Searching without permission.*)

> Don't request to search a patient's possessions unless you have clear evidence of contraband.

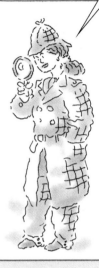

Art of the chart

Searching without permission

The notes below document a search conducted without the patient's permission.

5/1/09	1100	Cheryl Johnson, NP, reported seeing the pt. with a gun.
		Pt. refusing to allow staff or security officer to search belongings. Pt. states, "It's none of your business what I have.
		My stuff is my stuff." —————————————————————————————— K. Owens, RN
5/1/09	1110	Paula Lang, risk manager, and Robert O'Brien, administrator, notified of refusal to search belongings. —————
		—— K. Owens, RN
5/1/09	1130	Lang and O'Brien discussed personal safety concerns of all patients and staff. Initiated search of belongings without
		pt.'s permission. Retrieved black gun approximately 6" long placed in between folded pajamas. Pt. states, "It's none of
		your business. I always have a gun to protect myself." ——————————————————— K. Owens, RN
5/1/09	1140	Tom Jones, security, reported to room. Jones advised of need to turn over loaded gun. Gun disarmed by Jones and
		placed in hospital safe until discharge. ————————————————————————— K. Owens, RN
5/1/09	1200	Lang, Risk, and O'Brien reinforced hospital policy on firearms. Pt. stated, "Now I feel very unsafe since you took my
		gun." Safety and protection standards reviewed. —————————————————————— K. Owens, RN

Can I have a witness?

If a search is required, request to have someone present to witness the search and follow your facility's policy for searching for contraband. (See *Contraband search.*)

Search basics

Here are some guidelines to consider when searching for contraband:

• Searches should take place in a private setting if possible.
• A nurse should be present during the search.
• The persons conducting the search should be of the same gender as the patient.
• Safety of the person performing the search should be considered. For example, a pen or pencil should be used to sort through clothing to make sure no sharp objects are present.
• Unless an item poses a threat to the safety or well-being of the patient or staff, outside law enforcement agencies don't need to be contacted.

Take note

When documenting a search, include these items in the patient's record:

• identity of staff members present during the search
• reason for search

Art of the chart

Contraband search

Here's an example of how to document a situation requiring a search for contraband.

3/14/09	1800	Pt. stated, "Why don't you come back later to watch fireworks in my room?" Explained that fireworks aren't allowed in
		the hospital. Requested giving the fireworks to the staff. Stated, "I'm just kidding." ————— B. Hadley, RN
3/14/09	1815	Sally Smith, nurse-manager, and Tom Jones, security in attendance, made aware to search his person and personal
		belongings. Advised that fireworks aren't permitted in the hospital and the safety of the patients and staff is of
		primary concern. ————— B. Hadley, RN
3/14/09	1845	Search concluded. No evidence of fireworks found. Hospital policy regarding fireworks reviewed. Pt. able to verbalize
		understanding and stated, "I'm sorry for any inconvenience." ————— B. Hadley, RN

- reason for suspicion of contraband
- the contraband's potential for causing harm to the patient or others
- all items recovered during the search.

Equipment tampering

At times, a patient may tamper with equipment or misuse supplies without understanding the consequences. For example, the patient may press keys on a pump or monitor, detach tubing, or play with equipment switches. If your patient misuses equipment, explain that such misuse can harm him. Tell him to call for the nurse if he feels the equipment isn't working properly or is causing him discomfort or if he has other concerns.

> Documentation for equipment tampering should include what the patient did and how you handled the situation.

Write on

When tampering occurs, document in the progress notes what you saw the patient do (or what he told you he did) and what you did about the situation. Most medical equipment, including I.V. pumps and feeding pumps, have lock-out capabilities, which prevent the patient from manipulating the machine. (See *Patient tampering.*)

Art of the chart

Patient tampering

The notes below document a situation in which a patient tampered with equipment.

1/1/09	0930	1,000 ml of D₅W at 60 ml per hr infusing via pump in Ⓡ hand ———————————————— K. Connor, RN
1/1/09	1020	I.V. fluids assessed at 1000; 840 ml left in bag. Pt. stated, "I flicked the switch because I didn't see anything
		happening. Then I pressed the green button and the arrow." BP 110/82, P 89, T 98.4° F. No signs of fluid
		overload. Breath sounds clear bilaterally. Instructed pt. not to touch the pump or I.V. Repositioned pump to limit
		access. Dr. J. Wilder notified at 1015. ———————————————— K. Connor, RN

Situations related to personal safety

In some cases, you'll need to document situations that affect your own safety and well-being in the workplace. Such situations include:
• hostile advances
• harassment and sexual harassment.

Hostile advances

When a patient makes a hostile advance, the nurse's responsibility is to prevent harm to the patient and others. The nurse must assess the emotional crisis, provide emergency treatment to avoid worsening of the patient's condition, and objectively document the situation.

Take action

A sudden change in the patient's personality or behavior is a warning sign that he may turn hostile. If a patient makes hostile advances, take these steps to intervene:
• Contain the patient in a safe environment. This may require assistance from staff members trained in treating patients in crisis.
• Follow facility guidelines for the use of restraints if necessary.
• Modify the environment. For example, place the patient in a private room, if possible, or decrease external stimulation.
• Designate a family member or staff member to provide one-to-one care of the patient. This means that the patient should be within eyesight and arm's length at all times. However, remain aware of the patient's right to privacy, especially during procedures and when the patient has to use the bathroom or a urinal, commode, or bedpan. The patient shouldn't be left alone during these times but should be protected from being exposed unnecessarily.
• Make frequent attempts to converse with the patient.
• Identify specific problem behaviors. Set limits and redirect problem behavior.
• Set goals and reinforce appropriate behaviors.
• Consider requesting a psychiatric consult.

The write stuff

Documentation should include a description of the patient's behavior and whether one-to-one observation is needed. Record only the facts, not opinions. Avoid labeling the patient. Be specific and

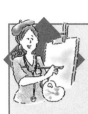

Art of the chart

One-to-one observation

This example illustrates correct documentation of one-to-one observation in response to hostile behavior.

1/2/09	0400	Pt. moving about in the bed, calling out loudly. Pt. attempted to get out of bed by himself. Unable to verbalize specific
		needs. Responds to verbal cues and touching of arm. ——————————————— M. Frank, RN
1/2/09	0415	One-to-one observation in place for safety and comfort. ——————————————— M. Frank, RN

objective in documentation. The need for ongoing one-to-one care should be documented each shift. (See *One-to-one observation*.)

Harassment and sexual harassment

Harassment is defined as verbal or physical conduct that denigrates or shows hostility or aversion toward another individual based on race, culture, color, religion, gender, sexual orientation, national origin, age, culture, or disability. Examples of harassing behaviors include:
• derogatory comments
• slurs
• negative stereotyping
• interference with an individual's normal work
• derogatory posters, cartoon drawings, or electronically submitted e-mails.

Sex in the facility

Sexual harassment is defined as offensive, unwelcome, or unwanted conduct of a sexual nature, which may include nonverbal, verbal, or physical behaviors. Examples of sexual harassment include:
• repeated sexually oriented teasing or jokes
• flirtations
• sexual advances or propositions
• commentary about an individual's body
• whistling
• touching, pinching, or brushing up against another's body
• displaying objects or pictures that are sexual in nature

• the explicit or implicit threat of sexual favors in return for continued employment or advancement in the workplace.

To be harassment free

Whether it originates from a patient, a doctor, another employee, an outside vendor, or a visitor, harassment in any form creates an intimidating and hostile work environment. Health care facilities have an obligation to provide an environment free from harassment, which is why documentation of such behavior is so important.

Sexual harassment and harassment from a patient can be disturbing to a nurse. Even if the offending patient is elderly or cognitively impaired, distrust can develop between the patient and the nurse. The key is to maintain a professional relationship with the patient. Providing quality patient care should be of utmost concern. This includes properly documenting the incident.

Focus on the facts

Documentation of the incident should include only the facts. Document the specific behavior of the patient. Don't include your perceptions, concerns, or thoughts regarding the patient's behavior. Additionally, don't include requests for reassignment in the patient's chart. (See *Inappropriate behavior*.) All incidents of sexual harassment involving patients should also be reported to the nurse-manager.

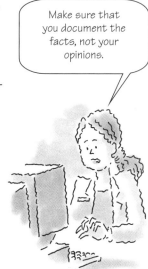

Make sure that you document the facts, not your opinions.

Art of the chart

Inappropriate behavior

This example illustrates how to document inappropriate behavior.

1/15/09	2100	Pt. pulled staff member onto bed and started kissing her. Discussed inappropriate behavior. Pt. unable to verbalize his understanding of conversation. ———————————————————————— L. Green, RN

That's a wrap!

Charting special situations review

Request to photograph a patient
• Photographs are commonly taken in cases involving accidents, child abuse, or rape.
• Signed consent must be obtained unless child abuse is suspected.
• Most states require photographs of suspected child abuse cases to be sent to child protection services along with a written report.
• The facility has the right to refuse permission for photographs if such actions interfere with delivery of patient care.

What to document
• Consent

Release of information to the media
• Anyone who comes in contact with a patient in a health care facility is obliged to maintain confidentiality.
• The patient and attending doctor must give permission for information to be released to the media.
• Information is releasable if the case is on the public record, a police or coroner case, or a situation involving an accident, fire, or disaster.

What to document
• Consent from the patient and doctor
• Whether the nurse assisted the facility spokesperson in obtaining information or consent
• Date, time, and name of the facility spokesperson

Searching for contraband
• Contraband is any item that's prohibited from being in a patient's possession, such as con-trolled substances, drug paraphernalia, alcohol, and weapons.
• If there's clear evidence of contraband, a search may be ordered.
• A nurse and a witness must be present during the search.
• The search must be performed by someone of the same gender as the patient.

What to document
• Staff members present at search
• Reason for search
• Reason for suspicion of contraband
• Contraband's potential for causing harm to the patient or others
• Items recovered during the search

Equipment tampering
• The patient misuses or tampers with equipment.

What to document
• What you saw the patient do (or what he told you he did)
• What you did about the situation

Hostile advances
• Safety of the patient and others is a priority.
• The patient must be contained in a safe environment.

What to document
• The behavior of the patient
• Whether one-to-one observation is needed
• The facts—not opinions, labels, or negative attitudes

Harassment and sexual harassment
• Harassment is verbal or physical conduct that denigrates or shows hostility or aversion toward another individual based on race,

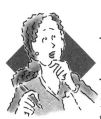

Quick quiz

1. When photographing a patient, what situation requires that
the documentation should go beyond the patient's chart?
  A. Rape
  B. Child abuse
  C. Research
  D. Accident

Answer: B. In most states, child abuse cases must be reported to
the authorities. Photographs and a written report should be sent
to child protective services.

2. When releasing information to the media about a patient's
status, the facility spokesperson describes his condition as seri-
ous, which means the patient is:
  A. stable with excellent indicators.
  B. stable with favorable indicators.
  C. unstable with questionable indicators.
  D. unstable with unfavorable indicators.

Answer: C. A patient whose condition is listed as serious is
unstable with questionable indicators.

3. What's the first intervention the nurse must perform when
confronted with a hostile patient?
  A. Call the nurse-manager.
  B. Call the doctor.
  C. Attempt to calm the patient.
  D. Contain the patient in a safe environment.

Answer: D. The first nursing priority is to contain the hostile
patient in a safe environment.

4. What information should be clearly documented in the patient's chart if a search for contraband is conducted?

    A.   Inventory of items recovered in search

    B.   Names of family members present

    C.   Patient's age

    D.   Reason for having the contraband

Answer: A. Documentation of a search for contraband should include an inventory of all items recovered during the search, the reason for the search, the reason contraband was suspected, and the staff members present during the search.

Scoring

☆☆☆ If you answered all four questions correctly, great work! You've probably been chart smart right from the start.

☆☆ If you answered three questions correctly, nice job! You're super savvy when it comes to special situations.

☆ If you answered fewer than three questions correctly, chin up. Document your trouble spots so you can review them later.

Part III Charting in health care settings

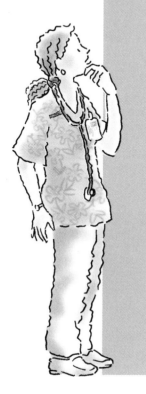

Acute care

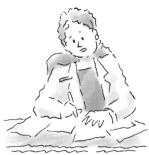

Just the facts

In this chapter, you'll learn:

♦ medical record forms used in acute care settings

♦ contents and organization of those forms

♦ advantages and disadvantages of each form

♦ more detailed information about critical pathways.

A look at acute care

Like many nurses working in acute care settings, you may feel discouraged — even overwhelmed — by the amount of information you have to document each day. You may also be baffled by some methods of documentation, such as computer charting, flow sheets, and critical pathways. Ironically, formats that are meant to save time for nurses may actually end up costing time. Nurses accustomed to writing long, handwritten notes may be uncomfortable taking advantage of shortcuts offered by newer methods, especially given today's litigious environment, in which documentation is strongly linked to liability. The result: Many nurses end up double documenting — for example, recording the information with a check mark on a flow sheet and then documenting it again in longhand in progress notes.

> I'd hate to have to document all this information twice. That's what can happen when nurses are uncomfortable with newer methods of charting.

Let familiarity (and this book) be your friend

To cope with the documentation chaos that characterizes contemporary nursing, your best weapon is familiarity with the various formats available, their advantages and disadvantages, and how you can use them to enhance your nursing practice.

Forms, forms, and more forms

The following forms — commonly used to create medical records in acute care settings — are explained in this chapter:

- admission database or admission assessment forms
- nursing care plans
- critical pathways
- patient care Kardexes
- graphic forms
- progress notes
- flow sheets
- discharge summary and patient discharge instruction forms.

Other forms include patient-teaching documents, dictated documentation, and patient self-documentation. Adapted or newly developed forms may also be used.

Yes, these forms *do* serve a purpose

A medical record with well-organized, completed forms serves three purposes:

It helps you communicate patient information to other members of the health care team.

It protects you and your employer legally by providing evidence of the nature and quality of care the patient received. (See *Didn't document, didn't do.*)

It's used by your facility to obtain accreditation and reimbursement for care.

In the long run, taking the time to carefully commit patient information to a standard, easy-to-use format frees you to spend more time on direct patient care.

Admission database form

The admission database form — also known as an *admission assessment* — is used to document your initial patient assessment. The scope of information documented at this stage is usually broad because you're establishing a comprehensive base of clinical information.

The clock is ticking

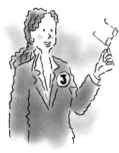

The Joint Commission requires that the admission assessment — including a health history and physical examination — be completed within 24 hours of admission; some facilities require a shorter time frame. To complete the admission database form, you must collect relevant information from various sources and analyze it. The finished form portrays a complete picture of the patient at admission.

Case in point

Didn't document, didn't do

In the case of *Pommier v. ABC Insurance Company* (1998), a 55-year-old patient with a fractured hip underwent surgery. During surgery, the patient was immobilized on the operating table. The operating room nurse noted that the patient was able to move her toes on both feet. The day after surgery, a nurse noted that the patient had good color, motion, and strength in both feet. However, while performing rounds, the doctor discovered that the patient had peroneal palsy in her left foot and leg. At the time of discharge, the patient was fitted with a left drop foot brace because of the condition.

The testimony

The patient and her family testified that immediately after the surgery the patient experienced significant pain in her left leg. The nurse's notes, however, didn't contain documentation of the patient's pain.

The verdict

Ultimately, the circulating nurse and other members of the surgical team were held responsible for failing to use proper padding during surgery and for failing to document the final position check of the patient. The nurse testified that it wasn't her usual practice to document all padding used during surgery and that she always used padding around the knee in such a surgery. However, given the inability to explain another reason for the injury, the nurse's failure to document the use of padding allowed for the jury to determine that proper padding wasn't used.

Finding form

The admission database form may be organized in different ways. Some facilities use a form organized by body system. Others use a format that groups information to reflect such principles of nursing practice as patient response patterns.

Get integrated! You'll be complimented for it

More and more facilities are using integrated admission database forms. On integrated admission database forms, nursing and medical assessments complement each other, reducing the need for repeated documentation. (See *Integrated admission database form*, pages 222 to 225.)

Charting with style

Regardless of how the form is organized, findings are documented in two basic styles:

standardized, open-ended style, which comes with preprinted headings and questions

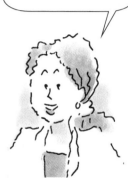

I feel like a million bucks! The wealth of information I gather during admission is invaluable.

(Text continues on page 226.)

Art of the chart

Integrated admission database form

Most health care facilities use a multidisciplinary admission form. The sample form below has spaces that can be filled in by the nurse, the doctor, and other health care providers.

Name _Beatrice Perry_
Address _2 Clayton Street_
Dallas, Texas 55532
Admission Date _2/21/09_ Time _1345_
Admitted per: ___ Ambulatory
_✓_ Stretcher ___ Wheelchair
T _97_ P _92_ R _24_ BP _98/52_
Ht. _5'2"_ Wt. _225 lb_
(estimated/actual)

ORIENTATION TO ROOM/UNIT POLICIES EXPLAINED
✓ Call light
✓ Bed oper.
✓ Phone
✓ Television
✓ Meals
___ Advance directive explained
___ Living will

___ Living will or
___ Valuables for
✓ Elec.
✓ Smoking
___ Side rails
✓ ID bracelet
___ Visiting hours

> Be time-efficient by asking technicians or nursing assistants to get some information, if your policy allows.

SECTION COMPLETED BY: _K. Crawford CCST_   **TIME:** _1350_

Name and phone numbers of two people to call if necessary:

NAME	RELATIONSHIP	PHONE #
Mary Ryan	daughter	665-2190
John Carr	son	665-4185

REASON FOR HOSPITALIZATION ___ (patient quote:) _I go numb in my (R) arm and leg_
ANTICIPATED DATE OF DISCHARGE: _3/2/09_
PREVIOUS HOSPITALIZATIONS: SURGERY/ILLNESS   DATE
TIA   _11/4/02_

HEALTH PROBLEM	Yes	No	?
Arthritis		✓	
Blood problem (anemia, sickle cell, clotting, bleeding)		✓	
Cancer		✓	
Diabetes	✓		
Eye problems (cataracts, glaucoma)		✓	
Heart problem		✓	
Liver problem		✓	
Hiatal hernia		✓	
High blood pressure	✓		
HIV/AIDS		✓	
Kidney problem		✓	
Comments: ___			

HEALTH PROBLEM	Yes	No	?
Lung problem (Emphysema) Asthma, Bronchitis, TB, Pneumonia, Shortness of breath)	✓		
Stroke		✓	
Ulcers		✓	
Thyroid problem		✓	
Psychological disorder		✓	
Alcohol abuse		✓	
Drug abuse			
Drug(s)___			
___		✓	
Smoking	✓		
Other ___			

ALLERGIES: ☐ TAPE ☐ IODINE ☐ LATEX ☐ no known allergies
☐ FOOD:___   ☑ DRUG: _Penicillin_ ___
☐ BLOOD REACTION:___   ☐ OTHER:___

MEDICATIONS: ___
HERBAL PREPARATIONS: ___

INFORMATION RECEIVED FROM: **SECTION COMPLETED BY:**
☑ Patient ☐ Relative___ ☐ Friend___ ☐ Other___   _N. O'Meara, RN_ Date _2/21/09_ Time _1405_

Integrated admission database form *(continued)*

All assessment sections are to be completed by a professional nurse.   Date 2/21/09

> This diagram allows you to map any impairment in skin integrity.

GENERAL PHYSICAL APPEARANCE

___✓___ Clean   _____ Disheveled

SKIN INTEGRITY: Indicate the location of any of the following on the chart to the right using the designated letter: a = rashes, b = lesions, c = significant bruises/abrasions, d = burns, e = pressure sores, f = recent scars, g = presence of tubes/appliances, h = other

Comments: _b: ischemic leg ulcer (2cm ~ healing)_

PRESSURE SORE POTENTIAL ASSESSMENT

PARAMETERS	0	1	2	3	Score
Mental status	(Alert)	Lethargic	Semicomatose	Comatose	0
			Count These Conditions As Double		
Activity	Ambulatory	(Needs help)	Chairfast	Bedfast	1
Mobility	Full	(Limited)	Very limited	Immobile	1
Incontinence	(None)	Occasional	Usually of urine	Total of urine and feces	0
Oral nutrition intake	Good	(Fair)	Poor	None	1
Oral fluid intake	(Good)	Fair	Poor	None	0
Predisposing diseases (diabetes, neuropathies, vascular disease, anemias)	Absent	Slight	Moderate	(Severe)	6
	Patients with scores of 10 or above should be considered at risk.			Total	9

FALL-RISK ASSESSMENT

Impaired: ____sensory function   ____general debility/weakness
            ____urinary/GI function   _✓_history of recent falls/dizziness/blackouts
            ____mobility function   (automatically designates patient as prone-to-fall)
            ____mental status   _✓_prone-to-fall risk (indicated on nursing Kardex___✓___)

NEUROLOGICAL

___Dizziness   ___Syncope   ___Headache   ___Blurred vision
___Recent seizure _✓_Numbness/tingling location: (R) arm and leg

CODE
Pupils: mm

LOC: _✓_Alert   ___Lethargic   ___Semicomatose   ___Comatose
Mental Status: _✓_Oriented   ___Confused   ___Disoriented
Speech: _✓_Clear   ___Slurred   ___Garbled   ___Aphasic

Extremities movement/strength
Pupil Reaction
 - Reactive
 - Nonreactive
D Dilated
C Constricted
> Greater than
< Less than
= Equal
= Sluggish

Neurological Checklist

Right Arm	Right Leg	Right Pupil	Pupil Reaction	Coma Scale				
Left Arm	Left Leg	Left Pupil		Eyes Open	Best Verbal Response	Best Motor Response	Total	
12/14	12/14	5/6	+	4	5	6	15	

COMA SCALE CODE	Response	1	2	3	4	5	6
	EYES OPEN	Never	To Pain	To Sound	Sponta- neously		
	VERBAL	None	Incompre- hensible Sounds	Inappro- priate words	Confused Conversa- tion	Oriented	
	MOTOR	None	Extension	Flexion Abnormal	Flexion Withdrawal	Localizes Pain	

+1:cannot move   +3:move against gravity
+2:cannot move against gravity   +4:move strongly against gravity

Comments: _numbness transient_   T. Jones, MD

BEHAVIORAL

Behavior: _✓_Cooperative   ___Uncooperative ___Depressed
           ___Restless   ___Other
           ___Combative   _✓_Anxious   ___Unresponsive

Comments: _____
Religious/Spiritual beliefs: _Lutheran_
P. request to contact minister/priest/rabbi? _✓_Y ___N
Name _Reverend Thomas Jones_ Phone # _559-4192_

PAIN

Pt. having pain at present? ___Y _✓_N
Pt. had pain in last several months? ___Y _✓_N
Rate pain on a scale of 0-10 (0 = no pain, 10 = severe pain) _____
Pain location_____ Quality_____

Radiation___Y ___N Duration_____
What aggravates pain?_____What alleviates pain?_____
Effects on ADLs_____
Pt. pain goals _____

> These circles will help you document pupil reaction accurately.

(continued)

Integrated admission database form *(continued)*

| Addressograph | Date _2/21/09_ |

CARDIOVASCULAR

Skin Color: ___Normal ___Flushed ___Pale ✓Cyanotic
Apical Pulse: ___Regular ✓Irregular ___Pacemaker: Type _____ Rate _____
Peripheral Pulses: ✓Present ___Equal ✓Weak ___Absent Comments: _bilat. weak lower extremities_
Specify: R____radial ___ pedal L ___radial ___pedal
Comments:_____
Edema: ___No ✓Yes _+l bilat. pretibial_ Numbness: ___No ✓Yes Site:___ _Rt. arm and leg_
Chest Pain: ✓No ___Yes   P_____ Q_____ R_____ S_____ T_____
Family Cardiac History: ___No ✓Yes Telemetry Monitor: ___No ✓Yes rhythm _normal sinus_
Comments:_____

PULMONARY

Respirations: ✓Regular ___Irregular ___Shortness of breath ___Dyspnea on exertion
O₂ use at home? ___Yes ✓No
Chest expansion: ✓Symmetrical ___Asymmetrical (explain: _____)
Breath sounds: ___Clear ___Crackles ___Rhonchi ✓Wheezing Location _bilat upper lobe, inspiratory_
Cough: None ✓Nonproductive ___Productive ___ Describe _____
Comments: _pulse oximetry 98% on 2 L; sleeps with 2 pillows_

GASTROINTESTINAL

Stool: ✓Formed   Diarrhea ___
___Loose   Constipation ___   Obese ✓   *NUTRITION:
___Liquid   Abdomen: thin ___   ✓Special Diet
___Mucus   ✓Soft   emaciated ___   _1800 ADA_
___Ostomy   ___Rigid   nourished ___   ___Tube feeding
___Incontinent   ✓Nontender   ___Chewing problem
Color: ✓Brown   ___Tender   ___Swallowing problems
___Black   ___(Location)   ___Nausea/vomiting
___Red tinged   Bowel Sounds ✓Present   ___Poor appetite
___Bloody   ___Absent   ___Wt. loss/gain ___ lb
___Hypoactive
___Hyperactive   *** Refer to dietitian if any ✓**

GENITOURINARY/ REPRODUCTIVE

Color of Urine: ✓Yellow ___Amber ___Pink/Red tinged ___Brown ___Orange ___Clear ___Cloudy
___Ileo-Conduit ___Incontinent ___Catheter in place ___Frequency ___Urgency
___Difficulty in initiating stream ___Pain ___Burning ___Oliguria ___Anuria
___Dialysis   Access site: _____   Date of last dialysis: _____
Comments:_____
Date of LMP _1977_ Date of last PAP _5/01_ Breast self-exam ___Yes ✓No
Use of contraceptives: ___Yes (type _____) ___No ✓N/A
    Vaginal Discharge: ___Yes (describe _____) ✓No
    Bleeding: ___Yes (amount _____) ✓No
Pregnancies: Pregnant ___Yes ___Weeks gravida _____ Para _____ ✓No
Date of last Prostate Exam _____ Testicular self-exam ___Yes ___No
Comments: _____

ACTIVITY/ MOBILITY PATTERNS

___Ambulates independently ___Full ROM ___Limited ROM (explain: _____)
✓Ambulates with assistance (explain:_____) ✓cane ___walker ___crutches
___Gait steady/unsteady ___Mobility in bed (ability to turn self) _____
Musculoskeletal ___Pain ___Weakness ___Contractures ___Joint swelling
___Paralysis ___Deformity ___Joint stiffness ___Cast ___Amputation
Describe: _____
Comments: _____

Note that the form contains room for additional comments.

REST/ SLEEP PATTERNS

___Use of sleeping aids _____ Sleeps _6_ hr/day
Comments:_____

Additional assessment comment: _On arrival, diaphoretic with hand tremors. vital signs stable. glucose 56 mg/dl._
Orange juice and lunch given to pt. 2 hr postprandial glucose 204. Symptoms subsided with juice. Nutritionist and diabetes
educator consulted _____ _N. O'Meara, R.N._
MRI shows no cerebral lesions. Carotid Doppler ultrasound pending. _____ _T. Jones, MD_

Integrated admission database form *(continued)*

> This final page deals with patient teaching and discharge planning.

EDUCATION/DISCHARGE SECTION
Instructions: Assessment sections must be completed within 8 hours of admission. Discharge planning and summary must be completed by day of discharge.

Addressograph

EDUCATIONAL ASSESSMENT

Yes	No	
✓		Patient understands current diagnosis
✓		Family/significant other understands diagnosis
✓		Patient able to read English
✓		Patient able to write English
✓		Patient able to communicate
	✓	Patient/family understands prehospital medication/treatment regimen

Yes	No	**Emotional Factors:**
✓		Patient appears to be cop~~i~~
✓		Family appears to be c~~o~~ing*
	✓	Any suspicion of fa~~m~~ly violence
	✓	Any suspicion of family abuse
	✓	Any suspicion of family neglect

Comment: _diabetes teaching_

Language spoken, written, and read (other than English): _____
Interpreter services needed: ✓No ___Yes
Are there any barriers to learning (e.g., emotional, physical, cognitive)? _No_
Religious or cultural practices that may alter care or teaching needs? ___Yes ✓No Describe: _____
Is pt/family motivated to learn? ✓Yes ___No describe: _____

> This assessment form is multidisciplinary. In this example, nurses and doctors provided information.

DISCHARGE ASSESSMENT

Living arrangements/caregiver (relationship): _lives alone_
Type of dwelling: ___Apartment ✓House ___ Nursing Home ___More than 1 floor? ✓Yes ___No Describe: _____
___Boarding Home ___Other _____
Physical barriers in home: ✓No ___Yes (explain: _____
Access to follow-up medical care: ✓Yes ___No (explain: _____
Ability to carry out ADL: ___Self-care ✓Partial assistance ___Total assistance
Needs help with: ✓Bathing ___Feeding ___Ambulation ___Other _____
Anticipated discharge destination: ___Home ___Rehab. ✓Nursing Home ___SNF ___Boarding H~~___~~
___Other _____
Currently receiving services from a community agency? ___ Yes ___No
If yes, check which one ___visiting nurses ___Meals on Wheels
Concerned about returning home? ___Being alone ___Financial problems ___Homemaking ___Meal prep.
___Managing ADLs ___Other _____
Assessment completed by: _N. O'Meara, RN_ Date _2/21/09_ Time _1430_
Assessment completed by: _T. Jones, MD_ Date _2/21/09_ Time _1445_

DISCHARGE PLANNING

Resources notified:	Name	Date	Time	Signature
Social worker				
Home care coordinator	M. Murphy, RN	2/28/09	0900	M. Murphy, RN
Other_____				

Equipment/Supplies needed: _stair chair_
Arranged for by: _M. Murphy, RN_ Date _2/28/09_ Time _0930_
Comment: _daughter to stay with pt at home_

DISCHARGE SUMMARY

Alterations in patterns: If yes, explain.	Yes	No	Explanation
Nutrition	✓		adherence to ADA diet regimen
Elimination		✓	
Self-care		✓	
Skin integrity		✓	
Mobility	✓		needs help with stairs
Comfort pain		✓	
Mental status/behavior		✓	
Vision/Hearing/Speech		✓	

Discharge instructions given (specify): _standard hosp. discharge instruction sheet_
Effects of illness on employment/lifestyle: _____
Central venous line removed: _N/A_ By whom: _____
Belongings sent with patient: ✓clothes ✓dentures ✓eyeglasses ___hearing aid ___prosthesis ___valuables
✓prescriptions ✓other _cane_
Follow-up medical supervision to be provided by: _Dr. W. Schran_
✓Patient/family instructed to call for follow-up appointment Discharge destination: _pt's home with daughter_
Section completed by: _C. Rafferty, RN_ Date _3/2/09_ Time _1215_

standardized, closed-ended style, which has preprinted headings, checklists, and questions with specific responses (you simply check off the appropriate response). Most facilities use a combination of styles in one form.

As you complete the admission database form, keep in mind that the information you chart is used by The Joint Commission, quality improvement groups, and other parties to continue accreditation, justify requests for reimbursement, and maintain or improve patient care standards.

Form and function

A carefully completed admission database form is extremely valuable. It contains physiologic, psychosocial, and cultural information that's useful throughout the patient's stay in your facility. It contains:
• baseline data that's used later for comparison with the patient's progress
• important information about the patient's current health status as well as clues about actual and potential health problems (for example, your admission assessment may turn up facts about prescription drugs, over-the-counter drugs, and herbal remedies the patient takes; possible drug and food allergies also may be revealed)
• insight into the patient's ability to comply with therapy and his expectations for treatments
• details about the patient's lifestyle, family relationships, and cultural influences. (During discharge planning, you'll need information about the patient's living arrangements, caregivers, resources, and support systems.)

How to use the admission database form

Conduct the patient interview and record the information on the admission form or progress notes as soon as possible, noting the date and time of the entry.

Acute illness, short hospital stays, and staff shortages can make it difficult to conduct a thorough and accurate initial interview. In some cases, you can ask the patient to complete a questionnaire about his past and present health status and use this to document his health history.

Ready, willing, and able?

Before completing the admission database form, consider the patient's ability and readiness to participate. For example, if he's sedated, confused, hostile, angry, or having pain or breathing problems, ask only the most essential questions. You can perform an in-depth interview later, when his condition improves.

Turning to friends and family

If the patient can't provide information, consider seeking help from friends or family members. Be sure to document your sources.

During your interview, try to alleviate as much of the patient's discomfort and anxiety as possible. Also, try to create a quiet, private environment for your talk.

If the patient is too ill to be interviewed and family members aren't available, base your initial assessment on your observations and physical examination. Be sure to document on the admission form why you couldn't obtain complete data and then obtain the rest of the information as soon as possible.

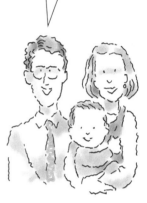

Don't forget that we can also be a source of information.

Potential problems

Admission database forms can present some difficulties. At times, through no fault of your own, you won't be able to complete some forms. The quality of recorded data depends in part on the ability of the patient or members of his family to provide accurate information.

Too many cooks...er, health care workers...can spoil the chart

Many other people will chart on the integrated admission database forms, increasing the risk of missing or incorrect information. You can't assume that colleagues collected the right information. You're responsible for verifying and correcting information gathered by nursing assistants and licensed practical nurses; likewise, the doctor is responsible for verifying information that you have collected. Remember, adding new information later may require you to revise the care plan accordingly.

Care plans and critical pathways

In acute care settings today, two different formats are being used to guide the process of care for a patient:

  traditional care plan

  critical pathway.

Stick with the traditional? Let's take a critical look...

Both formats offer important advantages and disadvantages. The traditional care plan, based on a nursing assessment and nursing diagnosis, provides a more precise account of the patient's individual nursing needs. The standardized critical pathway is a better tool for facilitating interdisciplinary communication and is perhaps more suited to the demands of the managed care environment.

Care plans

The full nursing care needs of any patient are unlikely to be documented on a critical pathway. For this reason, some acute care facilities are continuing to rely on the traditional format of a care plan as the chief mechanism for documenting each patient's nursing care. (See *Care plan requirements*.) (For more information on care plans, see chapter 3, Care plans.)

Critical pathways

Many acute care facilities are abandoning the traditional care plan in favor of a standardized critical pathway. Critical pathways are combinations of multidisciplinary care plans.

A time of transition

The changeover from plan to pathway has thrown nursing documentation into a transitional state. You may find yourself working in a facility that uses both formats. Many nurses aren't yet comfortable with critical pathways and are double-documenting — copying information from a pathway into a care plan.

Critical pathways are on the case

Critical pathways are used in health care facilities that employ case management systems for delivering care. In such a system, a registered nurse acting as case manager oversees a closely monitored and controlled system of multidisciplinary care.

Nurses, doctors, and other health care providers are responsible for establishing a care track, or case map, for each diagnosis-related group (DRG). A DRG is a way of classifying a patient according to his medical diagnosis for the purpose of obtaining reimbursement for hospital costs. The care track is used to determine a patient's daily care requirements and desired outcomes. The average length of stay for the patient's DRG is used in defining the care track. The case manager oversees achievement of outcomes, length of stay, and the use of equipment throughout the patient's illness.

Why take the pathway?

For acute care facilities, critical pathways work best with diagnoses that have fairly predictable outcomes — for example, hip

---

Care plan requirements

Although The Joint Commission no longer requires a specific care-planning format, it does require that this information be included in care plans in an acute care setting:
• ongoing assessments of the patient's illness and response to care, including patient needs, concerns, problems, capabilities, and limitations
• ongoing evaluation and modification of nursing diagnoses, interventions, and expected outcomes, based on identified patient needs and care priorities
• notation of nursing interventions, patient monitoring and surveillance, and patient responses
• reevaluation of patient progress compared with goals and the care plan
• documentation of the inability to meet patient care goals and the reason.

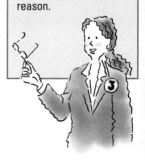

replacement, stroke, myocardial infarction, and open heart surgery. The pathway is a way to standardize and organize care for routine conditions. It makes it easier for the case manager to track data needed to streamline use of materials and human resources, ensure that patients receive quality care, improve coordination of care, and reduce the cost of care.

Health care facilities have a financial incentive to switch to critical pathway documentation. Well-developed critical pathways with demonstrated cost reductions may provide the facility with an advantage when negotiating contracts with managed care organizations.

Precautions along the pathway

Using a critical pathway doesn't eliminate the need for nurses to diagnose and treat human responses to health problems. Patients are individuals and commonly require nursing intervention beyond that specified in the critical pathway.

For example, a patient enters the hospital for a hip replacement and can't communicate verbally because of a previous stroke. The critical pathway wouldn't include measures to assist this patient in making his needs known. Therefore, you would develop a nursing care plan around the nursing diagnosis *Verbal communication impairment.* By using the critical pathway and developing a nursing care plan based on the patient's individual nursing diagnoses, you can provide the best in collaborative care. (For more information about critical pathways, see chapter 3, Care plans.)

Patient care Kardex

The patient care Kardex, sometimes called the *nursing Kardex,* gives a quick overview of basic patient care information. A Kardex can be computer-generated, or it may be a checklist on a large index card, on which the nurse can mark off items that apply to the patient. It also contains space for recording current orders for medications, patient care activities, treatments, and tests. (See *Considering the Kardex,* pages 230 and 231.)

A Kardex isn't a Joint Commission requirement. Some facilities have eliminated Kardexes, incorporating the information they contain into the patient's care plan.

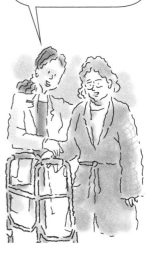

Critical pathways have their advantages, but you still must address your patient's individual needs.

(Text continues on page 232.)

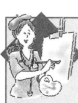

Art of the chart

Considering the Kardex

Here's an example of a patient care Kardex for a critical care unit. Remember that the categories, words, and phrases on a Kardex are brief and intended to trigger images of special circumstances, procedures, activities, or patient conditions.

Care status
Self-care ☐
Partial care with assistance ☐
Complete care ☑
Shower with assistance ☑
Tub ☐
Active exercises ☐
Passive exercises ☐

Special Care
Back care ☑
Mouth care ☑
Foot care ☐
Perineal care ☑
Catheter care ☐
Tracheostomy care ☐
Other (specify)_____ ☐

Condition
Satisfactory ☐
Fair ☐
Guarded ☑
Critical ☐
No code ☐
Advance directive?
  Yes ☑
  No ☐
Date___ 3/12/09

Prosthesis
Dentures
  upper ☑
  lower ☑
Contact lenses ☐
Glasses ☑
Hearing aid ☑
Other (specify)_____ ☐

Isolation
Strict ☐
Contact ☐
Airborne ☑
Neutropenic ☐
Droplet ☐
Other (specify)_____ ☐

Diet
Type: *low-fat, no conc. sweets*
Force fluids ☐
NPO ☐
Assist with feeding ☐
Isolation tray ☑
Calorie count ☐
Supplements_____

Tube feedings ☐
Type: _____
Rate: _____
Route: _____
  NG ☐
  G tube ☐
  J tube ☐

Admission
Height: *60"*
Weight: *145 lb (65.8 kg)*
BP: *124/72*
TPR: *100.4 T.P.O. - 92-24*

Frequency
BP: *q/hr*
TPR: *q/hr*
Apical pulses:
Peripheral pulses: *q/hr*
Weight:
Neuro check:
Monitor:
Strips:
Turn:
Cough: *q/hr*
Deep breathe: *q/hr*
Central venous
  pressure:
Other (specify)_____

GI tubes
Salem sump ☐
Levin tube ☐
Feeding tube ☐
Type (specify):_____
Other (specify):_____ ☐

Activity
Bed rest ☑
Chair t.i.d. ☐
Dangle ☐
Commode ☐
Commode with assist ☐
Ambulate ☐
BRP ☐
Fall-risk category (specify): ____ ☐
Other (specify):_____ ☐

Mode of transport
Wheelchair ☐
Stretcher ☑
With oxygen ☑

I.V. devices
Saline lock ☐
Peripheral I.V. ☐
Central venous access device ☐
Triple-lumen access device ☑
Hickman ☐
Jugular ☐
Peripherally inserted ☐
PICC ☐
Parenteral nutrition ☐
Irrigations:_____

Dressings
Type:
Change: *CVP*
    as needed

> The check marks are intended to alert you to important patient care considerations.

Considering the Kardex *(continued)*

> You can quickly find the information you need with this format.

...rapy
☐

Liters/minute _____
Method
- Nasal cannula ☐
- Face mask ☐
- Venturi (Venti) mask ☐
- Nonrebreather mask ☐
- Trach collar ☐
Nebulizer ☐
Chest PT ☐
Incentive spirometry ☐
T-piece ☐
Other (specify)_____ ☐

Drains
Type: _____
Number: _____
Location: _____

Urine Output
I&O ☑
Strain urine ☐
Indwelling catheter ☑
Date inserted _3/12/09_
Size: _16 Fr._
Intermittent catheter ☐
   Frequency: _____

Side rails
Constant ☐
PRN ☐
Nights ☐

Restraints
Date: _____
Type: _____

Specimens and tests
CBC daily
24-hour collection
Other (specify)_____

Stools

Special notes

Social services
consulted 3/12/09

Monitoring
Hardwire ☑
Telemetry ☐

Pulmonary artery catheter ☑
  Pulmonary artery
  pressure _q 1h_
  Pulmonary artery
  wedge pressure: _q 2h_
CVP _____
Arterial line ☐
Other (specify) _ICP_ ☑

Mechanical ventilation
Type: _____
Tidal volume: _700 ml_
FIO$_2$ _50%_
Mode: _AC_
Rate: _12_

> On an obstetrics unit, you might find additional information on the Kardex cover sheet.

Delivery
Date: _____
Time: _____
Type of delivery: _____

Special procedures
Perineal rinse ☐
Sitz bath ☐
Witch hazel compress ☐
Breast binders ☐
Ice ☐
Abdominal binders ☐
Other (specify)_____ ☐

Mother
Due date: _____
Gravida: _____
Para: _____
Rh: _____
Blood type: _____
Membranes ruptured: _____
Episiotomy ☐
Lacerations ☐
RhoGAM studies?
  Yes ☐
  No ☐
Rubella titer?
  Yes ☐
  No ☐

Infant
Male ☐
Female ☐
Full term ☐
Premature ☐
  Weeks ☐
Apgar score ☐
Nursing ☐
Formula ☐
Condition (specify): _____
Other (specify): _____

It's all in the Kardex

Refer to the Kardex during change-of-shift reports and throughout the day. The information it contains includes:
• patient's name, age, marital status, and religion
• medical diagnoses, listed by priority
• nursing diagnoses, listed by priority
• current doctors' orders for medication, treatments, diet, I.V. therapy, diagnostic tests, procedures, and other measures
• consultations
• results of diagnostic tests and procedures
• permitted activities, functional limitations, assistance that's needed, and safety precautions.

All shapes and sizes

Kardexes come in various shapes, sizes, and types and may be computer-generated. Some facilities use different Kardexes to document specific information, such as medication information, test results, and nonnursing data.

Computerized Kardex

Typically used to record laboratory or diagnostic test results and X-ray findings, a computerized Kardex usually includes information on medical orders, referrals, consultations, specimens (for culture and sensitivity tests or for blood glucose analysis, for example), vital signs, diet, and activity restrictions.

The Kardex can be all aces

The Kardex has some good points, including:
• It allows quick access to information about task-oriented interventions, such as specific patient care, medication administration, and I.V. therapy.
• The care plan may be added to the Kardex to provide all the necessary data for patient care, although this duplicates information.

A key Kardex kriticism

The Kardex has one major drawback: It's only as useful as nurses make it. It isn't an effective charting tool if there isn't enough space for appropriate information, if it isn't updated frequently, if it isn't completed, or if it isn't read before giving patient care.

In addition, Kardexes aren't usually part of the permanent record, so make sure that the information on the Kardex is also found elsewhere on the patient's chart.

Remember: The Kardex is only as useful as you make it!

How to use the Kardex

The Kardex is most effective when you tailor the information to the needs of a particular setting. For instance, an intensive care unit Kardex should include information on hardwire or telemetry monitoring and arterial pressure monitoring.

A Kardex a day keeps confusion away

Use the Kardex to record information that helps nurses plan daily interventions. For example, record the time a patient prefers to bathe, his food preferences before and during chemotherapy, and which analgesics or positions are usually required to ease pain.

The medication Kardex

If your facility uses a separate medication Kardex on acute care units, you'll find this document on the medication cart or other designated place. The medication Kardex may include the medication administration record (MAR), which lists medications, doses, and frequency and route of administration. Medication administration is documented on this form, which is a permanent part of the patient's record. (See *The medication Kardex*, pages 234 and 235.)

Getting the most out of your medication Kardex

When recording information on a medication Kardex, here are some tips:
- Include the date and administration time as well as the medication dose, route, and frequency. Don't forget to initial the entry.
- Indicate when you administer a stat dose of a medication and, if appropriate, the number of doses ordered and the stop date.
- Write legibly, using only standard abbreviations. When in doubt about how to abbreviate a term, spell it out. Remember, the MAR is a legal record, so any information entered there should be legible and above question.
- After giving the first dose of a medication, sign your full name, your licensure status, and your initials in the appropriate space.
- After withholding a medication dose, document which dose wasn't given (usually by circling the time it was scheduled). Also document the reason it was omitted—for example, withholding oral medications from a patient because he has surgery scheduled that day.

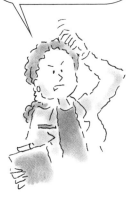

Now what does this say? I can't stress enough how important it is to write legibly!

How are things progressing? Need more space?

If you administer all medications according to the care plan, you don't need to document further. However, if your MAR doesn't

(Text continues on page 236.)

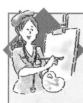

Art of the chart

The medication Kardex

One type of Kardex is the medication Kardex. It contains a permanent record of the patient's medications and may also include the patient's diagnosis and information about allergies and diet. A sample form is shown here.

NURSE'S FULL SIGNATURE, STATUS AND INITIALS

Nurse's signature	INIT.		INIT.		INIT.
Roy Charles, RN	RC				
Theresa Hopkins, RN	TH				

> Don't forget to sign your name.

DIAGNOSIS: *Heart failure, Atrial flutter*

ALLERGIES: *ASA*   **DIET:** *Cardiac*

ROUTINE/DAILY ORDERS/FINGERSTICKS/ INSULIN COVERAGE	DATE: 3/6/09	DATE:	DATE:	DATE:	DATE:	DATE:	DATE:	DATE:	DATE:	DATE:	DATE:

ORDER DATE INIT.	RE-NEWAL DATE INIT.	MEDICATIONS DOSE, ROUTE, FREQUENCY	TIME	SITE	INT.	SITE	INT.	SITE	INT.	SITE	INT.	SITE	INT.	SITE	INT.	SITE	INT.	SITE	INT.	SITE	INT.	SITE	INT.
3/6/09		*digoxin 0.125 mg*	0900	s.c.	RC																		
RC		*I.V. daily*	HR		72																		
3/6/09		*furosemide 40 mg*	0900	s.c.	RC																		
RC		*I.V. q/2h*	2100		TH																		
3/6/09		*enalaprilat*	0500	s.c.	TH																		
RC		*1.25 mg I.V. q/6h*	1100	s.c.	RC																		
			1100	s.c.	RC																		

> Initial in this column to verify that the dose, route, and frequency were checked against the doctor's orders.

The medication Kardex *(continued)*

PRN MEDICATION

ALLERGIES: ASA

Addressograph

INITIAL	SIGNATURE & STATUS	INITIAL	SIGNATURE & STATUS	INITIAL	SIGNATURE & STATUS	INITIAL	SIGNATURE & STATUS
RC	Roy Charles, RN						
TH	Theresa Hopkins, RN						

YEAR 20 _09_   P.R.N. MEDICATIONS

ORDER DATE: 3/6 RENEWAL DATE: / DISCONTINUED DATE: /	DATE	3/6						
MEDICATION: acetaminophen — DOSE 650 mg	TIME GIVEN	0930						
DIRECTION: p.r.n. mild pain — ROUTE: P.O.	DATA							
	INIT.	RC						
ORDER DATE: 3/6 RENEWAL DATE: 3/8 DISCONTINUED DATE: /	DATE	3/6						
MEDICATION: morphine sulphate — DOSE	TIME GIVEN	2 mg	0930					
DIRECTION: 15 minutes prior to changing (R) heel dressing — ROUTE: I.V.	DATA	(R)A						
	INIT.	RC						
ORDER DATE: 3/6 RENEWAL DATE: / DISCONTINUED DATE: /	DATE	3/6						
MEDICATION: Milk of Magnesia — DOSE 30ml	TIME GIVEN	2115						
DIRECTION: q.6h p.r.n. — ROUTE: P.O.	DATA							
	INIT.	TH						
ORDER DATE: 3/6 RENEWAL DATE: / DISCONTINUED DATE: /	DATE	3/6						
MEDICATION: prochlorperazine — DOSE 5 mg	TIME GIVEN	1100	2230					
DIRECTION: q.8h p.r.n. — ROUTE: I.M.	DATA	(R)glut.	(L)glut.					
prn nausea and vomiting	INIT.	RC	TH					
ORDER DATE: / RENEWAL DATE: / DISCONTINUED DATE: /	DATE							
MEDICATION: — DOSE	TIME GIVEN							
DIRECTION: — ROUTE:	DATA							
	INIT.							
ORDER DATE: / RENEWAL DATE: / DISCONTINUED DATE: /	DATE							
MEDICATION: — DOSE	TIME GIVEN							
DIRECTION: — ROUTE:	DATA							
	INIT.							
ORDER DATE: / RENEWAL DATE: / DISCONTINUED DATE: /	DATE							
MEDICATION: — DOSE	TIME GIVEN							
DIRECTION: — ROUTE:	DATA							
	INIT.							

I.M. sites must be charted.

have space for some information, such as the parenteral administration site, the patient's response to as-needed medications, or
deviations from the medication order, you'll need to record this

3/1/09	0900	Digoxin held per order of Dr. T. John because of pt's heart rate of 53. Digoxin level pending. ———————————————————— Dave Bevins, RN

information in the progress notes. For example, consider the
progress note shown above.

Graphic form

The graphic form is used to plot the patient's vital signs. Weight,
intake and output, appetite, and activity level also may be documented on the graphic form. (See *Plotting along: Using a graphic
form.*)

The graphic form usually has a column of data printed on the
left side of the page, times and dates written across the top, and
open blocks within the side and top borders.

Advantages — in graphic terms

The graphic form has two important advantages:
• It presents information at a glance, which allows more visual
comparison of data than is possible in narrative-style forms. For
example, if a patient's temperature goes up or down or fluctuates
over time, you can detect it much more readily on a graph than in
a narrative account of the patient's temperature.
• Unlicensed personnel, such as nursing assistants and technicians, are allowed to document measurements on graphic forms,
saving nurses valuable time.

Disadvantages — in graphic terms

Guess what? Graphic forms also have disadvantages:
• If data placed on the graph aren't accurate, legible, and complete, the form is useless. Every vital sign you take should be transcribed onto the form. For accuracy, double-check the graph after
transcribing information.
• If you use information from the graph alone, you won't get a
complete picture of the patient's clinical condition. You must combine the graph with narrative documentation.

Plotting along: Using a graphic form

Plotting information on a graphic form helps you visualize changes in your patient's temperature, blood pressure, heart rate, weight, and intake and output. Review the sample form below.

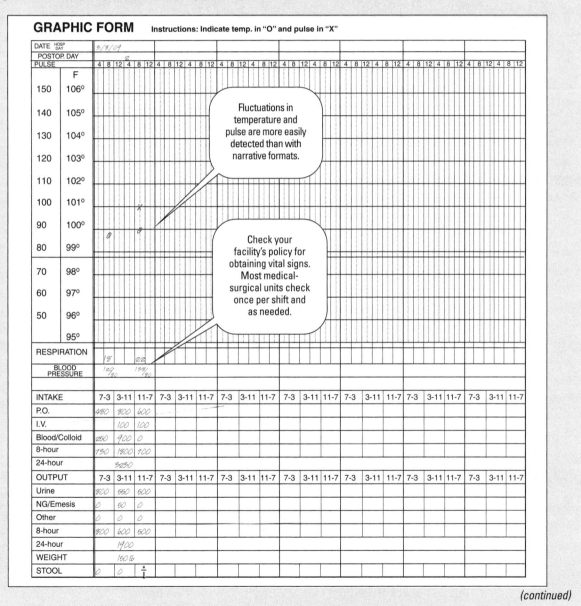

Plotting along: Using a graphic form (continued)

Additional space is usually provided for more frequently monitored vital signs.

DATE	TIME	BLOOD PRESSURE	PULSE	RESP.	MISCELLANEOUS
3/8/09	0800	130/80	96	20	T 99⁴ blood transfusion
3/8/09	0815	134/82	102	18	T 99⁸ no s/s of reaction
3/8/09	0830	128/84	91	16	T 99²

How to use a graphic form

To avoid transcription errors, document directly onto a graphic form when information is obtained.

A few more charting opportunities

If a medication (an antipyretic or antihypertensive, for example) precipitates a change in a particular vital sign, document this change in the progress notes as well as on the graphic form. Be specific about the relationship between the medication and its effect.

Make sure that you also document vital signs on the graphic form and the progress notes when a patient has an acute episode, such as chest pain or a seizure. Be sure to:
• chart legibly
• put data in the correct time line
• make the dots you plot on the graph large enough to be seen easily. (Connect the dots if your facility requires it.)

Progress notes and flow sheets

In the acute care setting, progress notes and flow sheets are used to record the patient's status and monitor changes in his condition.

Making progress with progress notes

Progress notes are written chronologically. The standard format for nursing progress notes has a column for the date and time and a column for detailed comments about:

> I love observing a patient's steady progress toward achieving outcomes!

- the patient's problems (the nursing diagnoses)
- the patient's needs
- pertinent nursing observations
- nursing reassessments and interventions
- the patient's responses to interventions
- evaluation of expected outcomes.

All members of the health care team can document integrated progress notes, which are in chronological order based on the date. (See *A group effort: Integrated progress notes.*)

Making good progress

Progress notes are helpful for the following reasons:
- They're written chronologically and reflect the nursing diagnoses.

Art of the chart

A group effort: Integrated progress notes

One key advantage of integrated progress notes: Every member of the health care team can document on them. Integrated progress notes are written in chronological order and dated, as in the sample below.

> Don't skip lines between entries.

INTEGRATED PROGRESS NOTES

3/8/09 0800 Nursing note	
Pt with temp. 102°F. Dr. R. Weber notified. No order at this time. ————————	—— P. Smith, RN
3/8/09 0830 MICU attending	
Pt continues to appear w/o change in status. Remains febrile and unresponsive. Will discuss code status with family.	
Prognosis poor. ———————————————————————————	—— R. Weber, MD
3/8/09 1030 Infectious disease attending	
Pt continues with fever of unknown origin. T max. 104°F. Acetaminophen ineffective. Cultures from 11/23 pending.	
Change all central line accesses and cond tips for culture. Continue vancomycin, gentamicin, and amikacin.	
Monitor trough levels and adj[...]ngly. Try to obtain HIV testing consent from family. Send	
fungal cultures. If positive fo[...]icin B. use test dose. Consult renal for worsening renal	
failure. ———————————————————————————————	—— J. Barry, MD
3/8/09 1545 Intern progress note	
HIV consent obtained. Labs to be drawn. ———————————————	—— J. Krimm, DO

> Make sure that you record the date and time.

• They contain narrative information that doesn't easily fit into the available space or format provided by other documentation forms.

Progress or pitfalls?

On the other hand, progress notes have these pitfalls:
• If they aren't well-organized, you may have to read through the entire form to find what you're looking for. To help prevent such a situation, some facilities require you to put a heading on each note.
• You may waste time recording information on progress notes that you have already recorded on other forms.

How to write progress notes

When writing progress notes, include the following information:
• date and time of the entry
• the patient's condition
• interventions
• the patient's response to care
• details of changes in the patient's condition
• evaluation of interventions.

A solid base of nursing diagnoses

Some progress notes are designed to focus on nursing diagnoses. If your facility uses this type of note, be sure to record the nursing diagnosis that relates to your entry. (See *Nursing diagnosis–based progress notes.*)

Set your watch

Every time you write a progress note, be sure to record the exact time you gave the care or noted the observation. Don't record entries in blocks of time such as 3:30 to 8:30. Years ago, when nurses were required to write progress notes every 2 hours, charting blocks of time was common. However, today, most nurses use a flow sheet to chart how often they check on a patient. Together, flow sheets and progress notes usually provide adequate evidence of nursing care.

Change in condition? Chart it.

Be sure to document new patient problems, such as onset of seizures, and the resolution of old problems such as no complaint of pain in 12 hours. Also, record deteriorations in the patient's condition—for example, *Pt has increasing dyspnea, causing him to remain on bed rest. ABG values show PaO_2 of 55. O_2 provided by rebreather mask as ordered.*

Art of the chart

Nursing diagnosis–based progress notes

Progress notes can be written using a nursing diagnosis, as the sample below shows.

Patient identification information
Robert Burns
131 Green Ave.
Tempe, AZ
(123) 666-7777

Memorial General, Tempe, AZ

Notes are directly related to the patient problem.

PROGRESS NOTES

Date and time	Nursing diagnosis and related problems	Notes
3/8/09 - 1100	Fluid volume, excess R/T chronic renal insufficiency	Bilat. +4 pretibial and pedal edema. #16 Fr. Foley with urimeter inserted to monitor hourly output. Furosemide 40 mg I.V. given at 1055. Head of bed elevated to 45 degrees; O₂ 2 L. Nasal cannula in place. ———————— P. Smith, RN
3/8/09 - 1130	Fluid volume, excess R/T chronic renal insufficiency	200 ml clear yellow urine in urimeter. Edema unchanged. Pt states: "It isn't as hard to catch my breath." ———————— P. Smith, RN

Document your observations of the patient's response to the care plan. If his behaviors are similar to agreed-upon objectives, document that the goals are being met. If not, document that they aren't being met.

Don't repeat yourself

Avoid including information that's already on the flow sheet, except when there's a sudden change in the patient's condition, such as a decreased level of consciousness, a change in skin condition, or swelling at an I.V. site.

Say what you did

Sometimes, nurses document a problem but fail to describe what they did about it. Outline your interventions clearly, including such information as notification of other health team members, interventions, and the patient's response. For example, *Patient*

Did I already document that? I have to remember not to repeat myself.

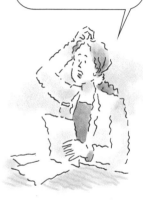

at 8 a.m. had oral temp of 102° F, Dr. P. Bard notified. Aceta-
minophen 650 mg given P.O. At 10 a.m. patient had oral temp.
of 100° F.

Avoid vague wording. Using a phrase like "appears to be" indicates uncertainty about what you're charting. Phrases like "no
problems" and "had a good day" are also ambiguous. Chart specific
observations instead. For example, *Patient reports his left hip*
has less pain, a 2 on a scale of 0 to 10. Yesterday it was a 5.

> Flow sheets
> are easy to prepare
> and easy to read!

Flow sheets

Flow sheets highlight specific patient information according to
preestablished parameters of nursing care. They have spaces for
recording dates, times, and specific interventions, which are set
by each facility.

Charting with a nice flow

Flow sheets are used to chart data related to physical assessment
of the patient and record routine aspects of patient care, such as
activities of daily living, fluid balance, nutrition, pain, and skin integrity. They're also useful for recording specific nursing interventions.

Many facilities also document I.V. therapy and patient education on flow sheets. The style and format of flow sheets may vary
to fit the needs of patients on particular units. Using flow sheets
doesn't exempt you from narrative charting to describe your observations, patient teaching, patient responses, detailed interventions, and unusual circumstances. (See *Let it flow.*)

Go flow sheets!

Flow sheets have many sterling qualities:
• You can insert nursing data quickly and concisely, preferably at
the time you give care or observe a change in the patient's condition.
• Because they provide an easy-to-read record of changes in the
patient's condition over time, flow sheets allow all members of the
health care team to compare data and assess the patient's
progress.
• The concise format enables you to evaluate patient trends at a
glance.
• They're less time-consuming to read because they tend to be
more legible than handwritten progress notes.
• The format reinforces standards of nursing care and facilitates
precise, less-fragmented nursing documentation.

Art of the chart

Let it flow

As this sample shows, a patient care flow sheet lets you quickly document routine interventions.

PATIENT CARE FLOW SHEET

> Be sure to initial your entry.

> Note the exact time.

Date: 3/8/09	2300-0700	0700-1500	1500-2300
RESPIRATORY			
Breath sounds	clear 2330 AS	Crackles LLL 0800 JM	clear 1600 HM
Treatments/Results		Nebulizer 0830 JM	
Cough/Results		Mod. amt. tenacious yellow mucus 0900 JM	
O₂ therapy	Nasal cannula at 2 L/min AS	Nasal cannula at 2 L/min JM	Nasal cannula at 2 L/min HM
CARDIAC			
Chest pain			
Heart sounds	Normal S₁ and S₂ AS	Normal S₁ and S₂ JM	S₂ HM
Telemetry	N/A	N/A	
PAIN			
Type and location	Ⓛ flank 0400 AS	Ⓛ flank 1000 JM	Ⓛ flank 1600 HM
Intervention	meperidine 0415 AS	reposition and meperidine 1010 JM	meperidine 1615 HM
Pt response	Improved from #9 to #3 in 1/2 hour AS	Improved from #8 to #2 in 1/2 hr JM	complete relief in 1 hr HM
NUTRITION			
Type		Regular JM	Regular HM
Toleration %		90% JM	80% HM
Supplement		1 can Ensure JM	
ELIMINATION			
Stool appearance			
Enema	N/A	N/A	N/A
Results			
Bowel sounds	present all quadrants 2330 AS	present all quadrants 0800 JM	hyperactive all quadrants 1600 HM
Urine appearance	clear amber 0400 AS	clear amber 1000 JM	Dark yellow 1500 HM
Indwelling urinary catheter	N/A	N/A	N/A
Catheter irrigations			

> Make sure that you document your patient's response to medications.

> Use the flow sheet to track changes in your patient's responses.

(continued)

Let it flow (continued)

PATIENT CARE FLOW SHEET

Date 3/8/09	2300-0700	0700-1500	1500-2300
TUBES			
Type	N/A	N/A	N/A
Irrigation	——————————	——————————	——————————
Drainage appearance	——————————	——————————	——————————
HYGIENE			
Self/partial/ complete	——————————	Partial 1000 JM	Partial 2100 HM
Oral care	——————————	1000 JM	2100 HM
Back care	0400 AF	1000 JM	2100 HM
Foot care	——————————	1000 JM	——————————
Remove/reapply elastic stockings	2330 AF	1000 JM	2100 HM
ACTIVITY			
Type	bed rest AF	Out of bed to chair x 20 min 1000 JM	Out of bed to chair x 20 min 1800 HM
Toleration	Turns self AF	T ol. well JM	Tol. well
Repositioned	2330 supine AF 0400 Ⓛ side AF	Ⓛ side 0800 JM Ⓡ side 1200 JM	self HM
ROM	——————————	1000 (active) JM 1400 (active) JM	1800 (active) HM 2200 (active) HM
SLEEP			
Sleeps well	0400 AF 0600 AF	N/A	N/A
Awake at intervals	2300 AF 0400 AF	——————————	——————————
Awake most of the time	——————————	——————————	——————————
SAFETY			
ID bracelet on	2330 AF 0200 AF	0800 JM 1200 JM 1500 JM	1600 HM 2100 HM
Call button in reach	2330 AF 0200 AF	0800 JM 1200 JM 1500 JM	1600 HM 2100 HM
Side rails up	2330 AF 0200 AF	0900 JM 1200 JM 1500 JM	1600 HM 2100 HM

Don't leave space blank. Write "none" or "N/A" or draw a line through the space.

Flow sheets encourage you to chart care promptly.

Flow sheet faults

Flow sheets also have some less-than-ideal qualities:
• They may not have enough space for recording unusual events.
• Overuse of these forms can lead to incomplete documentation that obscures the patient's clinical picture.
• They may cause legal hassles if they aren't consistent with the progress notes. What's checked off on the flow sheet needs to agree with what's documented on the progress notes.
• The format may fail to reflect the patients' needs as well as the nurses' documentation needs on each unit. Flow sheets can become a liability if they aren't tailored to each unit and revised as needed.

How to use flow sheets

Ideally, flow sheets are used to document all routine assessment data and nursing interventions. Some common examples of these are:
• repositioning or turning the patient
• range-of-motion exercises
• patient education
• wound care
• medication administration.

Charting routine assessment data this way allows you to focus on changes in the patient's condition, his complex needs, and his progress toward achieving expected outcomes.

Make sure that data on the flow sheet are consistent with data in your progress notes. Of course, all entries should accurately reflect the care given. Discrepancies can damage your credibility and increase your chance of liability. (See *Detail deficiency*, page 246.)

Completing the picture

Sometimes, recording only the information requested isn't enough to give a complete picture of the patient's health. In such a case, record additional information in the space provided on the flow sheet. If additional information isn't necessary, draw a line through the space to indicate this.

If your flow sheet doesn't have enough additional space and you need to record more information, use the progress notes. Write "see progress notes" in the space provided to indicate more in-depth data are elsewhere in the record.

Symbolic significance

Fill out flow sheets completely, using the specified symbols — such as check marks, "X"s, initials, circles, or the time — to indicate assessment of a parameter or performance of an intervention.

Case in point

Detail deficiency

Thomas v. Greenview Hospital, Inc. (2004) is an example of how a lack of specific documentation can lead to legal troubles.

Patient history
An elderly patient with various medical problems, including an amputated right leg and end-stage renal disease, underwent hemiarthroplasty and remained hospitalized to receive dialysis. After surgery, the patient was considered at risk for developing pressure ulcers. It was ordered that she be turned every 2 hours and as needed, which was consistent with the facility's written policies and procedures.

While in the facility, the patient developed a foul-smelling, stage III pressure ulcer that was approximately 6¾" × 5⅞" (17 cm × 15 cm). Although the patient ultimately died from chronic renal failure, the patient's family claimed that the patient developed the pressure ulcer as a direct result of the nursing staff's negligence and that such negligence lead to her death.

Let the record speak
There were no specific entries in the patient's chart documenting that she was turned at least every 2 hours. The nurses involved acknowledged that the chart lacked specific references to how often the patient was turned but maintained that the entries did state that safety rounds, which routinely included turning the patient, were performed every 2 hours.

The verdict
The court stated that even though there was evidence to suggest the nurses routinely turned patients as a part of their safety rounds, such evidence wasn't admissible to prove that they followed this practice when treating the patient.

When necessary, use the abbreviation "N/A" (not applicable) or another abbreviation recognized by your facility.

A ban on blanks

Don't leave blank spaces, which may imply that an intervention wasn't completed, wasn't attempted, or wasn't recognized. If you must omit something, document the reason for the omission.

Discharge summaries

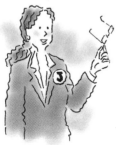

Discharge summaries reflect the reassessment and evaluation components of the nursing process. *To comply with The Joint Commission requirements, you must document your assessment of a patient's continuing care needs as well as any referrals for care and begin discharge planning early in the patient's stay.*

To help in this kind of documentation, many facilities combine discharge summaries and patient instructions in one form. This form contains sections for recording patient assessment, patient education, detailed special instructions, and the circumstances of discharge. It uses a narrative style along with open- and closed-ended styles. (See *Moving on: Discharge summaries.*)

Art of the chart

Moving on: Discharge summaries

By combining the patient's discharge summary with instructions for care after discharge, you can fulfill two requirements with a single form. When using this documentation method, be sure to give one copy to the patient and keep one for the record.

DISCHARGE INSTRUCTIONS

1. SUMMARY Tara Nicholas is a 55-year-old woman admitted with complaints of severe headache and hypertensive crisis.
Treatment: Apresoline I.V. drip for 24 hours
Started Lopressor for hypertension
Recommendation: Pt. to lose 10-15 lbs
Follow low-sodium, low-cholesterol diet

Have the patient or a family member read the medication instruction back to you.

2. ALLERGIES penicillin

3. MEDICATIONS (drug, dose time) Lopressor 25 mg orally at 6am and 6pm
temazepam 15 mg orally at 10pm

Write instructions clearly so the patient or family can easily understand them. This is the form they'll refer to when they're trying to remember your teaching.

4. DIET Low sodium, low cholesterol

5. ACTIVITY As tolerated

6. DISCHARGED TO Home

7. IF QUESTIONS ARISE, CONTACT DR. Pritchett   TELEPHONE NO. 555-1448

8. SPECIAL INSTRUCTIONS

9. RETURN VISIT DR. Pritchett   PLACE Health Care Clinic

ON DATE 3/15/09   TIME 8:45 am

Tara Nicholas
SIGNATURE OF PATIENT FOR RECEIPT
OF INSTRUCTIONS FROM DOCTORS

JE Pritchett MD
SIGNATURE OF DOCTOR GIVING
INSTRUCTIONS

In sum, discharge summaries are all good

We have only good things to say about discharge summary forms:
• The combined form provides useful data about additional teaching needs and points out whether the patient has the information he needs to care for himself or to get further help.

• The form establishes compliance with The Joint Commission requirements and helps safeguard you from malpractice accusations.

How to use discharge summaries

After completing your discharge summary form, give one copy to the patient and put another copy in the medical record for future reference. Make sure that the completed form outlines the patient's care, provides useful information for further teaching and evaluation, and documents that the patient has the information he needs to care for himself or to get further help.

Taking note of narrative discharge notes

Not all facilities use combined forms — some use narrative discharge notes. (See *Parting words: Narrative discharge notes.*) If your facility uses these notes, be sure to include the following information on the form:
• the patient's status at admission and discharge
• significant information about the patient's stay in the facility, including resolved and unresolved patient problems and referrals for continuing care
• instructions given to the patient, his family members, and other caregivers about medications, treatments, activity, diet, referrals, follow-up appointments, and other special instructions.

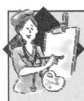

Art of the chart

Parting words: Narrative discharge notes

Some health care facilities use a narrative-style discharge summary, which is similar to a progress note. Here's a sample.

Date	Time	Progress notes
3/9/09	Discharge	68 y.o. black male admitted 3/6/09 with chest pain, hypertension; BP 190/100, and shortness of
	1530	breath. MI ruled out. Chest pain relieved with sublingual nitroglycerin and O₂. Persantine thallium performed
	(summary)	11/30. Tolerated procedure well. Has been ambulating in the hallway without chest pain or shortness of
		breath since 11/30. BP remains stable (144/86 at 1215). Drug regimen includes daily aspirin 325 mg,
		and Captopril 25 mg orally b.id. Verbalized understanding of medication times, dosages, and adverse effects.
		Will call Dr. T. Harris for 10-day postdischarge appointment. Discharge instruction sheet given.
		———————— B. McCort, RN

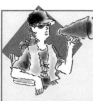

That's a wrap!

Acute care documentation review

Admission database form
- Documents patient's initial assessment
- Must be completed within 24 hours of admission
- May be integrated with nursing and medical assessments
- Contains physiologic, psychosocial, and cultural information that's used throughout hospitalization

Care plan
- Outlines the patient's nursing care
- Includes ongoing assessments, nursing diagnoses, expected outcomes, nursing interventions, and evaluation of care

Critical pathway
- Is a multidisciplinary care plan that helps standardize care for routine conditions
- Determines the patient's daily care requirements and desired outcomes

Patient care Kardex
- Gives a quick overview of basic patient care information
- Allows quick access to information about task-oriented interventions, such as specific patient care, medication administration, and I.V. therapy
- Isn't usually a part of the permanent record, so information must also be recorded in another part of the chart

Graphic form
- Is used to plot vital signs and other standard data
- Presents information at a glance
- Saves the nurse time because unlicensed personnel are allowed to record data on it

Progress notes
- Are used to record the patient's status and monitor his condition
- Reflect the nursing process in a format that's arranged chronologically, making it easy to follow

- Allow the nurse to record information that doesn't fit into other documentation forms

Flow sheets
- Are used to record the routine aspects of care as well as specific nursing interventions, allowing you to focus on changes in the patient's condition
- Highlight specific information according to preestablished parameters of nursing care
- Commonly used to document I.V. therapy and patient education

Discharge summary
- Reflects the reassessment and evaluation components of the nursing process
- Commonly combined with patient discharge instruction forms
- Provides useful data about additional teaching needs and the patient's ability to care for himself
- Establishes compliance with The Joint Commission requirements

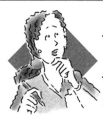

Quick quiz

1. An admission database is a:
   A. collection of computer information about your patient's psychosocial status.
   B. form that documents the initial patient assessment data.
   C. collection of data printed by a computer.
   D. form that documents ongoing physical assessments.

   Answer: B. It's also known as an *admission assessment form.*

2. In discharge planning, the staff nurse is responsible for:
   A.   initiating a referral for home health services.
   B.   evaluating the patient's mental status when his compe-
        tence is an issue.
   C.   deciding when the patient should be discharged.
   D.   making sure the patient's prescriptions are filled.

Answer: A. Initiating a referral for home health services is within the nurse's scope of practice.

3. A care track is an important part of a:
   A.   computer-generated Kardex.
   B.   critical pathway.
   C.   flow sheet.
   D.   graphic form.

Answer: B. The care track, or *case map*, defines a patient's daily care requirements and desired outcomes, consistent with the average length of stay for a specified DRG.

4. Progress notes are organized according to what order?
   A.   Alphabetical
   B.   Numerical
   C.   Chronological
   D.   No order

Answer: C. Progress notes chronologically record the patient's status and track changes in his condition.

5. Which of the following actions does The Joint Commission require nurses to do?
   A.   Begin discharge planning early in the patient's stay.
   B.   Use critical pathways.
   C.   Complete an admission assessment within 48 hours of
        admission.
   D.   Include a patient care Kardex in the medical record.

Answer: A. The Joint Commission requires that discharge planning begin early in the patient's stay.

Scoring

☆☆☆   If you answered all five questions correctly, amazing! You're destined to be acclaimed for accurate observation of acute care.

☆☆   If you answered four questions correctly, wonderful! Your progress is well noted.

☆   If you answered fewer than four questions correctly, don't worry! You can take the test as many times as you want and record your scores on a flow sheet.

Home health care

Just the facts

In this chapter, you'll learn:

♦ current and future trends in home health care

♦ risks and responsibilities in documenting home health care

♦ forms used for home health care documentation

♦ requirements for documenting patient teaching in home health care.

A look at home health care

The purpose of home health nursing is to restore, maintain, or promote health and function for patients and their families at home. A home health agency plans, coordinates, and supplies care based on the needs of the patient and family and the resources available to them. Think of the home health agency as a hospital without walls. Home care is one component of comprehensive health care.

An emerging health care powerhouse

Recent trends have contributed to the growth of the home health care industry, including:
• development of a prospective payment system (PPS) for home health agencies
• use of the Outcome and Assessment Information Set (OASIS), a tool used to help assess the patient's condition
• increasing number of patients of advanced age
• increased availability of sophisticated home care equipment
• use of electronic claim processing and surveillance of the Centers for Medicare and Medicaid Services (CMS) and fiscal intermediaries.

The Balanced Budget Act of 1997 required the development of a PPS for Medicare home health services and the implementation of this system in October 2000. Under this system, Medicare pays home health agencies a predetermined base payment. The payment is adjusted for the health care needs and conditions of the patient.

Quicker has equaled sicker

Managed care organizations have identified sophisticated methods of performing utilization review, causing a decrease in the average length of stay. Therefore, patients are typically sicker when they're discharged to home.

Because support services in the home and community cost less than institutional care, government and private insurance payers are expanding their coverage of home health care. In the future, the home health industry may become the primary supplier of health care in the United States.

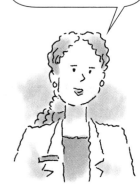

Home health services are expanding in part because they cost less than institutional care.

Not your traditional patient

Traditionally, homebound Medicare recipients have constituted the major portion of the home health caseload. Agencies have expanded services to new populations, representing all age-groups and a variety of medical conditions. This expansion has led to the emergence of home health subspecialties, such as home infusion agencies and high-tech cancer-related home care, including stem cell transplants. These agencies may be offshoots of parent organizations or stand-alone agencies. (See *The hospice alternative*.)

Documentation requirements

Although Medicare has tied reimbursement to the OASIS assessment, all patients older than age 18, excluding women receiving maternal-child services, must have an OASIS evaluation. OASIS regulations require that nurses complete an assessment and that agencies transmit the assessment and other data within strict time frames.

Patient assessment must be completed:
• within 5 days of the initiation of care and at 60 days and 120 days (if needed)
• when the patient is transferred to another agency
• when the patient is discharged from home care
• when there's a significant change in the patient's condition.

Creating opportunities for care

Before receiving care from a home health care agency, patients with private insurance must obtain authorization from their insurance providers. In many cases, insurance limitations restrict treatment options.

The hospice alternative

Many home health care agencies provide hospice care services. Hospice programs provide palliative care to terminally ill patients in both homes and hospitals.

Medicare coverage

Since 1983, patients who have met specific admission criteria can qualify for the hospice Medicare benefit instead of the traditional Medicare benefit, allowing greater freedom to choose the hospice alternative for terminal care. The patient receives noncurative medical and support service not otherwise covered by Medicare.

Medicare coverage for hospice care is available if:

• the patient is eligible for Medicare Part A, which covers skilled nursing home and hospital care; people eligible for Medicare include those who are age 65 or older, long-term disabled patients, and people with end-stage renal disease.

• the patient's doctor and the hospice medical director certify that the patient is terminally ill with a life expectancy of 6 months or less.

• the patient receives care from a Medicare-approved hospice program.

A Medicare-approved hospice program will usually provide care in the patient's home. The hospice team and the patient's doctor establish a care plan for medical and support services for the management of a terminal illness.

A patient without coverage for hospice benefits may be eligible for free or reduced-cost care through local programs or foundations. Alternatively, a patient may pay privately for hospice services.

Understanding and acceptance of treatment

With hospice care, the patient and primary caregiver must complete documentation, indicating their understanding of hospice care. The patient and caregiver must sign an informed consent form that outlines everyone's responsibilities. The patient and primary caregiver must also sign a form indicating understanding and acceptance of the role of the primary caregiver. The form below is an example of this type of document.

REEDSVILLE HOME HEALTH AND HOSPICE
ACCEPTANCE OF PRIMARY CAREGIVER ROLE

I have been offered the opportunity to ask questions regarding the Hospice program and Hospice care of this patient. I understand that the Hospice program provides palliative, or comfort, measures and services, but not aggressive, invasive, or life-sustaining procedures.

I also understand that the Hospice concept of care is based upon the active participation of a primary care person who is not provided through the Hospice benefit, who is and will be willing to assist this patient with personal care and with activities of daily living as well as with safety precautions when Hospice personnel are not scheduled to be in the home. I accept the responsibility of being primary caregiver, and I agree to make appropriate arrangements to provide this role to this patient.

If, for any reason, I am unable to serve in this capacity at a time as deemed necessary for the safety and care of this patient, I agree to make other arrangements to fulfill the responsibilities of primary caregiver that are acceptable to Reedsville Home Health and Hospice. I further understand that Reedsville Home Health and Hospice will assist in making the arrangements but that I will be financially responsible for any costs associated with them.

Name of patient: ___Joan Powell___
Signature of patient: ___Joan Powell___
Date: ___2/25/09___
Name of primary caregiver: ___Joseph Powell___
Date: ___2/25/09___
Signature of primary caregiver: ___Joseph Powell___
Relationship: ___husband___
Witness: ___Cathy Melvin, RN___
Date: ___2/25/09___

> When the patient and caregiver sign this form, it indicates that they understand the purpose and goals of hospice care and agree to comply with regulations for hospice eligibility.

In this cost-conscious environment, nurses take on an especially important role in helping patients get coverage by educating them about local, state, and federal benefit programs. When you help a patient identify a program for which he qualifies — such as veteran's benefits or Meals On Wheels — you help him get the services he needs while ensuring that your agency receives proper reimbursement.

Legal risks and responsibilities

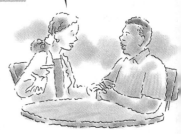

I'll help you find programs that augment your health coverage. That way, we both win.

Home health agencies are licensed and regulated by state governments and accredited by private agencies such as the Community Health Accreditation Program (CHAP), which is administered through the National League for Nursing (NLN) and The Joint Commission. In many cases, obtaining state licensure hinges on having accreditation. Home health agencies must also adhere to Medicare and Medicaid regulations administered by CMS and its agencies and carriers.

Meeting standards

Home health agencies are evaluated for such factors as accurate and complete documentation and adherence to standards, particularly establishing eligibility for services and quality of care. If standards aren't met, a home health agency may fail to earn licensure or accreditation, may have its current license and accreditation revoked, or may have reimbursement privileges withheld or revoked.

Risks of poor documentation

Home health agencies must maintain complete and legally sound documentation. For reimbursable services, nurses must document each instance that the specified service is provided. Nurses must also document the services the agency refuses to provide. Inadequate or incomplete documentation can have serious consequences.

Evaluating admissions

Since the inception of PPS for home health agencies, agencies have had to carefully evaluate admissions. Because of this evaluation process, not all patients who are referred for home health care qualify. If a patient has no caregiver or has a complex chronic medical condition, the cost of his care may quickly exceed the allotted reimbursement. Therefore, home health care agencies are unable to admit these patients.

Let's admit it: Admission assessment is crucial

A complete admission assessment and detailed documentation of this assessment are crucial in determining the appropriateness of each patient referred for admission.

Liability

After a nurse or home health agency is named in a lawsuit, it's too late to correct inaccurate documentation. For example, a nurse fails to record the patient's apical pulse and rhythm before administering digoxin. Later, the family sues the home health agency, alleging the staff caused the patient to go into complete heart block by failing to recognize signs of digoxin toxicity.

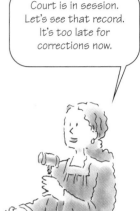

Court is in session. Let's see that record. It's too late for corrections now.

No record, no proof

Without a documented record, the agency is unable to prove that the patient wasn't experiencing excessive slowing of the pulse, a classic sign of digoxin toxicity.

Financial losses

Inadequate or incomplete documentation may result in refusal by third-party payers or fiscal intermediaries to cover services.

A bad business practice

Insurance companies who negotiate preferred provider contracts may refuse to do business with home health agencies that provide incomplete documentation.

Documentation guidelines

Documentation of care and discharge planning begins when you evaluate a new patient for service. (See *Does the patient qualify?* page 256.) You may use a referral form to document the patient's needs. (See *Referral form*, pages 257 and 258.) Patients and caregivers also fill out several forms during the initial home visit. (See *Paperwork for patients*, page 256.)

Be sure to begin at the beginning

When you start caring for a patient, always document activities completed during your nursing visit: assessments, interventions, the patient's response to treatment, and whether he had complications. Also, record your communications with other members of the health care team and the date of the next visit. Use your agency's flow sheets.

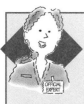

Advice from the experts

Does the patient qualify?

Careful screening, which is done at the initial evaluation, is critical when determining what clinical services a patient needs. When evaluating a new patient for service, look for the following criteria.

Clinical criteria
- Homebound status
- Skilled care needed; medically necessary
- Appropriately prescribed therapies that can be done in the home
- Ability to progress from therapies
- Caregiver available to assist patient

Technical criteria (patient or caregiver)
- Senses intact
- Ability to learn and follow procedures

- Ability to recognize complications and initiate emergency medical procedures

Environmental criteria
- Access to a telephone
- Access to electricity
- Access to water
- Clean living environment

Financial criteria
- Verification of insurance coverage
- Full knowledge of copayment or out-of-pocket expenses
- Agreement to comply with the conditions of participation

The information you provide gets around

The information you provide is used by third-party payers during utilization review to evaluate each claim in accordance with criteria for coverage. It may also be used by the government and oversight agencies to determine the validity of services.

Documentation details

Home care documentation should cover:
- OASIS
- evidence that the home environment is safe for the procedure or treatment or can be safely adapted; findings about the home and measures taken to ensure safe delivery of care
- rationale for treatment and patient response
- *emergency and resource numbers given to the patient or caregiver (The Joint Commission requires that the patient or caregiver have 24-hour emergency telephone access to the agency or nurse.)*
- patient's or caregiver's ability to perform steps in home care procedures, including the ability to perform return demonstration
- patient's or caregiver's ability to troubleshoot equipment, including a backup plan for a power failure

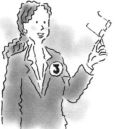

(Text continues on page 259.)

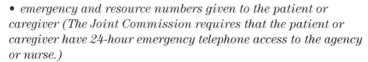

Paperwork for patients

During your initial home visit, you'll ask the patient or caregiver to read and sign many forms. These required forms include:
- patient rights and responsibilities
- advance directives, including a do-not-resuscitate option
- consent for services
- medical information authorization and release
- privacy statement
- assignment of benefits
- equipment acceptance
- medication reconciliation list
- patient-teaching checklist
- emergency preparedness plan.

If an I.V. infusion is required, the forms also include:
- consent for vascular access
- infusion treatment service agreement.

Feeling validated
In addition, your agency may require the patient to cosign the Outcome and Assessment Information Set form and the nurses' notes or a time sheet to validate your visit in the home.

Art of the chart

Referral form

Also called an intake form, a referral form is used to document the patient's needs when you begin your evaluation of a new patient. Use the form shown here as a guide.

Date of referral: _2/26/09_   Branch ⟨⟨This form provides an overview of the patient's condition, required treatment, and psychosocial and cultural concerns.⟩⟩ #: _91-413_   H ✔

Info taken by: _Beth Isham, RN_   _North_   date: _2/27/09_

Patient's name: _Geraldine Rush_

Address: _66 Newton St._

City: _Burlington_   State: _VT_   Zip: _05402_

Phone: _(802) 123-4561_   Date of birth: _4/3/25_

Primary caregiver name & phone number: _husband (Dennis) (802) 123-4561_

Insurance name: _Medicare_   Ins. #: _123-45-6189_

Is this a managed care policy (HMO)? _no_

Primary Dx: (Code _162.5_)   _lung cancer_   Date: _2/20/09_

(Code _877_)   _pressure ulcer (coccyx)_   Date: _2/22/09_

(Code _714.0_)   _rheumatoid arthritis_   Date: _1980_

Procedure: (Code _86.28_)   _pressure ulcer_   Date: _2/10/09_

Referral source: _J. Silva, hospital SW_   Phone: _165-2813_

Doctor name & phone #: _Frank Crabbe_   Phone: _165-4321_

Doctor address: _9073 Parkway Drive, Burlington_

Hospital _University Hospital_   Admit _2/10/09_   Discharge _2/25/09_

Functional limitations: Pain management, _nonambulatory, poor fine motor skills due to rheumatoid arthritis_

ORDERS/SERVICES: (specify amount, frequency, and duration)

⟨SN:⟩ _SN visits 3x/week & p.r.n. x 2 months_

⟨AL⟩ _CNA visits 4 hours daily 5 days/week x 2 months_

⟨PT, OT⟩ ST: _PT & OT evaluations and visits 2-3 x/week & p.r.n. x 2 months_   ⟨⟨Check out this part of the form to determine what services the patient needs.⟩⟩

⟨MSW:⟩ _MSW evaluation & weekly vs x 2 months_

Spiritual coordinator: _Rev. Carlson, St. Paul's Lutheran Church_

Counselor: _JoAnne Knowlton, MSW_

Volunteer: _Rosalie Marshall - niece will provide care on weekends_

Other services provided: _shopping, laundry, meal prep_

Goals: _wound care, pain management, terminal care at home_

Equipment: _needs: commode, hospital bed, bedpan, Hoyer lift, side rail w/c_

Company & Phone number: _Scott Medical Equipment 165-9931_

Safety Measures _side rails ↑_   Nutritional req _diet as tolerated_

FUNCTIONAL LIMITATIONS: (Circle Applicable) | ACTIVITIES PERMITTED: (Circle Applicable)

1 Amputation	5 Paralysis	9 Legally blind	1. Complete bedrest	6. Partial wgt bearing	Ⓐ Wheelchair
2 Bowel/Bladder	⑥ Endurance	A Dyspnea with	2. Bedrest BRP	7. Independent at home	B. Walker
3 Contracture	⑦ Ambulation	minimal exer	3. Up as tolerated	8. Crutches	C. No restriction
4 Hearing	8 Speech	Ⓑ Other _R.A._	④ Transfer bed/chair	9. Cane	D. Other—specify

Accessibility to bath Y - Ⓝ   Shower Y - Ⓝ   Bathroom Y - Ⓝ   Exit Y - Ⓝ

Mental status: (Circle) Oriented Comatose Forgetful ⟨Depressed⟩ Disoriented Lethargic Agitated Other

(continued)

Referral form *(continued)*

Allergies: _____none known_____

• Hospice appropriate meds   • Med company: _____Walker Pharmacy_____

MEDICATIONS:

morphine sulfate liq. 20 mg/ml 40 mg P.O. q6h p.r.n. pain

Reglan 10 mg P.O. q.i.d. p.r.n. nausea/vomiting

Colace 200 mg P.O. daily p.r.n. constipation

Benadryl 25-50 mg P.O. at bedtime p.r.n. sleeplessness

Living will   yes ✔   no _____   obtained _____   Family to mail to office _____

Guardian, POA, or responsible person: _____husband_____

Address & phone number: _____same_____

Other family members: _____

ETOH ___0___   Drug Use: ___0___   Smoker _2 ppd x 40 years quit 2 yrs ago_

History: ___Other than problems associated with arthritis, was in general good health until 12/07, Dx: lung CA - husband cared for___
___at home until 11/08.___

Social history (place of birth, education, jobs, retirement, etc.): ___Born & raised in Toronto, became U.S.___
___citizen when married in 1951. 2 yrs. college - majored in music. Retired church organist.___

ADMISSION NOTES: VS: T _98° P.O._   AP _86_   RR _18_   BP _140/72_

Lungs: _decreased breath sounds LLL._   Extremities: _cool to touch Pedal pulses present._

Wgt _118_   Recent wgt (loss)/gain of _40 lb over 6 months_

Admission narrative: _visit made to pt/husband in hospital before discharge. Both have been told that she is failing rapidly,_
___and would like her to return home with Hospice services. Niece willing to help 2 days/week. Pt apprehensive; husband blames___
___himself for the coccygeal decubitus that developed under his care.___

Psychosocial issues: ___Pt has always cared for husband. Describes self as depressed that she is no longer able to do so;___
___worries who will care for him after she dies.___

Environmental concerns: _(need smoke detectors)_

Are there any cultural or spiritual customs or beliefs of which we should be aware before providing Hospice services? _Pt would like Holy Communion just before death (& weekly)_

Funeral home: _____not yet chosen_____   Contact made? yes _____ no __x__

DIRECTIONS: _corner Newton/Elm duplex, white with green trim. Door on (L) says 66. Bell broken - knock loudly._

Agency Representative Signature: ___Beth Isham, R.N___   Date: ___2/21/09___
Home Care Supervisor

• patient's or caregiver's ability to recognize potential complications, respond appropriately, and get help when necessary.

Home health care forms

Key forms used to document home health care include:
• agency assessment and OASIS forms
• care plan
• progress notes
• patient-teaching sheets
• nursing and discharge summaries
• Medicare-mandated forms, including home health certification and care plan, medical update, and patient information.

Agency assessment and OASIS forms

When a patient is referred to your home health care agency, you must complete a thorough and specific assessment and chart the information on a patient assessment form.

Assess the patient's:
• physical status
• functional status
• mental and emotional status
• home environment in relation to safety and support services
• knowledge of his disease or current condition, prognosis, and treatment plan
• potential for complying with the treatment plan.

Guidelines for use

As with any setting, be thorough during home health care. A thorough patient assessment provides the information you need to plan appropriate care.

Consider the following guidelines:
• Obtain information about the patient's past and current health. Organize the interview by body system, and ask open-ended questions.
• When taking a physical assessment, use a systematic approach, as is appropriate in any setting. For example, you may take a body-system or head-to-toe approach.
• When assessing functional abilities, have the patient demonstrate his ability in addition to answering the questions.
• When assessing the home environment, consider such factors as the presence of a caregiver, structural barriers, access to a telephone, and safety and hygiene practices.

- When assessing the patient's potential for complying with the treatment plan, consider such factors as history of psychiatric disorders, developmental status, substance abuse, comprehension, ability to read and write, and the presence of language barriers.
- OASIS isn't a substitute for a thorough assessment; it's an addition. Some agencies have integrated their assessment forms and OASIS. (See *Using the OASIS-B1 form.*)
- OASIS guidelines specify the questions to be asked. All must be asked, even though the patient may decline to answer some. Note the questions he declines to answer on your record, and report the situation to your supervisor.

Care plan

Professional standards dictated by CHAP in 1993 — under the guidance of NLN — require you to develop a comprehensive care plan in cooperation with the patient and his caregivers.

Family counsel

In many aspects of care, the patient and family become the decision makers. This fact must be taken into account when developing your care plan; adjust your interventions, patient goals, and teaching accordingly. Reimbursement must also be considered.

Don't go astray — without documenting it, at least

Legally speaking, a care plan is the most direct evidence of your nursing judgment. If you outline a care plan and then deviate from it, a court may decide that you strayed from a reasonable standard of care. So be sure to update your care plan and make sure it fits the patient's needs.

Collating care

Some agencies use the home health certification form and care plan form (required for Medicare reimbursement) as the official care plan for Medicare patients. Most home health agencies, however, require a separate care plan.

Agencies use a multidisciplinary, integrated care plan for those patients receiving more than one service such as physical or occupational therapy. (See *Interdisciplinary care plan*, page 276.)

Guidelines for use

To document most effectively on your care plan, follow these suggestions:
- Keep a copy of the care plan in the patient's home for easy reference by him and his family.

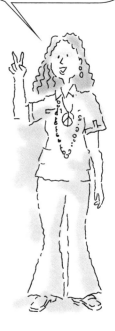

Change of plans? Just document it, man. Don't get caught out of date!

(Text continues on page 275.)

Art of the chart

Using the OASIS-B1 form

The OASIS-B1 form includes more than 80 topics, such as socioeconomic, physiologic, and functional data; service utilization information; and neurological, emotional, and behavioral data.

<u>Items to be Used at Specific Time Points</u>

<u>Start of Care</u> - Home Health Patient Tracking Sheet, M0080-M0826
   Start of care—further visits planned

<u>Resumption of Care</u> - M0080-M0826
   Resumption of care (after inpatient stay)

<u>Follow-Up</u> - M0080-M0110, M0230-M0250, M0390, M0420, M0440, M0450, M0460, M0470,
   Recertification (follow-up) assessment   M0474, M0476, M0488, M0490, M0520-M0550, M0650-M0700, M0800, M0826
   Other follow-up assessment

<u>Transfer to an Inpatient Facility</u> - M0080-M0100, M0830-M0855, M0890-M0906
   Transferred to an inpatient facility—patient not discharged from an agency
   Transferred to an inpatient facility—patient discharged from agency

<u>Discharge from Agency — Not to an Inpatient Facility</u>
   Death at home - M0080-M0100, M0906
   Discharge from agency - M0080-M0100, M0200-M0220, M0250, M0280-M0380, M0410-M0820,
                                          M0830-M0880, M0903-M0906

Note: For items M0640-M0800, please note special instructions at the beginning of the section.

CLINICAL RECORD ITEMS

(M0080)   Discipline of Person Completing Assessment:

       [X] 1-RN   ☐ 2-PT   ☐ 3-SLP/ST   ☐ 4-OT

(M0090)   Date Assessment Completed: <u>02 /02 /2009</u>
                                  month   day   year

(M0100)   This Assessment is Currently Being Completed for the Following Reason:

       <u>Start/Resumption of Care</u>
   [X] 1 – Start of care—further visits planned
   ☐ 3 – Resumption of care (after inpatient stay)

       <u>Follow-Up</u>
   ☐ 4 – Recertification (follow-up) reassessment [Go to *M0110*]
   ☐ 5 – Other follow-up [Go to *M0110*]

       <u>Transfer to an Inpatient Facility</u>
   ☐ 6 – Transferred to an inpatient facility—patient not discharged from agency [Go to *M0830*]
   ☐ 7 – Transferred to an inpatient facility—patient discharged from agency [Go to *M0830*]

       <u>Discharge from Agency — Not to an Inpatient Facility</u>
   ☐ 8 – Death at home [Go to *M0906*]
   ☐ 9 – Discharge from agency [Go to *M0200*]

(continued)

Using the OASIS-B1 form *(continued)*

(M0110)   **Episode Timing:** Is the Medicare home health payment episode for which this assessment will define a case mix group an "early" episode or a "later" episode in the patient's current sequence of adjacent Medicare home health payment episodes?

☐ 1 – Early
☐ 2 – Later
☐ UK – Unknown
☐ NA – Not Applicable: No Medicare case mix group to be defined by this assessment.
At follow-up go to M0230

DEMOGRAPHICS AND PATIENT HISTORY

(M0175)   From which of the following **Inpatient Facilities** was the patient discharged <u>during the past 14 days</u>? **(Mark all that apply.)**

☐ 1 – Hospital
☐ 2 – Rehabilitation facility
☐ 3 – Skilled nursing facility
☐ 4 – Other nursing home
☐ 5 – Other (specify) _____
☒ NA – Patient was not discharged from an inpatient facility **[If NA, go to *M0200*]**

(M0180)   **Inpatient Discharge Date** (most recent):

__ __ / __ __ / __ __ __ __
month   day   year
☐ UK – Unknown

(M0190)   List each **Inpatient Diagnosis** and ICD 9 CM code at the level of highest specificity for only those conditions treated during an inpatient stay within the last 14 days (no surgical, E codes, or V codes):

Inpatient Facility Diagnosis	ICD-9-CM
a. _____	(__ __ __ • __ __)
b. _____	(__ __ __ • __ __)

(M0200)   **Medical or Treatment Regimen Change Within Past 14 Days:** Has this patient experienced a change in medical or treatment regimen (e.g., medication, treatment, or service change due to new or additional diagnosis, etc.) within the last 14 days?

☐ 0 – No **[If No, go to *M0220*; if No at Discharge, go to *M0250*]**
☒ 1 – Yes

(M0210)   List the patient's **Medical Diagnoses** and ICD 9 CM codes at the level of highest specificity for those conditions requiring changed medical or treatment regimen (no surgical, E codes, or V codes):

Changed Medical Regimen Diagnosis	ICD-9-CM
a. *open wound Ⓛ ankle*	(*8 9 1* • *0 0*)
b. _____	(__ __ __ • __ __)
c. _____	(__ __ __ • __ __)
d. _____	(__ __ __ • __ __)

(M0220)   **Conditions Prior to Medical or Treatment Regimen Change or Inpatient Stay Within Past 14 Days:** If this patient experienced an inpatient facility discharge or change in medical or treatment regimen within the past 14 days, indicate any conditions which existed <u>prior to</u> the inpatient stay or change in medical or treatment regimen. **(Mark all that apply.)**

☐ 1 – Urinary incontinence
☐ 2 – Indwelling/suprapubic catheter
☐ 3 – Intractable pain
☐ 4 – Impaired decision-making
☐ 5 – Disruptive or socially inappropriate behavior
☐ 6 – Memory loss to the extent that supervision required
☒ 7 – None of the above
☐ NA – No inpatient facility discharge <u>and</u> no change in medical or treatment regimen in past 14 days
☐ UK – Unknown

Using the OASIS-B1 form *(continued)*

M0230/240/246   **Diagnoses, Severity Index, and Payment Diagnoses:** List each diagnosis for which the patient is receiving home care (Column 1) and enter its ICD-9-CM code at the level of highest specificity (no surgical/procedure codes) (Column 2) . Rate each condition (Column 2) using the severity index. (Choose one value that represents the most severe rating appropriate for each diagnosis.) V codes (for M0230 or M0240) or E codes (for M0240 only) may be used. ICD-9-CM sequencing requirements must be followed if multiple coding is indicated for any diagnoses. If a V code is reported in place of a case mix diagnosis, then M0246 Payment Diagnoses may be completed. A case mix diagnosis is a diagnosis that determines the Medicare PPS case mix group.

Code each row as follows:

Column 1:   Enter the description of the diagnosis.

Column 2:   Enter the ICD-9-CM code for the diagnosis described in Column 1;
Rate the severity of the condition listed in Column 1 using the following scale:
0 – Asymptomatic, no treatment needed at this time
1 – Symptoms well controlled with current therapy
2 – Symptoms controlled with difficulty, affecting daily functioning; patient needs ongoing monitoring
3 – Symptoms poorly controlled; patient needs frequent adjustment in treatment and dose monitoring
4 – Symptoms poorly controlled; history of re-hospitalizations

(M0230) Primary Diagnosis & (M0240) Other Diagnoses	
(1)	(2)
	ICD-9-CM and severity rating for each condition
Description	ICD-9-CM / Severity Rating
(M0230) Primary Diagnosis	**(V codes are allowed)**
a. *open wound @ ankle*	a. (8 9 1 • 0 0) ☐0 ☐1 ☒2 ☐3 ☐4
(M0240) Other Diagnoses	**(V or E codes are allowed)**
b. *Type 2 diabetes*	b. (2 5 0 • 7 2) ☐0 ☐1 ☒2 ☐3 ☐4
c. *Peripheral Vascular Disease*	c. (_ 4 4 3 • 8 9) ☐0 ☐1 ☐2 ☒3 ☐4
d. _____	d. (_ _ _ _ • _ _) ☐0 ☐1 ☐2 ☐3 ☐4
e. _____	e. (_ _ _ _ • _ _) ☐0 ☐1 ☐2 ☐3 ☐4
f. _____	f. (_ _ _ _ • _ _) ☐0 ☐1 ☐2 ☐3 ☐4

(M0250)   Therapies the patient receives <u>at home</u>: (Mark all that apply.)
☐   1 – Intravenous or infusion therapy (excludes TPN)
☐   2 – Parenteral nutrition (TPN or lipids)
☐   3 – Enteral nutrition (nasogastric, gastrostomy, jejunostomy, or any other artificial entry into the alimentary canal)
☒   4 – None of the above

(continued)

Using the OASIS-B1 form *(continued)*

(M0260) **Overall Prognosis:** BEST description of patient's overall prognosis for <u>recovery from this episode of illness.</u>
- ☐ 0 – Poor: little or no recovery is expected and/or further decline is imminent
- ☒ 1 – Good/Fair: partial to full recovery is expected
- ☐ UK – Unknown

(M0270) **Rehabilitative Prognosis:** BEST description of patient's prognosis for <u>functional status</u>.
- ☒ 0 – Guarded: minimal improvement in functional status is expected; decline is possible
- ☐ 1 – Good: marked improvement in functional status is expected
- ☐ UK – Unknown

(M0280) **Life Expectancy:** (Physician documentation is not required.)
- ☐ 0 – Life expectancy is greater than 6 months
- ☒ 1 – Life expectancy is 6 months or fewer

(M0290) **High Risk Factors** characterizing this patient: **(Mark all that apply.)**
- ☒ 1 – Heavy smoking
- ☐ 2 – Obesity
- ☐ 3 – Alcohol dependency
- ☐ 4 – Drug dependency
- ☐ 5 – None of the above
- ☐ UK – Unknown

LIVING ARRANGEMENTS

(M0300) **Current Residence:**
- ☒ 1 – Patient's owned or rented residence (house, apartment, or mobile home owned or rented by patient/couple/significant other)
- ☐ 2 – Family member's residence
- ☐ 3 – Boarding home or rented room
- ☐ 4 – Board and care or assisted living facility
- ☐ 5 – Other (specify) _____

(M0340) **Patient Lives With: (Mark all that apply.)**
- ☐ 1 – Lives alone
- ☒ 2 – With spouse or significant other
- ☐ 3 – With other family member
- ☐ 4 – With a friend
- ☐ 5 – With paid help (other than home care agency staff)
- ☐ 6 – With other than above

SUPPORTIVE ASSISTANCE

(M0350) **Assisting Person(s) Other than Home Care Agency Staff: (Mark all that apply.)**
- ☐ 1 – Relatives, friends, or neighbors living outside the home
- ☒ 2 – Person residing in the home (EXCLUDING paid help)
- ☐ 3 – Paid help
- ☐ 4 – None of the above [**If None of the above, go to** *M0390*]
- ☐ UK – Unknown [**If Unknown, go to** *M0390*]

(M0360) **Primary Caregiver** taking <u>lead</u> responsibility for providing or managing the patient's care, providing the most frequent assistance, etc. (other than home care agency staff):
- ☐ 0 – No one person [**If No one person, go to** *M0390*]
- ☒ 1 – Spouse or significant other
- ☐ 2 – Daughter or son
- ☐ 3 – Other family member
- ☐ 4 – Friend or neighbor or community or church member
- ☐ 5 – Paid help
- ☐ UK – Unknown [**If Unknown, go to** *M0390*]

Using the OASIS-B1 form *(continued)*

(M0370) How Often does the patient receive assistance from the primary caregiver?
- [X] 1 – Several times during day and night
- [ ] 2 – Several times during day
- [ ] 3 – Once daily
- [ ] 4 – Three or more times per week
- [ ] 5 – One to two times per week
- [ ] 6 – Less often than weekly
- [ ] UK – Unknown

(M0380) Type of Primary Caregiver Assistance: (Mark all that apply.)
- [X] 1 – ADL assistance (e.g., bathing, dressing, toileting, bowel/bladder, eating/feeding)
- [X] 2 – IADL assistance (e.g., meds, meals, housekeeping, laundry, telephone, shopping, finances)
- [ ] 3 – Environmental support (housing, home maintenance)
- [X] 4 – Psychosocial support (socialization, companionship, recreation)
- [X] 5 – Advocates or facilitates patient's participation in appropriate medical care
- [ ] 6 – Financial agent, power of attorney, or conservator of finance
- [ ] 7 – Health care agent, conservator of person, or medical power of attorney
- [ ] UK – Unknown

SENSORY STATUS

(M0390) Vision with corrective lenses if the patient usually wears them:
- [X] 0 – Normal vision: sees adequately in most situations; can see medication labels, newsprint.
- [ ] 1 – Partially impaired: cannot see medication labels or newsprint, but <u>can</u> see obstacles in path, and the surrounding layout; can count fingers at arm's length.
- [ ] 2 – Severely impaired: cannot locate objects without hearing or touching them or patient nonresponsive.

(M0400) Hearing and Ability to Understand Spoken Language in patient's own language (with hearing aids if the patient usually uses them):
- [X] 0 – No observable impairment. Able to hear and understand complex or detailed instructions and extended or abstract conversation.
- [ ] 1 – With minimal difficulty, able to hear and understand most multi-step instructions and ordinary conversation. May need occasional repetition, extra time, or louder voice.
- [ ] 2 – Has moderate difficulty hearing and understanding simple, one-step instructions and brief conversation; needs frequent prompting or assistance.
- [ ] 3 – Has severe difficulty hearing and understanding simple greetings and short comments. Requires multiple repetitions, restatements, demonstrations, additional time.
- [ ] 4 – <u>Unable</u> to hear and understand familiar words or common expressions consistently, or patient nonresponsive.

(M0410) Speech and Oral (Verbal) Expression of Language (in patient's own language):
- [X] 0 – Expresses complex ideas, feelings, and needs clearly, completely, and easily in all situations with no observable impairment.
- [ ] 1 – Minimal difficulty in expressing ideas and needs (may take extra time; makes occasional errors in word choice, grammar or speech intelligibility; needs minimal prompting or assistance).
- [ ] 2 – Expresses simple ideas or needs with moderate difficulty (needs prompting or assistance, errors in word choice, organization or speech intelligibility). Speaks in phrases or short sentences.
- [ ] 3 – Has severe difficulty expressing basic ideas or needs and requires maximal assistance or guessing by listener. Speech limited to single words or short phrases.
- [ ] 4 – <u>Unable</u> to express basic needs even with maximal prompting or assistance but is not comatose or unresponsive (e.g., speech is nonsensical or unintelligible).
- [ ] 5 – Patient nonresponsive or unable to speak.

(M0420) Frequency of Pain interfering with patient's activity or movement:
- [ ] 0 – Patient has no pain or pain does not interfere with activity or movement
- [ ] 1 – Less often than daily
- [X] 2 – Daily, but not constantly
- [ ] 3 – All of the time

(M0430) Intractable Pain: Is the patient experiencing pain that is <u>not easily relieved</u>, occurs at least daily, and affects the patient's sleep, appetite, physical or emotional energy, concentration, personal relationships, emotions, or ability or desire to perform physical activity?
- [X] 0 – No
- [ ] 1 – Yes

(continued)

Using the OASIS-B1 form (continued)

INTEGUMENTARY STATUS

(M0440) Does this patient have a **Skin Lesion** or an **Open Wound**? This excludes "OSTOMIES."

    ☐   0 – No [**If No, go to** *M0490*]
    ☒   1 – Yes

(M0445) Does this patient have a **Pressure Ulcer?**

    ☒   0 – No [**If No, go to** *M0468*]
    ☐   1 – Yes

(M0450) **Current Number of Pressure Ulcers at Each Stage:** (Circle one response for each stage.)

Pressure Ulcer Stages	Number of Pressure Ulcers				
a) Stage 1: Nonblanchable erythema of intact skin; the heralding of skin ulceration. In darker-pigmented skin, warmth, edema, hardness, or discolored skin may be indicators.	0	1	2	3	4 or more
b) Stage 2: Partial thickness skin loss involving epidermis and/or dermis. The ulcer is superficial and presents clinically as an abrasion, blister, or shallow crater.	0	1	2	3	4 or more
c) Stage 3: Full-thickness skin loss involving damage or necrosis of subcutaneous tissue which may extend down to, but not through, underlying fascia. The ulcer presents clinically as a deep crater with or without undermining of adjacent tissue.	0	1	2	3	4 or more
d) Stage 4: Full-thickness skin loss with extensive destruction, tissue necrosis, or damage to muscle, bone, or supporting structures (e.g., tendon, joint capsule, etc.)	0	1	2	3	4 or more
e) In addition to the above, is there at least one pressure ulcer that cannot be observed due to the presence of eschar or a nonremovable dressing, including casts? ☐ 0 – No ☐ 1 – Yes					

(M0460) [At follow-up, skip to M0470 if patient has no pressure ulcers]

Stage of Most Problematic (Observable) Pressure Ulcer:

    ☐   1 – Stage 1
    ☐   2 – Stage 2
    ☐   3 – Stage 3
    ☐   4 – Stage 4
    ☐   NA – No observable pressure ulcer

(M0464) **Status of Most Problematic (Observable) Pressure Ulcer:**

    ☐   1 – Fully granulating
    ☐   2 – Early/partial granulation
    ☐   3 – Not healing
    ☐   NA – No observable pressure ulcer

(M0468) Does this patient have a **Stasis Ulcer?**

    ☐   0 – No [**If No, go to** *M0482*]
    ☒   1 – Yes

(M0470) **Current Number of Observable Stasis Ulcer(s):**

    ☐   0 – Zero
    ☒   1 – One
    ☐   2 – Two
    ☐   3 – Three
    ☐   4 – Four or more

Using the OASIS-B1 form (continued)

(M0474) Does this patient have at least one **Stasis Ulcer that Cannot be Observed** due to the presence of a nonremovable dressing?
- [x] 0 – No
- [ ] 1 – Yes

(M0476) [At follow-up, skip to M0488 if patient has no stasis ulcers]
Status of Most Problematic (Observable) Stasis Ulcer:
- [ ] 1 – Fully granulating
- [x] 2 – Early/partial granulation
- [ ] 3 – Not healing
- [ ] NA – No observable stasis ulcer

(M0482) Does this patient have a **Surgical Wound**?
- [x] 0 – No [**If No, go to** *M0490*]
- [ ] 1 – Yes

(M0484) **Current Number of (Observable) Surgical Wounds:** (If a wound is partially closed but has <u>more</u> than one opening, consider each opening as a separate wound.)
- [ ] 0 – Zero
- [ ] 1 – One
- [ ] 2 – Two
- [ ] 3 – Three
- [ ] 4 – Four or more

(M0486) Does this patient have at least one **Surgical Wound that Cannot be Observed** due to the presence of a nonremovable dressing?
- [ ] 0 – No
- [ ] 1 – Yes

(M0488) [At follow-up, skip to M0490 if patient has no surgical wounds]
Status of Most Problematic (Observable) Surgical Wound:
- [ ] 1 – Fully granulating
- [ ] 2 – Early/partial granulation
- [ ] 3 – Not healing
- [ ] NA – No observable surgical wound

RESPIRATORY STATUS

(M0490) When is the patient dyspneic or noticeably **Short of Breath**?
- [x] 0 – Never; patient is not short of breath
- [ ] 1 – When walking more than 20 feet, climbing stairs
- [ ] 2 – With moderate exertion (e.g., while dressing, using commode or bedpan, walking distances less than 20 feet)
- [ ] 3 – With minimal exertion (e.g., while eating, talking, or performing other ADLs) or with agitation
- [ ] 4 – At rest (during day or night)

(M0500) **Respiratory Treatments** utilized at home: **(Mark all that apply.)**
- [ ] 1 – Oxygen (intermittent or continuous)
- [ ] 2 – Ventilator (continually or at night)
- [ ] 3 – Continuous positive airway pressure
- [ ] 4 – None of the above

ELIMINATION STATUS

(M0510) Has this patient been treated for a **Urinary Tract Infection** in the past 14 days?
- [x] 0 – No
- [ ] 1 – Yes
- [ ] NA – Patient on prophylactic treatment
- [ ] UK – Unknown

(continued)

Using the OASIS-B1 form *(continued)*

(M0520)   **Urinary Incontinence or Urinary Catheter Presence:**
- [X] 0 – No incontinence or catheter (includes anuria or ostomy for urinary drainage) [**If No, go to** *M0540*]
- [ ] 1 – Patient is incontinent
- [ ] 2 – Patient requires a urinary catheter (i.e., external, indwelling, intermittent, suprapubic) [**Go to** *M0540*]

(M0530)   When does **Urinary Incontinence** occur?
- [ ] 0 – Timed-voiding defers incontinence
- [ ] 1 – During the night only
- [ ] 2 – During the day and night

(M0540)   **Bowel Incontinence Frequency:**
- [X] 0 – Very rarely or never has bowel incontinence
- [ ] 1 – Less than once weekly
- [ ] 2 – One to three times weekly
- [ ] 3 – Four to six times weekly
- [ ] 4 – On a daily basis
- [ ] 5 – More often than once daily
- [ ] NA – Patient has ostomy for bowel elimination
- [ ] UK – Unknown

(M0550)   **Ostomy for Bowel Elimination:** Does this patient have an ostomy for bowel elimination that (within the last 14 days): a) was related to an inpatient facility stay, <u>or</u> b) necessitated a change in medical or treatment regimen?
- [X] 0 – Patient does <u>not</u> have an ostomy for bowel elimination.
- [ ] 1 – Patient's ostomy was <u>not</u> related to an inpatient stay and did <u>not</u> necessitate change in medical or treatment regimen.
- [ ] 2 – The ostomy <u>was</u> related to an inpatient stay or <u>did</u> necessitate change in medical or treatment regimen.

NEURO/EMOTIONAL/BEHAVIORAL STATUS

(M0560)   **Cognitive Functioning:** (Patient's current level of alertness, orientation, comprehension, concentration, and immediate memory for simple commands.)
- [ ] 0 – Alert/oriented, able to focus and shift attention, comprehends and recalls task directions independently.
- [X] 1 – Requires prompting (cuing, repetition, reminders) only under stressful or unfamiliar conditions.
- [ ] 2 – Requires assistance and some direction in specific situations (e.g., on all tasks involving shifting of attention), or consistently requires low stimulus environment due to distractibility.
- [ ] 3 – Requires considerable assistance in routine situations. Is not alert and oriented or is unable to shift attention and recall directions more than half the time.
- [ ] 4 – Totally dependent due to disturbances such as constant disorientation, coma, persistent vegetative state, or delirium.

(M0570)   **When Confused (Reported or Observed):**
- [X] 0 – Never
- [ ] 1 – In new or complex situations only
- [ ] 2 – On awakening or at night only
- [ ] 3 – During the day and evening, but not constantly
- [ ] 4 – Constantly
- [ ] NA – Patient nonresponsive

(M0580)   **When Anxious (Reported or Observed):**
- [ ] 0 – None of the time
- [ ] 1 – Less often than daily
- [X] 2 – Daily, but not constantly
- [ ] 3 – All of the time
- [ ] NA – Patient nonresponsive

(M0590)   **Depressive Feelings Reported or Observed in Patient: (Mark all that apply.)**
- [ ] 1 – Depressed mood (e.g., feeling sad, tearful)
- [ ] 2 – Sense of failure or self reproach
- [X] 3 – Hopelessness
- [ ] 4 – Recurrent thoughts of death
- [ ] 5 – Thoughts of suicide
- [ ] 6 – None of the above feelings observed or reported

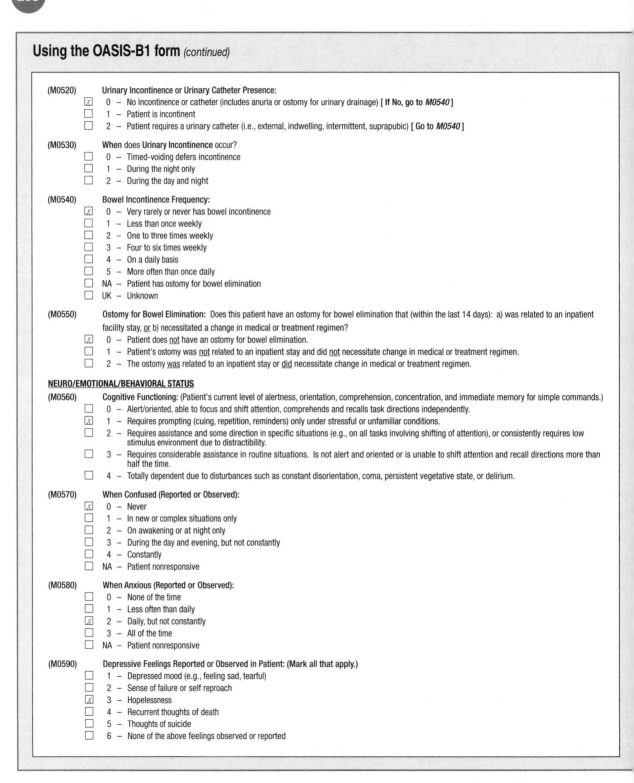

Using the OASIS-B1 form *(continued)*

(M0610) Behaviors Demonstrated <u>at Least Once a Week</u> (Reported or Observed): (Mark all that apply.)

☐ 1 – Memory deficit: failure to recognize familiar persons/places, inability to recall events of past 24 hours, significant memory loss so that supervision is required

☐ 2 – Impaired decision-making: failure to perform usual ADLs or IADLs, inability to appropriately stop activities, jeopardizes safety through actions

☐ 3 – Verbal disruption: yelling, threatening, excessive profanity, sexual references, etc.

☐ 4 – Physical aggression: aggressive or combative to self and others (e.g., hits self, throws objects, punches, dangerous maneuvers with wheelchair or other objects)

☐ 5 – Disruptive, infantile, or socially inappropriate behavior (**excludes** verbal actions)

☐ 6 – Delusional, hallucinatory, or paranoid behavior

☒ 7 – None of the above behaviors demonstrated

(M0620) Frequency of Behavior Problems (Reported or Observed) (e.g., wandering episodes, self abuse, verbal disruption, physical aggression, etc.):

☒ 0 – Never

☐ 1 – Less than once a month

☐ 2 – Once a month

☐ 3 – Several times each month

☐ 4 – Several times a week

☐ 5 – At least daily

(M0630) Is this patient receiving **Psychiatric Nursing Services** at home provided by a qualified psychiatric nurse?

☒ 0 – No

☐ 1 – Yes

ADL/IADLs

For M0640-M0800, complete the "Current" column for all patients. For these same items, complete the "Prior" column only at start of care and at resumption of care; mark the level that corresponds to the patient's condition 14 days prior to start of care date (M0030) or resumption of care date (M0032). In all cases, record what the patient is *able to do.*

(M0640) Grooming: Ability to tend to personal hygiene needs (i.e., washing face and hands, hair care, shaving or makeup, teeth or denture care, fingernail care).

Prior Current

☒   ☐   0 – Able to groom self unaided, with or without the use of assistive devices or adapted methods.

☐   ☐   1 – Grooming utensils must be placed within reach before able to complete grooming activities.

☐   ☒   2 – Someone must assist the patient to groom self.

☐   ☐   3 – Patient depends entirely upon someone else for grooming needs.

☐   UK – Unknown

(M0650) Ability to Dress <u>Upper</u> Body (with or without dressing aids) including undergarments, pullovers, front-opening shirts and blouses, managing zippers, buttons, and snaps:

Prior Current

☒   ☐   0 – Able to get clothes out of closets and drawers, put them on and remove them from the upper body without assistance.

☐   ☒   1 – Able to dress upper body without assistance if clothing is laid out or handed to the patient.

☐   ☐   2 – Someone must help the patient put on upper body clothing.

☐   ☐   3 – Patient depends entirely upon another person to dress the upper body.

☐   UK – Unknown

(M0660) Ability to Dress <u>Lower</u> Body (with or without dressing aids) including undergarments, slacks, socks or nylons, shoes:

Prior Current

☒   ☐   0 – Able to obtain, put on, and remove clothing and shoes without assistance.

☐   ☐   1 – Able to dress lower body without assistance if clothing and shoes are laid out or handed to the patient.

☐   ☒   2 – Someone must help the patient put on undergarments, slacks, socks or nylons, and shoes.

☐   ☐   3 – Patient depends entirely upon another person to dress lower body.

☐   UK – Unknown

(continued)

Using the OASIS-B1 form *(continued)*

(M0670)   Bathing: Ability to wash entire body. <u>Excludes</u> grooming (washing face and hands only).

Prior	Current		
☐	☐	0 –	Able to bathe self in <u>shower or tub</u> independently.
☒	☐	1 –	With the use of devices, is able to bathe self in shower or tub independently.
☐	☐	2 –	Able to bathe in shower or tub with the assistance of another person:
			(a) for intermittent supervision or encouragement or reminders, <u>OR</u>
			(b) to get in and out of the shower or tub, <u>OR</u>
			(c) for washing difficult-to-reach areas.
☐	☒	3 –	Participates in bathing self in shower or tub, <u>but</u> requires presence of another person throughout the bath for assistance or supervision.
☐	☐	4 –	<u>Unable</u> to use the shower or tub and is bathed in <u>bed or bedside chair</u>.
☐	☐	5 –	Unable to effectively participate in bathing and is totally bathed by another person.
☐		UK –	Unknown

(M0680)   Toileting: Ability to get to and from the toilet or bedside commode.

Prior	Current		
☒	☒	0 –	Able to get to and from the toilet independently with or without a device.
☐	☐	1 –	When reminded, assisted, or supervised by another person, able to get to and from the toilet.
☐	☐	2 –	<u>Unable</u> to get to and from the toilet but is able to use a bedside commode (with or without assistance).
☐	☐	3 –	<u>Unable</u> to get to and from the toilet or bedside commode but is able to use a bedpan/urinal independently.
☐	☐	4 –	Is totally dependent in toileting.
☐		UK –	Unknown

(M0690)   Transferring: Ability to move from bed to chair, on and off toilet or commode, into and out of tub or shower, and ability to turn and position self in bed if patient is bedfast.

Prior	Current		
☐	☐	0 –	Able to independently transfer.
☒	☒	1 –	Transfers with minimal human assistance or with use of an assistive device.
☐	☐	2 –	<u>Unable</u> to transfer self but is able to bear weight and pivot during the transfer process.
☐	☐	3 –	Unable to transfer self and is <u>unable</u> to bear weight or pivot when transferred by another person.
☐	☐	4 –	Bedfast, unable to transfer but is able to turn and position self in bed.
☐	☐	5 –	Bedfast, unable to transfer and is <u>unable</u> to turn and position self.
☐		UK –	Unknown

(M0700)   Ambulation/Locomotion: Ability to <u>SAFELY</u> walk, once in a standing position, or use a wheelchair, once in a seated position, on a variety of surfaces.

Prior	Current		
☒	☐	0 –	Able to independently walk on even and uneven surfaces and climb stairs with or without railings (i.e., needs no human assistance or assistive device).
☐	☒	1 –	Requires use of a device (e.g., cane, walker) to walk alone <u>or</u> requires human supervision or assistance to negotiate stairs or steps or uneven surfaces.
☐	☐	2 –	Able to walk only with the supervision or assistance of another person at all times.
☐	☐	3 –	Chairfast, <u>unable</u> to ambulate but is able to wheel self independently.
☐	☐	4 –	Chairfast, unable to ambulate and is <u>unable</u> to wheel self.
☐	☐	5 –	Bedfast, unable to ambulate or be up in a chair.
☐		UK –	Unknown

(M0710)   Feeding or Eating: Ability to feed self meals and snacks. Note: This refers only to the process of <u>eating</u>, <u>chewing</u>, and <u>swallowing</u>, <u>not preparing</u> the food to be eaten.

Prior	Current		
☒	☐	0 –	Able to independently feed self.
☐	☒	1 –	Able to feed self independently but requires:
			(a) meal set-up; <u>OR</u>
			(b) intermittent assistance or supervision from another person; <u>OR</u>
			(c) a liquid, pureed or ground meat diet.
☐	☐	2 –	<u>Unable</u> to feed self and must be assisted or supervised throughout the meal/snack.
☐	☐	3 –	Able to take in nutrients orally <u>and</u> receives supplemental nutrients through a nasogastric tube or gastrostomy.
☐	☐	4 –	<u>Unable</u> to take in nutrients orally and is fed nutrients through a nasogastric tube or gastrostomy.

Using the OASIS-B1 form *(continued)*

☐ ☐ 5 – Unable to take in nutrients orally or by tube feeding.
☐ UK – Unknown

(M0720) **Planning and Preparing Light Meals** (e.g., cereal, sandwich) or reheat delivered meals:

Prior Current
☒ ☐ 0 – (a) Able to independently plan and prepare all light meals for self or reheat delivered meals; <u>OR</u>
     (b) Is physically, and mentally able to prepare light meals on a regular basis but has not routinely performed light meal preparation in the past (i.e., prior to this home care admission).
☐ ☒ 1 – <u>Unable</u> to prepare light meals on a regular basis due to physical, cognitive, or mental limitations.
☐ ☐ 2 – Unable to prepare any light meals or reheat any delivered meals.
☐ UK – Unknown

(M0730) **Transportation:** Physical and mental ability to <u>safely</u> use a car, taxi, or public transportation (bus, train, subway).

Prior Current
☐ ☐ 0 – Able to independently drive a regular or adapted car; <u>OR</u> uses a regular or handicap-accessible public bus.
☒ ☒ 1 – Able to ride in a car only when driven by another person; <u>OR</u> able to use a bus or handicap van only when assisted or accompanied by another person.
☐ ☐ 2 – <u>Unable</u> to ride in a car, taxi, bus, or van, and requires transportation by ambulance.
☐ UK – Unknown

(M0740) **Laundry:** Ability to do own laundry—to carry laundry to and from washing machine, to use washer and dryer, to wash small items by hand.

Prior Current
☐ ☐ 0 – (a) Able to independently take care of all laundry tasks; <u>OR</u>
     (b) Physically, cognitively, and mentally able to do laundry and access facilities, <u>but</u> has not routinely performed laundry tasks in the past (i.e., prior to this home care admission).
☒ ☐ 1 – Able to do only light laundry, such as minor hand wash or light washer loads. Due to physical, cognitive, or mental limitations, needs assistance with heavy laundry such as carrying large loads of laundry.
☐ ☒ 2 – <u>Unable</u> to do any laundry due to physical limitation or needs continual supervision and assistance due to cognitive or mental limitation.
☐ UK – Unknown

(M0750) **Housekeeping:** Ability to safely and effectively perform light housekeeping and heavier cleaning tasks.

Prior Current
☐ ☐ 0 – (a) Able to independently perform all housekeeping tasks; <u>OR</u>
     (b) Physically, cognitively, and mentally able to perform <u>all</u> housekeeping tasks but has not routinely participated in housekeeping tasks in the past (i.e., prior to this home care admission).
☐ ☐ 1 – Able to perform only <u>light</u> housekeeping tasks (e.g., dusting, wiping kitchen counters) independently.
☐ ☐ 2 – Able to perform housekeeping tasks with intermittent assistance or supervision from another person.
☐ ☐ 3 – <u>Unable</u> to consistently perform any housekeeping tasks unless assisted by another person throughout the process.
☒ ☒ 4 – Unable to effectively participate in any housekeeping tasks.
☐ UK – Unknown

(M0760) **Shopping:** Ability to plan for, select, and purchase items in a store and to carry them home or arrange delivery.

Prior Current
☐ ☐ 0 – (a) Able to plan for shopping needs and independently perform shopping tasks, including carrying packages; <u>OR</u>
     (b) Physically, cognitively, and mentally able to take care of shopping, but has not done shopping in the past (i.e., prior to this home care admission).
☐ ☐ 1 – Able to go shopping, but needs some assistance:
     (a) By self is able to do only light shopping and carry small packages, but needs someone to do occasional major shopping; <u>OR</u>
     (b) <u>Unable</u> to go shopping alone, but can go with someone to assist.
☒ ☒ 2 – <u>Unable</u> to go shopping, but is able to identify items needed, place orders, and arrange home delivery.
☐ ☐ 3 – Needs someone to do all shopping and errands.
☐ UK – Unknown

(M0770) **Ability to Use Telephone:** Ability to answer the phone, dial numbers, and <u>effectively</u> use the telephone to communicate.

Prior Current
☒ ☒ 0 – Able to dial numbers and answer calls appropriately and as desired.
☐ ☐ 1 – Able to use a specially adapted telephone (i.e., large numbers on the dial, teletype phone for the deaf) and call essential numbers.

(continued)

Using the OASIS-B1 form *(continued)*

☐ ☐ 2 – Able to answer the telephone and carry on a normal conversation but has difficulty with placing calls.
☐ ☐ 3 – Able to answer the telephone only some of the time or is able to carry on only a limited conversation.
☐ ☐ 4 – <u>Unable</u> to answer the telephone at all but can listen if assisted with equipment.
☐ ☐ 5 – Totally unable to use the telephone.
☐ ☐ NA – Patient does not have a telephone.
☐ UK – Unknown

MEDICATIONS

(M0780) Management of Oral Medications: <u>Patient's ability</u> to prepare and take <u>all</u> prescribed oral medications reliably and safely, including administration of the correct dosage at the appropriate times/intervals. <u>Excludes</u> injectable and I.V. medications. (NOTE: This refers to ability, not compliance or willingness.)

Prior Current
☒ ☒ 0 – Able to independently take the correct oral medication(s) and proper dosage(s) at the correct times.
☐ ☐ 1 – Able to take medication(s) at the correct times if:
    (a) individual dosages are prepared in advance by another person; <u>OR</u>
    (b) given daily reminders; <u>OR</u>
    (c) someone develops a drug diary or chart.
☐ ☐ 2 – <u>Unable</u> to take medication unless administered by someone else.
☐ ☐ NA – No oral medications prescribed.
☐ UK – Unknown

(M0790) Management of Inhalant/Mist Medications: <u>Patient's ability</u> to prepare and take <u>all</u> prescribed inhalant/mist medications (nebulizers, metered dose devices) reliably and safely, including administration of the correct dosage at the appropriate times/intervals. <u>Excludes</u> all other forms of medication (oral tablets, injectable and I.V. medications).

Prior Current
☐ ☐ 0 – Able to independently take the correct medication and proper dosage at the correct times.
☐ ☐ 1 – Able to take medication at the correct times if:
    (a) individual dosages are prepared in advance by another person, <u>OR</u>
    (b) given daily reminders.
☐ ☐ 2 – <u>Unable</u> to take medication unless administered by someone else.
☒ ☒ NA – No inhalant/mist medications prescribed.
☐ UK – Unknown

(M0800) Management of Injectable Medications: <u>Patient's ability</u> to prepare and take <u>all</u> prescribed injectable medications reliably and safely, including administration of correct dosage at the appropriate times/intervals. <u>Excludes</u> I.V. medications.

Prior Current
☒ ☒ 0 – Able to independently take the correct medication and proper dosage at the correct times.
☐ ☐ 1 – Able to take injectable medication at correct times if:
    (a) individual syringes are prepared in advance by another person, <u>OR</u>
    (b) given daily reminders.
☐ ☐ 2 – <u>Unable</u> to take injectable medications unless administered by someone else.
☐ ☐ NA – No injectable medications prescribed.
☐ UK – Unknown

EQUIPMENT MANAGEMENT

(M0810) Patient Management of Equipment (includes <u>ONLY</u> oxygen, I.V./infusion therapy, enteral/parenteral nutrition equipment or supplies): <u>Patient's ability</u> to set up, monitor and change equipment reliably and safely, add appropriate fluids or medication, clean/store/dispose of equipment or supplies using proper technique. (NOTE: This refers to ability, not compliance or willingness.)
☐ 0 – Patient manages all tasks related to equipment completely independently.
☐ 1 – If someone else sets up equipment (i.e., fills portable oxygen tank, provides patient with prepared solutions), patient is able to manage all other aspects of equipment.

Using the OASIS-B1 form *(continued)*

☐ 2 – Patient requires considerable assistance from another person to manage equipment, but independently completes portions of the task.

☐ 3 – Patient is only able to monitor equipment (e.g., liter flow, fluid in bag) and must call someone else to manage the equipment.

☐ 4 – Patient is completely dependent on someone else to manage all equipment.

☒ NA – No equipment of this type used in care [**If NA, go to** *M0826*]

(M0820) Caregiver Management of Equipment (includes <u>ONLY</u> oxygen, I.V./infusion equipment, enteral/parenteral nutrition, ventilator therapy equipment or supplies): <u>Caregiver's ability</u> to set up, monitor, and change equipment reliably and safely, add appropriate fluids or medication, clean/store/dispose of equipment or supplies using proper technique. **(NOTE: This refers to ability, not compliance or willingness.)**

☐ 0 – Caregiver manages all tasks related to equipment completely independently.

☐ 1 – If someone else sets up equipment, caregiver is able to manage all other aspects.

☐ 2 – Caregiver requires considerable assistance from another person to manage equipment, but independently completes significant portions of task.

☐ 3 – Caregiver is only able to complete small portions of task (e.g., administer nebulizer treatment, clean/store/dispose of equipment or supplies).

☐ 4 – Caregiver is completely dependent on someone else to manage all equipment.

☐ NA – No caregiver

☐ UK – Unknown

THERAPY NEED

(M0826) Therapy Need: In the home health plan of care for the Medicare payment episode for which this assessment will define a case mix group, what is the indicated need for therapy visits (total of reasonable and necessary physical, occupational, and speech-language pathology visits combined)? **(Enter zero ["000"] if no therapy visits indicated.)**

(*0 0 0*) Number of therapy visits indicated (total of physical, occupational and speech-language pathology combined).

☒ NA – Not Applicable: No case mix group defined by this assessment.

EMERGENT CARE

(M0830) Emergent Care: Since the last time OASIS data were collected, has the patient utilized any of the following services for emergent care (other than home care agency services)? **(Mark all that apply.)**

☒ 0 – No emergent care services [**If no emergent care, go to** *M0855*]

☐ 1 – Hospital emergency room (includes 23-hour holding)

☐ 2 – Doctor's office emergency visit/house call

☐ 3 – Outpatient department/clinic emergency (includes urgicenter sites)

☐ UK – Unknown [**If UK, go to** *M0855*]

(M0840) Emergent Care Reason: For what reason(s) did the patient/family seek emergent care? **(Mark all that apply.)**

☐ 1 – Improper medication administration, medication side effects, toxicity, anaphylaxis

☐ 2 – Nausea, dehydration, malnutrition, constipation, impaction

☐ 3 – Injury caused by fall or accident at home

☐ 4 – Respiratory problems (e.g., shortness of breath, respiratory infection, tracheobronchial obstruction)

☐ 5 – Wound infection, deteriorating wound status, new lesion/ulcer

☐ 6 – Cardiac problems (e.g., fluid overload, exacerbation of CHF, chest pain)

☐ 7 – Hypo/Hyperglycemia, diabetes out of control

☐ 8 – GI bleeding, obstruction

☐ 9 – Other than above reasons

☐ UK – Reason unknown

DATA ITEMS COLLECTED AT INPATIENT FACILITY ADMISSION OR AGENCY DISCHARGE ONLY

(M0855) To which **Inpatient Facility** has the patient been admitted?

☐ 1 – Hospital [**Go to** *M0890*]

☐ 2 – Rehabilitation facility [**Go to** *M0903*]

☐ 3 – Nursing home [**Go to** *M0900*]

☐ 4 – Hospice [**Go to** *M0903*]

☒ NA – No inpatient facility admission

(continued)

Using the OASIS-B1 form *(continued)*

(M0870)   Discharge Disposition: Where is the patient after discharge from your agency? **(Choose only one answer.)**

- [X]   1 – Patient remained in the community (not in hospital, nursing home, or rehab facility)
- [ ]   2 – Patient transferred to a noninstitutional hospice [Go to *M0903*]
- [ ]   3 – Unknown because patient moved to a geographic location not served by this agency [Go to *M0903*]
- [ ]   UK – Other unknown [Go to *M0903*]

(M0880)   After discharge, does the patient receive health, personal, or support **Services or Assistance? (Mark all that apply.)**

- [ ]   1 – No assistance or services received
- [X]   2 – Yes, assistance or services provided by family or friends
- [X]   3 – Yes, assistance or services provided by other community resources (e.g., meals-on-wheels, home health services, homemaker assistance, transportation assistance, assisted living, board and care)

    [Go to M0903]

(M0890)   If the patient was admitted to an acute care **Hospital**, for what **Reason** was he/she admitted?

- [ ]   1 – Hospitalization for <u>emergent</u> (unscheduled) care
- [ ]   2 – Hospitalization for <u>urgent</u> (scheduled within 24 hours of admission) care
- [ ]   3 – Hospitalization for <u>elective</u> (scheduled more than 24 hours before admission) care
- [ ]   UK – Unknown

(M0895)   Reason for Hospitalization: **(Mark all that apply.)**

- [ ]   1 – Improper medication administration, medication side effects, toxicity, anaphylaxis
- [ ]   2 – Injury caused by fall or accident at home
- [ ]   3 – Respiratory problems (SOB, infection, obstruction)
- [ ]   4 – Wound or tube site infection, deteriorating wound status, new lesion/ulcer
- [ ]   5 – Hypo/Hyperglycemia, diabetes out of control
- [ ]   6 – GI bleeding, obstruction
- [ ]   7 – Exacerbation of CHF, fluid overload, heart failure
- [ ]   8 – Myocardial infarction, stroke
- [ ]   9 – Chemotherapy
- [ ]   10 – Scheduled surgical procedure
- [ ]   11 – Urinary tract infection
- [ ]   12 – I.V. catheter-related infection
- [ ]   13 – Deep vein thrombosis, pulmonary embolus
- [ ]   14 – Uncontrolled pain
- [ ]   15 – Psychotic episode
- [ ]   16 – Other than above reasons

    [Go to M0903]

(M0900)   For what **Reason(s)** was the patient **Admitted** to a **Nursing Home? (Mark all that apply.)**

- [ ]   1 – Therapy services
- [ ]   2 – Respite care
- [ ]   3 – Hospice care
- [ ]   4 – Permanent placement
- [ ]   5 – Unsafe for care at home
- [ ]   6 – Other
- [ ]   UK – Unknown

(M0903)   Date of Last (Most Recent) Home Visit:

    0 2 / 0 2 / 2 0 0 9
    month   day   year

(M0906)   Discharge/Transfer/Death Date: Enter the date of the discharge, transfer, or death (at home) of the patient.

    _ _ / _ _ / _ _ _ _
    month   day   year

Source: The Outcome and Assessment Information Set (OASIS) is the intellectual property of the Center for Health Services and Policy Research, Denver. Used with permission.

• Make sure the plan is comprehensive by including more than the patient's physiologic problems. Also chart about the home environment, the resources needed, and the attitudes of the patient, family, and caregiver.

• Document physical changes that must be made in the patient's home for him to receive proper care. Help the family find the resources to implement them.

• Describe the primary caregiver, including whether he lives with the patient, their relationship, his age and physical ability, and his willingness to help the patient. The patient's well-being may depend on this person's abilities.

• Show in your documentation how you made the most of the patient's strengths and resources. Strengths include support systems, good health habits and coping behaviors, a safe and healthful environment, and financial security. Resources include the doctor, pharmacy, and medical equipment supplier.

• Document patient teaching given and the patient's or caregiver's response.

• Continually identify progress toward goals. If the patient isn't able to make progress, discharge may be considered.

• If the patient is homebound, make sure this is documented at every visit and state the reason why. Medicare requires a patient receiving skilled home care to be homebound; however, some commercial insurers don't.

• Make sure that documentation reflects consistent adherence by all caregivers to the care plan. Have caregivers demonstrate the procedures they use for the care they provide, and document their skill level.

• Keep the record updated, noting changes in the patient's condition or care plan, and document that you reported these changes to the doctor. Medicare, Medicaid, and certain other third-party payers won't reimburse for skilled services not reported to the doctor.

• Interdisciplinary care must be documented on an ongoing basis. Collaboration on patient care problems and changes to the care plan are described in detail on the patient's chart.

With each visit, you should add a new progress note to your records.

Progress notes

The home care progress note, as with notes in the acute care setting, is a place to document the patient's condition and significant events that occur while he's under your care. The progress note is written in chronological order based on each home visit. (See *Progress note*, page 277.)

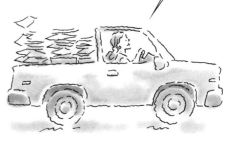

Art of the chart

The care plan is individualized for each patient. An example of an interdisciplinary care plan, on which other providers also record notes, is shown below.

> Note that this care plan is focused on patient problems.

Patient name:	Mary Long	Init. cert. period: _____
		Recert period #1: _____
Primary nurse:	N. Smith, RN	Init. cert. period: _____

PROBLEM	GOAL	APPROACH	INITIAL CERT	RECERT #1	RECERT #2
Atrial fibrillation (2/20/09)	Maintain optimal cardiac output.	1. Meds as ordered 2. Monitor vs, inc. apical rhythm and rate 3. Observe for chest pain, dyspnea, palpitations, anxiety, etc.	GOAL MET? Y N INIT:_____	GOAL MET? Y N INIT:_____	GOAL MET? Y N INIT:_____
Heart failure (2/26/09)	1. Maintain fluid and electrolyte balance. 2. Promote optimal gas exchange.	1. Meds as ordered 2. Nebulizer as ordered 3. Draw labs as ordered 4. I & O daily 5. Monitor edema 6. ✔ for shortness of breath, dyspnea, congestion (lung sounds) 7. amb. as tol 8. semi Fowler's when sitting	GOAL MET? Y N INIT:_____	GOAL MET? Y N INIT:_____	GOAL MET? Y N INIT:_____
Gastrostomy tube insertion (2/28/09)	1. Maintain optimal nutritional status. 2. Prevent skin breakdown.	1. Magnacal 80 ml per hr 2. Follow G-tube protocol, including site care & oral hygiene. 3. Weekly weights 4. I&O daily 5. ✔ for N/V, diarrhea	GOAL MET? Y N INIT:_____	GOAL MET? Y N INIT:_____	GOAL MET? Y N INIT:_____

> Set realistic goals.

Intervention Codes
(please circle all that apply)

A1. Skilled observation
A2. Foley insertion
A3. Bladder installation
A4. Irrigation care (wd. dsg.)
A5. Irrigation decub. care - meds.
A6. Venipuncture
A7. Restorative nursing
A8. Postcataract care
A9. Bowel/Bladder training

A10. Chest physical (incl. postural drainage)
A11. Administer vit. B_{12}
A12. Prepare/Administer insulin
A13. Administer other
A14. Administer I.V.
A15. Teach ostomy care
A16. Teach nasogastric feeding
A17. Reposition nasogastric feeding tube

A18. Teach gastrostomy
A19. Teach parenteral nutrition
A20. Teach care of trach
A21. Administer care of trach
A22. Teach inhalation Rx
A23. Administer inhalation Rx
A24. Teach administration of injections
A25. Teach diabetic care
A26. Disimpaction/enema
A27. Other
    Foot care (diabetic)
    Teach diet

Teach disease process
Teach use of O_2
Instruct re: Medication child
A28. Wound care/dsg - closed
A29. Decubitus care - simple
A30. Teach care of indwelling catheter
A31. Management and evaluation of patient care plan
A32. Teaching and training (other)

> Interventions are coded to allow for rapid documentation.

Work in progress

Every time you visit a patient, you must write a progress note. These notes document:
• changes in the patient's condition
• skilled nursing interventions you performed related to the care plan
• the patient's responses to the interventions
• events or incidents in the home that might affect the treatment plan
• patient's vital signs and pain assessment
• what you taught the patient and caregiver, including written instructional materials and brochures
• communication with other team members since the previous visit
• discharge plans
• time you arrived in the home and time you left the home.

Guidelines for use

The guidelines here will help you chart safely and efficiently on progress notes:
• Chart all events in chronological order.
• Avoid addendums.
• Provide a heading for each entry because many members of the health care team use the progress notes.
• Use flow sheets and checklists to record vital signs, intake and output measurements, and nutritional data. Encourage the patient or caregiver to fill out these forms when appropriate to get him involved and increase his feeling of control.

Art of the chart

Progress note

Use this sample progress note as a guide when charting in home care settings.

Date	Problem no.	Problem title — subjective, objective, assessment, plan
2/6/09	#2	A: ① foot stasis ulcer showing no improvement in size or amount of drainage since 2/1/09
		P: Dr. T. Miller notified. Wound culture ordered and collected; sent specimen to lab
		————————————— M. A. Ford, RN

• When possible, take time to complete your charting in the home while the patient sleeps or is otherwise occupied.

• Involve the patient in his own care and documentation by making statements like, "Here's what I've written about how your wound is healing. Is there anything else you want me to put in the notes?"

• If the patient has a medical emergency while you're there, contact emergency medical services and stay until the paramedics take over. Call the doctor for transport orders. Notify your supervisor, who'll arrange coverage for your other patients, if necessary. Record all assessments and interventions performed until you're relieved. Note the date and time of transfer and the name of the caregiver who assumes responsibility.

Patient teaching

Correct documentation will help justify to your agency and to third-party payers your visits to teach the patient or caregiver. Find out about the patient's and family's needs, resources, and support systems to help you outline the basic teaching plan.

Keeping continuity

Remember that teaching is usually an ongoing process requiring more than one visit. Until the patient becomes independent, your documentation will help other nurses continue the teaching and identify additional areas of teaching. (See *Certification of instruction.*)

Keep a list of teaching and reference materials you have supplied to the patient or caregiver. Also document modifications made to accommodate the patient's or caregiver's literacy skills and native language.

Being there

If the patient isn't physically or mentally able to perform the skills himself and no caregiver is available, report this in your documentation. The patient most likely isn't an appropriate candidate for home care. Never leave a patient alone to perform a procedure until he can express understanding of it and perform it competently.

Setting the terms (on the packages)

Be careful to call equipment by the same names used on the packages and in teaching literature. Consider providing a glossary of terms and labeling machines to match your instructions. Make sure that the patient can identify devices when speaking on the telephone. Document all teaching materials given to the patient,

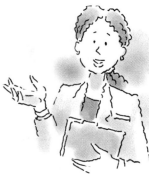

Be there for a patient until he can perform a procedure adequately on his own.

Art of the chart

Certification of instruction

The model patient-teaching form below shows what was taught to a home-care patient with an I.V. catheter. This type of form will help you document your teaching sessions clearly and completely.

CONTENT (check all that apply; fill in blanks as indicated)

1. ☐ Reason for therapy

2. Drug/Solution
   - ☐ Dose
   - ☐ Schedule
   - ☐ Label accuracy
   - ☐ Storage
   - ☐ Container integrity

3. Aseptic technique
   - ☐ Hand washing
   - ☐ Prepping caps/connections
   - ☐ Tubing/cap/needs
   - ☐ Needless adaptor changes

4. Access device maintenance
   Type/Name: _____
   - ☒ Device/Site Inspection
   - ☐ Site care/Dsg. changes
   - ☐ Catheter clamping
   - ☒ Maintaining patency
     - ☒ Saline flushing
     - ☐ Heparin locking
     - ☐ Fdg. Tube /declogging
     - ☐ Self insertion of device

5. Drug preparation
   - ☒ Premixed containers
   - ☐ Compounding
   - ☐ Client additives
   - ☐ Piggyback lipids

This document helps ensure continuity of patient teaching.

6. Method of administration
   - ☐ Gravity
   - ☒ Pump (name): _CADD pump_
   - ☐ Continuous   ☒ Intermittent
   - ☐ Cycle/Taper:

7. Administration technique
   - ☒ Pump rate/calibration
   - ☐ Priming tubing   ☐ Filter
   - ☐ Filling syringe
   - ☐ Loading pump
   - ☒ Access device hookup/disconnect

8. Potential complications/Adverse effects
   - ☐ Patient drug information sheet reviewed
   - ☒ Pump alarms/troubleshooting
   - ☒ Phlebitis/infiltration
   - ☐ Clotting/dislodgment
   - ☒ Infection   ☐ Air embolus
   - ☐ Breakage/cracking
   - ☐ Electrolyte imbalance
   - ☐ Fluid balance
   - ☐ Glucose intolerance
   - ☐ Aspiration
   - ☐ N / V / D / Cramping
   - ☐ Other: _____

9. Self-monitoring:
   - ☐ Weight   ☒ Temperature   ☐ P   ☐ PB
   - ☐ Urine S & A   ☐ Fingersticks
   - ☐ Other: _____

10. Supply handling/disposal
    - ☒ Disposal of sharps/supplies ☐ Opioids
    - ☐ Cleaning pump
    - ☒ Changing batteries
    - ☐ Blood/fluid precautions
    - ☐ Chemo/spill precautions

11. Information given to client re:
    - ☐ Pharmacy counseling
    - ☐ Advance directives
    - ☐ Inventory checks _____
    - ☐ Deliveries
    - ☒ 24-hour on-call staff _____
    - ☒ Reimbursement _____
    - ☐ Service complaints _____

12. Safety/Disaster plan
    - ☐ Back up pump batteries _____
    - ☒ Emergency room use _____
    - ☐ Electrical _____
    - ☒ Disaster _____
    - ☐ Other: _____

13. Written instructions
    - ☒ Yes ☐ No If, no why? _____

☐ Client or caregiver demonstrates or verbalizes competency to perform home infusion therapy.

COMMENTS: _Wife incorrectly changed pump battery. Procedure reviewed. Wife then demonstrated correct procedure. Wife also concerned about frequency of dressing changes. Access site nonreddened and not edematous. Protocol reviewed. Pt states he is satisfied with waiting until scheduled dressing change tomorrow._

The form provides room to comment and document individual instructions.

Theory/Skill reviewed/Return demonstration completed:

Chris Banner, RN _____   2/14/09
Signature of RN Educator   **Date**

CERTIFICATION OF INSTRUCTION

I agree that I have been instructed as described above and understand that the above functions will be performed in the home by myself and caregiver, outside a hospital or medically supervised environment.

Robert Burns _____   2/14/09
Client/Caregiver signature   **Date**

In this part of the form, the patient acknowledges responsibility for self-care activities.

and keep copies of teaching materials in your records. You may want to videotape your instructions in the home if more than one caregiver will be providing care.

Signing off

Most agencies require patients to sign a teaching documentation record indicating that they accept responsibility for learning self-care activities. This documentation is a critical piece of the home care chart.

Nursing and discharge summaries

As a home health nurse, you must submit a regular patient progress report to the attending doctor and the reimburser to confirm the need for continuing services. You must also complete a summary of the patient's progress and a discharge summary.

Summing it all up

When writing a summary of the patient's progress, include:
• current problems, treatments, interventions, and instructions
• home care provided by other health care professionals, such as a physical therapist or speech pathologist
• the reason for a change in services
• patient outcomes and responses—physical and emotional—to the services provided
• discharge plan.

Guidelines for use

You'll prepare a discharge summary to get the doctor's approval to discharge a patient, to notify third-party payers that services have been terminated, and to officially close the case. The discharge summary also serves as a brief history for quick review if the patient is readmitted at a later date.

When writing these summaries, record:
• time frame covered
• services provided and the names and titles of assigned staff
• clinical and psychosocial conditions of the patient at discharge
• recommendations for further care
• caregiver involvement in care
• interruptions in home care such as readmissions to the hospital
• referrals to community agencies
• OASIS discharge information
• patient's response to and comprehension of patient-teaching efforts
• outcomes attained.

> In your summary of the patient's progress, document his physical and emotional responses to care.

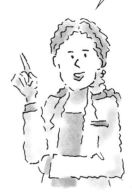

Medicare-mandated forms

CMS, the federal watchdog agency that oversees Medicare and Medicaid programs, requires home health agencies that receive Medicare funding to standardize their record keeping and documentation methods. Home health agencies must maintain the following forms for each qualified Medicare recipient:
- OASIS
- home health certification and plan of care (see *Home Health Certification and Plan of Care form*, page 282)
- medical update and patient information (see *Medical Update and Patient Information form*, page 283)
- notice of nondiscrimination
- privacy notice.

Doctor calls

In addition, home care nurses must document a doctor's telephone orders. The Joint Commission requires that you write the doctor's order verbatim, note the date and time, and write "V.T.O." (verified telephone order) on the order form, which means that you read back the order and received confirmation that it's correct. (See *Doctor's telephone orders*.)

Fill out and sign, please...

Medicare, via the fiscal intermediary, won't pay unless the required forms are properly completed, signed, and submitted. Forms are usually filled out by the nurse assigned to the patient, although some agencies have an admission team and a care team.

Future developments

Several major trends are emerging as the home health care industry continues to evolve:
- More private insurers require preauthorization for home health care services, which increases the paperwork burden for nurses.
- Fewer visits per episode of care are allowed. More focused reimbursement will dramatically alter the amount of home care patients will receive.
- The depth and breadth of federal regulations have placed increasing demands on care providers, and agencies will need to computerize record keeping.
- Telehealth technology is being used by home health agencies to monitor patients in their homes via telephone lines. Nurses

(Text continues on page 284.)

Art of the chart

Home Health Certification and Plan of Care form

The form below is the official form for authorizing Medicare coverage for home care (also known as form 485). It includes space for assessing functional abilities and documenting care plan information.

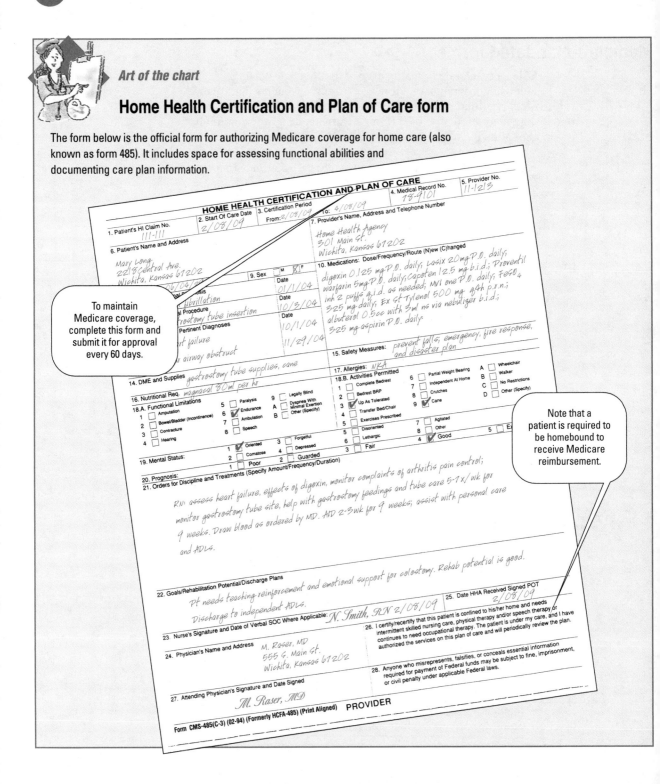

To maintain Medicare coverage, complete this form and submit it for approval every 60 days.

Note that a patient is required to be homebound to receive Medicare reimbursement.

Art of the chart

Medical Update and Patient Information form

To continue providing reimbursable skilled nursing care to a patient at home, Medicare requires you to complete the Medical Update and Patient Information form (also known as form 486).

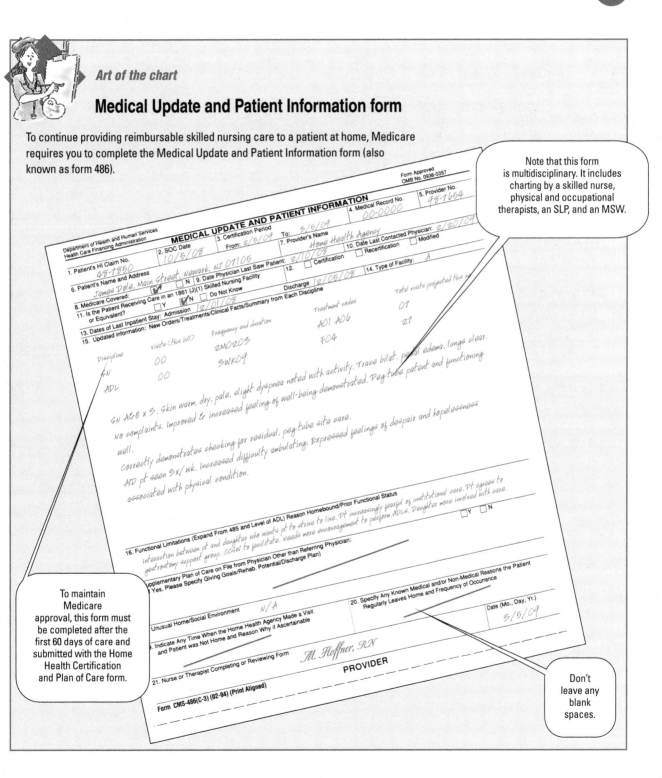

Note that this form is multidisciplinary. It includes charting by a skilled nurse, physical and occupational therapists, an SLP, and an MSW.

To maintain Medicare approval, this form must be completed after the first 60 days of care and submitted with the Home Health Certification and Plan of Care form.

Don't leave any blank spaces.

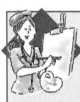

Art of the chart

Doctor's telephone orders

Home health nurses rely heavily on the use of telephone orders. The agency must follow guidelines established by the Centers for Medicare and Medicaid Services and The Joint Commission for taking and documenting these orders. Below is an example of a form used by one agency to fulfill documentation requirements.

Facility name		Address	
Suburban Home Health Agency		*123 Main Street*	
Last name	**First name**	**Attending doctor**	**Admission no.**
Smith	*Kevin*	*Dr. Michael Baker*	*141-111-471*

Date ordered	Date discontinued	ORDERS
2/10/09	*2/13/09*	*Tylenol 650 mg P.O. q 6h p.r.n*

> The order must be signed by the doctor within 48 hours.

Signature of nurse receiving order	Time	Signature of doctor	Date
V.T.O/ Mary Reo, RN	*1820*		

are able to help patients with chronic conditions using twice-per-week "visits" to identify the need for or help avoid hospitalization. Telehealth offers an ideal way to care for patients at home.

One predicted outcome: More reliance on outcomes

Increased reliance on disease-specific management programs will eventually lead to the use of critical pathways that incorporate patient outcomes in home health care. Both CMS and The Joint Commission are focused on outcomes. State departments of health services surveyors also have access to data. In addition, an agency's data are compared with data from similar agencies.

Blazing new trails with computers — Yee-ha!

Increasingly, home health care nurses are using laptop computers or handheld devices equipped with software designed to speed clinical documentation. Many of these programs are designed to help nurses develop a care plan, formulate goals, monitor patient progress, update medications, and generate visit notes.

This technology expedites the exchange of data between care providers and third-party payers. Nurses inexperienced in using computers should be aware that documentation may take longer until they adjust to the new equipment.

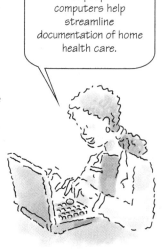

Laptop computers help streamline documentation of home health care.

Keeping it confidential

New technology raises new concerns about confidentiality. For example, e-mail and faxes can easily end up in the wrong hands. When using either method to transmit information about a patient, consider blacking out identifying data. Arrange for the recipient of a fax to wait at the other end for the fax to print.

Confidentiality when transmitting OASIS data on patients who aren't Medicare recipients continues to be a source of concern. Legislators and lawmakers will ultimately reconcile the parameters of government access to non-Medicare patients' clinical data.

In many cases, a home health agency will supply its nurses with laptop computers to streamline documentation. Laptop computers shouldn't be used by anyone other than agency personnel. You may be tempted to allow a computer-savvy spouse, friend, or child to add programs or manipulate data with all good intentions, but this is no more appropriate than it would be to let him read a patient's record. Finally, access to computer files should be protected by a password to prevent unauthorized individuals from entering files.

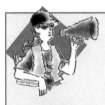

That's a wrap!

Home health care documentation review

The basics
You must become familiar with many forms unique to home care. For each visit, documentation includes:
• assessment
• interventions
• patient's treatment and response to treatment
• teaching and complications.

Legal risks and responsibilities
• Risks of poor documentation or inadequate documentation may result in a lawsuit or refusal by third-party payers to cover services.

Documentation guidelines
• Careful screening will determine what services the patient needs.
• Document activities completed during your nursing visits, including assessments, interventions, patient's response, and complications.
• Include evidence that the home environment is safe.
• Document emergency and resource numbers given to the patient or caregiver.
• Document the patient's or caregiver's ability to perform procedures, troubleshoot equipment, and recognize potential complications and respond appropriately.

Home health care forms
• *Agency assessment and OASIS forms* provide information on a thorough patient assessment needed to plan appropriate care.

• *A care plan* is required by professional standards and is the most direct evidence of your nursing judgment.
• *Progress notes* are written in chronological order and are the place to document the patient's condition and significant events that occur.
• *Patient teaching* is an ongoing process until the patient becomes independent. Correct documentation will help justify your visits.
• *Nursing and discharge summaries* are summaries of the patient's progress. A discharge summary must be submitted to the doctor and the reimburser.
• *Medicare-mandated forms* include an OASIS form, a Home Health Care Certification form, a care plan, and a Medical Update and Patient Information form.

Future developments
• Major charting trends continue to evolve, including preauthorization for services, fewer visits allowed per episode, increasing federal regulations, and use of telehealth technology.
• Increased reliance on disease-specific management programs can lead to critical pathways and outcomes incorporation.
• Laptop computers and handheld devices speed documentation and increase concerns about confidentiality.

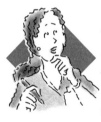

Quick quiz

1. Which agency requires standardized record keeping and documentation for Medicare recipients?
- A. The Joint Commission
- B. CMS
- C. CHAP
- D. CMC

Answer: B. CMS requires that documentation and record keeping be standardized for Medicare reimbursement.

2. Medicare requires that an OASIS patient assessment be completed within how many days from the initiation of care?
- A. 1 day
- B. 3 days
- C. 5 days
- D. 7 days

Answer: C. Patient assessment must be completed within 5 days of the initiation of care.

3. Changes in the patient's condition should be documented in:
- A. progress notes.
- B. intake and output record.
- C. order sheet.
- D. medication record.

Answer: A. Significant events that occur during your care of the patient should be documented in the progress notes.

4. What documentation form is the most legally direct evidence of your nursing judgment?
- A. Progress notes
- B. Order sheet
- C. Medication record
- D. Care plan

Answer: D. Legally speaking, the care plan is the most direct evidence of your nursing judgment.

Scoring

☆☆☆ If you answered all four questions correctly, relax on an island OASIS! You're home-free when it comes to documentation.

☆☆ If you answered three questions correctly, good for you! You meet all review requirements; now you can go on to the next chapter.

☆ If you answered fewer than three questions correctly, keep at it! You'll make better progress in the next chapter.

Long-term care

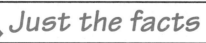

Just the facts

In this chapter, you'll learn:

♦ about agencies that regulate documentation in long-term care settings

♦ specific forms required in long-term care settings and how to complete them

♦ guidelines for correct documentation in long-term care.

A look at charting in long-term care

A long-term care facility provides continuing care for chronically ill or disabled patients. The purpose of care is to promote the highest level of functioning possible for the patient. Long-term care is an increasingly important form of health care delivery, especially because the elderly segment of the population is rapidly growing. (See *Elder power*, page 290.)

Maintaining accurate, complete documentation in long-term care is vital. Consider the following points:

• Long-term care facilities are highly regulated by state and federal agencies and therefore must adhere to high standards of documentation.

• Information in your records may be used to defend you and your facility in court.

• Your employer views documentation records as evidence of standardized, high-quality nursing care.

• Good record keeping ensures certification, licensure, reimbursement, and accreditation.

Elder power

According to the 2005 U.S. Census, 35.9 million people — 12% of the total population — were age 65 or older in 2003. Among the older population, 18.3 million people were ages 65 to 74, 12.9 million people were ages 75 to 84, and 4.7 million people were 85 or older. The older population will continue to increase; the older-than-85 population is estimated to reach 8.9 million by 2030.

Chances are, you're caring for many elderly patients right now. Studies show that people age 65 and older require health care services more often than any other age-group. Most older people have at least one chronic condition, and many have multiple conditions. That's why we need to increase focus on the needs of elderly patients, not only in long-term care but in all health care settings.

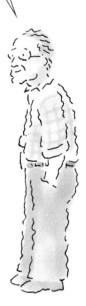

There's strength in numbers!

Documentation distinctions

Two key differences exist between documenting in long-term care settings and documenting in other settings:

Patients stay at long-term care facilities for weeks, months, or even years, so documentation isn't done as often, which takes the emphasis off charting and puts it on helping the patient relearn basic skills.

Some of the government forms used in long-term facilities are long and involved. So, even though charting isn't emphasized, it can still be extensive.

Categories of care

Long-term care facilities usually offer two levels of care: skilled and intermediate. The level of care administered to your patient should be your primary consideration when documenting.

Care may be complex...

In a skilled care facility, patient care involves specialized nursing skills, such as I.V. therapy, parenteral nutrition, respiratory care, and mechanical ventilation.

...or not so complex

An intermediate care facility deals with patients who have chronic illnesses and need less complex care. For example, they may simply need assistance with activities of daily living (ADLs), such as bathing and dressing.

Patients at both levels may need short- or long-term care and may move from one level to another according to their progress or decline. Living arrangements, geography, family and community support networks, and other factors determine the patient's length of stay.

Regulatory agencies

Documentation in long-term care facilities is regulated by federal and state agencies. Documentation is influenced by:
- federal programs, such as Medicare and Medicaid
- government agencies such as the Centers for Medicare and Medicaid Services (CMS)
- laws such as the Omnibus Budget Reconciliation Act (OBRA) of 1987
- state regulations for each facility
- accrediting agencies, such as The Joint Commission and the Commission for Accreditation for Rehabilitation Facilities (CARF).

Most elderly patients entering long-term care facilities pay for the services privately. When their funds become exhausted, they apply to Medicaid for coverage. If the patient requires services and is unable to pay initially, he can apply to receive Medicaid.

Medicare

Few of the services provided in long-term care facilities are eligible for Medicare reimbursement. However, Medicare does provide reimbursement for patients requiring skilled care, such as chemotherapy, tube feeding, and certain types of wound care. For these patients, Medicare requires certain minimum daily documentation to prove that a service was needed. If the patient's status changes, you must supply a revised care plan within 7 days.

Making reimbursement a reality

Be sure to document changes in status because a patient who isn't improving or expected to improve according to his care plan is ineligible for coverage. You must also document the need for new or continuing skilled services you provide. Medicare also requires documentation of your evaluations for expected outcomes.

According to Medicare guidelines, charting must clearly show that a patient needed care by a professional or technical staff member. To verify the need for skilled rehabilitative care, you must describe a reasonable expectation of improvement or services needed to establish a maintenance program. The amount, duration, and frequency of services must be reasonable and necessary.

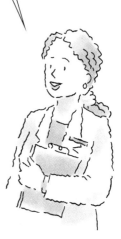

Medicare does cover some skilled services in long-term care, but daily documentation is required.

Medicaid

Most patients who receive skilled care in long-term care facilities either pay for it themselves or are on Medicaid. To ensure Medicaid reimbursement for these patients, document patient care once per day.

Reimbursement for intermediate care

To secure payment for patients receiving intermediate care, medications and treatments are documented daily. Document other types of care weekly, unless the patient's status changes and he requires a change in services. In this case, chart the change and document his status more frequently. Also, perform a monthly reevaluation for these patients and an evaluation of expected outcomes for all Medicaid patients.

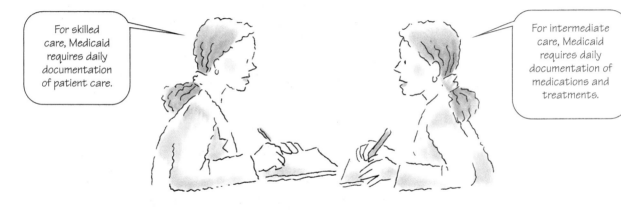

For skilled care, Medicaid requires daily documentation of patient care.

For intermediate care, Medicaid requires daily documentation of medications and treatments.

CMS

A branch of the Department of Health and Human Services, CMS regulates compliance with federal Medicare and Medicaid standards. CMS regulations are usually enforced at the state level.

To comply with CMS regulations, staff members at a long-term care facility must complete a lengthy form called the Minimum Data Set (MDS) for Resident Assessment and Care Screening, review the patient's status every 3 months, and perform a comprehensive reassessment annually.

OBRA

In 1987, Congress enacted OBRA, which imposed dozens of new requirements on long-term care facilities and home health agencies to protect the rights of patients receiving long-term care. OBRA requires that a comprehensive assessment be performed within 4 days of a patient's admission to a long-term care facility and then be charted on the MDS form. The assessment and care screening process must be reviewed every 3 months and repeated annually—more often if the patient's condition changes.

In addition, a comprehensive nursing assessment and a formulated care plan must be completed. The comprehensive care plan must be completed within 7 days of the completion of the MDS. This date may vary depending on whether it's a Medicare Prospective Payment System (PPS) or an intermediate assessment.

The Joint Commission

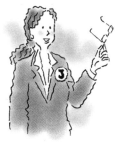

The Joint Commission accredits long-term care facilities using standards developed in conjunction with health care experts. Standard performance is documented in assessments, progress notes, care plans, and discharge plans. The ORYX initiative, begun in 1997, is another part of the accreditation process. It focuses on outcomes and other performance measurement data. The purpose of the initiative is to support quality improvements, not just in long-term care but in all health care organizations.

Forms used in long-term care

Many forms are used in acute care and home health care settings as well as in long-term care; others are used only in long-term care. Forms discussed in this chapter include:
* MDS
* Resident Assessment Protocol (RAP)
* Preadmission Screening and Annual Resident Review (PASARR)
* initial nursing assessment form
* nursing summaries
* ADL checklists or flow sheets
* care plans
* discharge and transfer forms.

In addition, many long-term care facilities have their own strict and comprehensive protocols. Typical protocols are those for bowel and bladder monitoring, physical and chemical restraints, safety, and infection control. Charting requirements when using these protocols vary, so check your facility's policies.

MDS

Mandated by OBRA, the MDS is a federal regulatory form that must be filled out for every patient admitted to a long-term care facility. (See *Minimum Data Set form.*)

The MDS form proves compliance with quality improvement and reimbursement requirements, standardizes information, and helps health care team members and agencies communicate. Doctors, nurses, social workers, and other staff members complete and sign different sections of the form.

The requirements for completion of the MDS vary with the type of admission. For skilled care residents under PPS, Medicare requires completion at these times:
- 5-day assessment
- 14-day assessment
- 30-day assessment
- 60-day assessment
- 90-day assessment
- readmission or return assessment.

For intermediate care residents, the MDS is completed at these times:
- admission assessment—required by day 14
- annual assessment
- significant change in status assessment
- quarterly review assessment—performed every 3 months.

A revised MDS — version 3.0 — will be in use beginning in 2009.

RAP

When an MDS form is completed, coded, computed, and processed, the patient's primary problems can be identified. These problems provide the basis for the patient's care plan. Another federally mandated form, the RAP summary, lists identified problem areas and documents the existence of a corresponding care plan. For example, if the patient has a stage II pressure ulcer documented in the MDS, the RAP summary indicates the need for a care plan to treat the pressure ulcer.

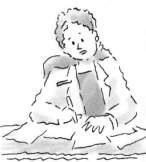

Here's the rap. The RAP summary documents patient problems and the existence of a care plan.

PASARR

For a patient to qualify for Medicare or Medicaid reimbursement, his mental status must also be documented. Federal regulations require that a long-term care facility performs a complete mental

(Text continues on page 304.)

Art of the chart

Minimum Data Set form

Patients in long-term care facilities that receive federal funds must have their health status evaluated at admission, and a care plan must be devised. The patient's health status and care plan are revised every 7 days.

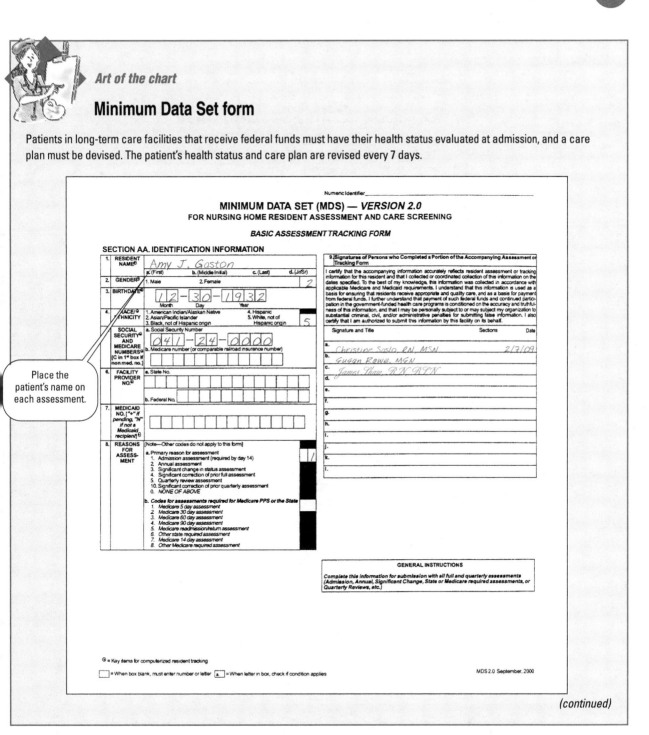

(continued)

Minimum Data Set form (continued)

Resident **Amy J. Gaston**   Numeric Identifier _____

MINIMUM DATA SET (MDS) — *VERSION 2.0*
FOR NURSING HOME RESIDENT ASSESSMENT AND CARE SCREENING
BACKGROUND (FACE SHEET) INFORMATION AT ADMISSION

The patient's name goes at the top of each page.

SECTION AB. DEMOGRAPHIC INFORMATION

1. DATE OF ENTRY — Date the stay began. Note — Does not include readmission if record was closed at time of temporary discharge to hospital, etc. In such cases, use prior admission date

`0 2` – `0 3` – `2 0 0 9`
Month   Day   Year

2. ADMITTED FROM (AT ENTRY)
1. Private home/apt. with no home health services
2. Private home/apt. with home health services
3. Board and care/assisted living/group home
4. Nursing home
5. Acute care hospital
6. Psychiatric hospital, MR/DD facility
7. Rehabilitation hospital
8. Other   `1`

3. LIVED ALONE (PRIOR TO ENTRY)
0. No
1. Yes
2. In other facility   `0`

4. ZIP CODE OF PRIOR PRIMARY RESIDENCE   `1 9 0 0 0`

5. RESIDENTIAL HISTORY 5 YEARS PRIOR TO ENTRY (Check all settings resident lived in during 5 years prior to date of entry given in item AB1 above)
- Prior stay at this nursing home   a.
- Stay in other nursing home   b.
- Other residential facility—board and care home, assisted living, group home   c.
- MH/psychiatric setting   d.
- MR/DD setting   e.
- NONE OF ABOVE   f. ✓

6. LIFETIME OCCUPATION(S) [Put "/" between two occupations]   `TEACHER`

7. EDUCATION (Highest Level Completed)
1. No schooling
2. 8th grade/less
3. 9-11 grades
4. High school
5. Technical or trade school
6. Some college
7. Bachelor's degree
8. Graduate degree   `8`

8. LANGUAGE (Code for correct response)
a. Primary Language
0. English   1. Spanish   2. French   3. Other   `0`
b. If other, specify

9. MENTAL HEALTH HISTORY — Does resident's RECORD indicate any history of mental retardation, mental illness, or developmental disability problem?
0. No   1. Yes   `0`

10. CONDITIONS RELATED TO MR/DD STATUS (Check all conditions that are related to MR/DD status that were manifested before age 22, and are likely to continue indefinitely)
- Not applicable—no MR/DD (Skip to AB11)   a. ✓
- MR/DD with organic condition   b.
- Down's syndrome   c.
- Autism   d.
- Epilepsy   e.
- Other organic condition related to MR/DD   f.
- MR/DD with no organic condition

11. DATE BACKGROUND INFORMATION COMPLETED

`0 2` – `0 7` – `2 0 0 9`
Month   Day   Year

SECTION AC. CUSTOMARY ROUTINE

1. CUSTOMARY ROUTINE (Check all that apply. If all information UNKNOWN, check last box only)
(In year prior to DATE OF ENTRY to this nursing home, or year last in community if now being admitted from another nursing home)

CYCLE OF DAILY EVENTS
- Stays up late at night (e.g., after 9 pm)   a.
- Naps regularly during day (at least 1 hour)   b. ✓
- Goes out 1+ days a week   c.
- Stays busy with hobbies, reading, or fixed daily routine   d. ✓
- Spends most of time alone or watching TV   e.
- Moves independently indoors (with appliances, if used)   f.
- Use of tobacco products at least daily   g.
- NONE OF ABOVE   h.

EATING PATTERNS
- Distinct food preferences   i.
- Eats between meals all or most days   j. ✓
- Use of alcoholic beverage(s) at least weekly   k.
- NONE OF ABOVE   l.

ADL PATTERNS
- In bedclothes much of day   m.
- Wakens to toilet all or most nights   n. ✓
- Has irregular bowel movement pattern   o.
- Showers for bathing   p.
- Bathing in PM   q. ✓
- NONE OF ABOVE   r.

INVOLVEMENT PATTERNS
- Daily contact with relatives/close friends   s. ✓
- Usually attends church, temple, synagogue (etc.)   t.
- Finds strength in faith   u. ✓
- Daily animal companion/presence   v.
- Involved in group activities   w.
- NONE OF ABOVE   x.
- UNKNOWN—Resident/family unable to provide information   y.

Use check marks to identify relevant information.

SECTION AD. FACE SHEET SIGNATURES

SIGNATURES OF PERSONS COMPLETING FACE SHEET:

a. *Christine Saslo, RN, MSN*
Signature of RN Assessment Coordinator   Date
James Shaw, RN, BSN 2/07/09

I certify that the accompanying information accurately reflects resident assessment or tracking information for this resident and that I collected or coordinated collection of this information on the dates specified. To the best of my knowledge, this information was collected in accordance with applicable Medicare and Medicaid requirements. I understand that this information is used as a basis for ensuring that residents receive appropriate and quality care, and as a basis for payment from federal funds. I further understand that payment of such federal funds and continued participation in the government-funded health care programs is conditioned on the accuracy and truthfulness of this information, and that I may be personally subject to or may subject my organization to substantial criminal, civil, and/or administrative penalties for submitting false information. I also certify that I am authorized to submit this information by this facility on its behalf.

Signature and Title	Sections	Date
b.		
c. *Susan Rowe, MSN 2/07/09*		
d.		
e.		
f.		
g.		

☐ = When box blank, must enter number or letter   `a.` = When letter in box, check if condition applies

MDS 2.0 September, 2000

Minimum Data Set form (continued)

Resident **Amy J. Gaston**   Numeric Identifier _____

MINIMUM DATA SET (MDS) — VERSION 2.0
FOR NURSING HOME RESIDENT ASSESSMENT AND CARE SCREENING
FULL ASSESSMENT FORM
(Status in last 7 days, unless other time frame indicated)

SECTION A. IDENTIFICATION AND BACKGROUND INFORMATION

1. RESIDENT NAME
Amy / J. / Gaston
a. (First)   b. (Middle Initial)   c. (Last)   d. (Jr/Sr)

2. ROOM NUMBER — 402

3. ASSESSMENT REFERENCE DATE
a. Last day of MDS observation period
02 - 07 - 2009
Month Day Year
b. Original (0) or corrected copy of form (enter number of correction)

4a. DATE OF REENTRY Date of reentry from most recent temporary discharge to a hospital in last 90 days (or since last assessment or admission if less than 90 days)
Month — Day — Year

5. MARITAL STATUS
1. Never married   3. Widowed   5. Divorced
2. Married   4. Separated   — 3

6. MEDICAL RECORD NO. — MM00099 22681

7. CURRENT PAYMENT SOURCES FOR N.H. STAY (Billing Office to indicate; check all that apply in last 30 days)
- Medicaid per diem — a.
- Medicare per diem — b. X
- Medicare ancillary part A — c.
- Medicare ancillary part B — d.
- CHAMPUS per diem — e.
- VA per diem — f.
- Self or family pays for full per diem — g. X
- Medicaid resident liability or Medicare co-payment — h.
- Private insurance per diem (including co-payment) — i.
- Other per diem — j.

8. REASONS FOR ASSESSMENT
a. Primary reason for assessment
1. Admission assessment (required by day 14)
2. Annual assessment
3. Significant change in status assessment
4. Significant correction of prior full assessment
5. Quarterly review assessment
6. Discharged—return not anticipated
7. Discharged—return anticipated
8. Discharged prior to completing initial assessment
9. Reentry
10. Significant correction of prior quarterly assessment
0. NONE OF ABOVE   — 1

[Note—If this is a discharge or reentry assessment, only a limited subset of MDS items need be completed]

b. Codes for assessments required for Medicare PPS or the State
1. Medicare 5 day assessment
2. Medicare 30 day assessment
3. Medicare 60 day assessment
4. Medicare 90 day assessment
5. Medicare readmission/return assessment
6. Other state required assessment
7. Medicare 14 day assessment
8. Other Medicare required assessment

9. RESPONSIBILITY/ LEGAL GUARDIAN (Check all that apply)
- Legal guardian — a.
- Other legal oversight — b.
- Durable power of attorney/health care — c. X
- Durable power attorney/financial — d.
- Family member responsible — e.
- Patient responsible for self — f.
- NONE OF ABOVE — g.

10. ADVANCED DIRECTIVES (For those items with supporting documentation in the medical record, check all that apply)
- Living will — a. X
- Do not resuscitate — b.
- Do not hospitalize — c.
- Organ donation — d.
- Autopsy request — e.
- Feeding restrictions — f.
- Medication restrictions — g.
- Other treatment restrictions — h.
- NONE OF ABOVE — i.

SECTION B. COGNITIVE PATTERNS

1. COMATOSE (Persistent vegetative state/no discernible consciousness)
0. No   1. Yes   (If yes, skip to Section G) — 0

2. MEMORY (Recall of what was learned or known)
a. Short-term memory OK—seems/appears to recall after 5 minutes
0. Memory OK   1. Memory problem — 1
b. Long-term memory OK—seems/appears to recall long past
0. Memory OK   1. Memory problem — 1

3. MEMORY/ RECALL ABILITY (Check all that resident was normally able to recall during last 7 days)
- Current season — a.
- Location of own room — b.
- Staff names/faces — c.
- That he/she is in a nursing home — d.
- NONE OF ABOVE are recalled — e. X

4. COGNITIVE SKILLS FOR DAILY DECISION-MAKING (Made decisions regarding tasks of daily life)
0. INDEPENDENT—decisions consistent/reasonable
1. MODIFIED INDEPENDENCE—some difficulty in new situations only
2. MODERATELY IMPAIRED—decisions poor; cues/supervision required
3. SEVERELY IMPAIRED—never/rarely made decisions   — 2

5. INDICATORS OF DELIRIUM—PERIODIC DISORDERED THINKING/ AWARENESS (Code for behavior in the last 7 days.) [Note: Accurate assessment requires conversations with staff and family who have direct knowledge of resident's behavior over this time].
0. Behavior not present
1. Behavior present, not of recent onset
2. Behavior present, over last 7 days appears different from resident's usual functioning (e.g., new onset or worsening)
a. EASILY DISTRACTED—(e.g., difficulty paying attention; gets sidetracked) — 1
b. PERIODS OF ALTERED PERCEPTION OR AWARENESS OF SURROUNDINGS—(e.g., moves lips or talks to someone not present; believes he/she is somewhere else; confuses night and day) — 0
c. EPISODES OF DISORGANIZED SPEECH—(e.g., speech is incoherent, nonsensical, irrelevant, or rambling from subject to subject; loses train of thought) — 0
d. PERIODS OF RESTLESSNESS—(e.g., fidgeting or picking at skin, clothing, napkins, etc; frequent position changes; repetitive physical movements or calling out) — 0
e. PERIODS OF LETHARGY—(e.g., sluggishness; staring into space; difficult to arouse; little body movement) — 0
f. MENTAL FUNCTION VARIES OVER THE COURSE OF THE DAY—(e.g., sometimes better, sometimes worse; behaviors sometimes present, sometimes not) — 0

6. CHANGE IN COGNITIVE STATUS Resident's cognitive status, skills, or abilities have changed as compared to status of 90 days ago (or since last assessment if less than 90 days)
0. No change   1. Improved   2. Deteriorated — 0

SECTION C. COMMUNICATION/HEARING PATTERNS

1. HEARING (With hearing appliance, if used)
0. HEARS ADEQUATELY—normal talk, TV, phone
1. MINIMAL DIFFICULTY when not in quiet setting
2. HEARS IN SPECIAL SITUATIONS ONLY—speaker has to adjust tonal quality and speak distinctly
3. HIGHLY IMPAIRED/absence of useful hearing — 1

2. COMMUNICATION DEVICES/ TECHNIQUES (Check all that apply during last 7 days)
- Hearing aid, present and used — a.
- Hearing aid, present and not used regularly — b.
- Other receptive comm. techniques used (e.g., lip reading) — c.
- NONE OF ABOVE — d. X

3. MODES OF EXPRESSION (Check all used by resident to make needs known)
- Speech — a. X
- Writing messages to express or clarify needs — b.
- American sign language or Braille — c.
- Signs/gestures/sounds — d.
- Communication board — e.
- Other — f.
- NONE OF ABOVE — g.

4. MAKING SELF UNDERSTOOD (Expressing information content—however able)
0. UNDERSTOOD
1. USUALLY UNDERSTOOD—difficulty finding words or finishing thoughts
2. SOMETIMES UNDERSTOOD—ability is limited to making concrete requests
3. RARELY/NEVER UNDERSTOOD — 1

5. SPEECH CLARITY (Code for speech in the last 7 days)
0. CLEAR SPEECH—distinct, intelligible words
1. UNCLEAR SPEECH—slurred, mumbled words
2. NO SPEECH—absence of spoken words — 0

6. ABILITY TO UNDERSTAND OTHERS (Understanding verbal information content—however able)
0. UNDERSTANDS
1. USUALLY UNDERSTANDS—may miss some part/intent of message
2. SOMETIMES UNDERSTANDS—responds adequately to simple, direct communication
3. RARELY/NEVER UNDERSTANDS — 2

7. CHANGE IN COMMUNICATION/ HEARING Resident's ability to express, understand, or hear information has changed as compared to status of 90 days ago (or since last assessment if less than 90 days)
0. No change   1. Improved   2. Deteriorated — 0

☐ = When box blank, must enter number or letter   a̲ = When letter in box, check if condition applies

MDS 2.0 September, 2000

This section is for your assessment of the patient's mental status.

(continued)

Minimum Data Set form (continued)

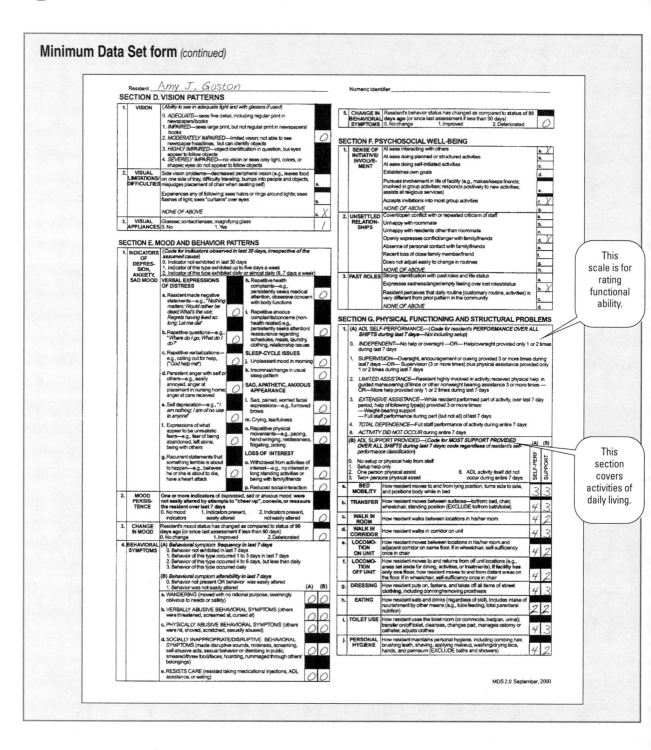

Resident **Amy J. Gaston**   Numeric Identifier _____

SECTION D. VISION PATTERNS

1. VISION *(Ability to see in adequate light and with glasses if used)*
0. ADEQUATE—sees fine detail, including regular print in newspapers/books
1. IMPAIRED—sees large print, but not regular print in newspapers/books
2. MODERATELY IMPAIRED—limited vision; not able to see newspaper headlines, but can identify objects
3. HIGHLY IMPAIRED—object identification in question, but eyes appear to follow objects
4. SEVERELY IMPAIRED—no vision or sees only light, colors, or shapes; eyes do not appear to follow objects   → **0**

2. VISUAL LIMITATIONS/ DIFFICULTIES
a. Side vision problems—decreased peripheral vision (e.g., leaves food on one side of tray, difficulty traveling, bumps into people and objects, misjudges placement of chair when seating self)
b. Experiences any of following: sees halos or rings around lights; sees flashes of light; sees "curtains" over eyes
c. NONE OF ABOVE → **X**

3. VISUAL APPLIANCES Glasses; contact lenses; magnifying glass 0. No 1. Yes → **1**

SECTION E. MOOD AND BEHAVIOR PATTERNS

1. INDICATORS OF DEPRESSION, ANXIETY, SAD MOOD *(Code for indicators observed in last 30 days, irrespective of the assumed cause)*
0. Indicator not exhibited in last 30 days
1. Indicator of this type exhibited up to five days a week
2. Indicator of this type exhibited daily or almost daily (6, 7 days a week)

VERBAL EXPRESSIONS OF DISTRESS
a. Resident made negative statements—e.g., "Nothing matters; Would rather be dead; What's the use; Regrets having lived so long; Let me die" → **0**
b. Repetitive questions—e.g., "Where do I go; What do I do?" → **0**
c. Repetitive verbalizations—e.g., calling out for help, ("God help me") → **0**
d. Persistent anger with self or others—e.g., easily annoyed, anger at placement in nursing home; anger at care received → **0**
e. Self deprecation—e.g., "I am nothing; I am of no use to anyone" → **0**
f. Expressions of what appear to be unrealistic fears—e.g., fear of being abandoned, left alone, being with others → **0**
g. Recurrent statements that something terrible is about to happen—e.g., believes he or she is about to die, have a heart attack

h. Repetitive health complaints—e.g., persistently seeks medical attention, obsessive concern with body functions → **0**
i. Repetitive anxious complaints/concerns (non-health related)—e.g., persistently seeks attention/reassurance regarding schedules, meals, laundry, clothing, relationship issues

SLEEP-CYCLE ISSUES
j. Unpleasant mood in morning → **0**
k. Insomnia/change in usual sleep pattern → **0**

SAD, APATHETIC, ANXIOUS APPEARANCE
l. Sad, pained, worried facial expressions—e.g., furrowed brows → **0**
m. Crying, tearfulness → **0**
n. Repetitive physical movements—e.g., pacing, hand wringing, restlessness, fidgeting, picking → **0**

LOSS OF INTEREST
o. Withdrawal from activities of interest—e.g., no interest in long standing activities or being with family/friends
p. Reduced social interaction

2. MOOD PERSISTENCE One or more indicators of depressed, sad or anxious mood were not easily altered by attempts to "cheer up," console, or reassure the resident over last 7 days
0. No mood indicators 1. Indicators present, easily altered 2. Indicators present, not easily altered

3. CHANGE IN MOOD Resident's mood status has changed as compared to status of 90 days ago (or since last assessment if less than 90 days)
0. No change 1. Improved 2. Deteriorated → **0**

4. BEHAVIORAL SYMPTOMS
(A) Behavioral symptom frequency in last 7 days
0. Behavior not exhibited in last 7 days
1. Behavior of this type occurred 1 to 3 days in last 7 days
2. Behavior of this type occurred 4 to 6 days, but less than daily
3. Behavior of this type occurred daily
(B) Behavioral symptom alterability in last 7 days
0. Behavior not present OR behavior was easily altered
1. Behavior was not easily altered

	(A)	(B)
a. WANDERING (moved with no rational purpose, seemingly oblivious to needs or safety)	0	0
b. VERBALLY ABUSIVE BEHAVIORAL SYMPTOMS (others were threatened, screamed at, cursed at)	0	0
c. PHYSICALLY ABUSIVE BEHAVIORAL SYMPTOMS (others were hit, shoved, scratched, sexually abused)	0	0
d. SOCIALLY INAPPROPRIATE/DISRUPTIVE BEHAVIORAL SYMPTOMS (made disruptive sounds, noisiness, screaming, self-abusive acts, sexual behavior or disrobing in public, smeared/threw food/feces, hoarding, rummaged through others' belongings)	0	0
e. RESISTS CARE (resisted taking medications/ injections, ADL assistance, or eating)	0	0

5. CHANGE IN BEHAVIORAL SYMPTOMS Resident's behavior status has changed as compared to status of 90 days ago (or since last assessment if less than 90 days) 0. No change 1. Improved 2. Deteriorated → **0**

SECTION F. PSYCHOSOCIAL WELL-BEING

> This scale is for rating functional ability.

1. SENSE OF INITIATIVE/ INVOLVEMENT
a. At ease interacting with others → **X**
b. At ease doing planned or structured activities
c. At ease doing self-initiated activities
d. Establishes own goals
e. Pursues involvement in life of facility (e.g., makes/keeps friends; involved in group activities; responds positively to new activities; assists at religious services)
f. Accepts invitations into most group activities → **X**
g. NONE OF ABOVE

2. UNSETTLED RELATIONSHIPS
a. Covert/open conflict with or repeated criticism of staff
b. Unhappy with roommate
c. Unhappy with residents other than roommate
d. Openly expresses conflict/anger with family/friends
e. Absence of personal contact with family/friends
f. Recent loss of close family member/friend
g. Does not adjust easily to change in routines
h. NONE OF ABOVE

3. PAST ROLES
a. Strong identification with past roles and life status
b. Expresses sadness/anger/empty feeling over lost roles/status
c. Resident perceives that daily routine (customary routine, activities) is very different from prior pattern in the community
d. NONE OF ABOVE

SECTION G. PHYSICAL FUNCTIONING AND STRUCTURAL PROBLEMS

> This section covers activities of daily living.

1. (A) ADL SELF-PERFORMANCE—(Code for resident's PERFORMANCE OVER ALL SHIFTS during last 7 days—Not including setup)
0. INDEPENDENT—No help or oversight —OR— Help/oversight provided only 1 or 2 times during last 7 days
1. SUPERVISION—Oversight, encouragement or cueing provided 3 or more times during last 7 days —OR— Supervision (3 or more times) plus physical assistance provided only 1 or 2 times during last 7 days
2. LIMITED ASSISTANCE—Resident highly involved in activity; received physical help in guided maneuvering of limbs or other nonweight bearing assistance 3 or more times — OR—More help provided only 1 or 2 times during last 7 days
3. EXTENSIVE ASSISTANCE—While resident performed part of activity, over last 7-day period, help of following type(s) provided 3 or more times:
   —Weight-bearing support
   —Full staff performance during part (but not all) of last 7 days
4. TOTAL DEPENDENCE—Full staff performance of activity during entire 7 days
8. ACTIVITY DID NOT OCCUR during entire 7 days

(B) ADL SUPPORT PROVIDED—(Code for MOST SUPPORT PROVIDED OVER ALL SHIFTS during last 7 days; code regardless of resident's self-performance classification)
0. No setup or physical help from staff
1. Setup help only
2. One person physical assist   8. ADL activity itself did not occur during entire 7 days
3. Two+ persons physical assist

		(A) SELF-PERF	(B) SUPPORT
a. BED MOBILITY	How resident moves to and from lying position, turns side to side, and positions body while in bed	3	3
b. TRANSFER	How resident moves between surfaces—to/from: bed, chair, wheelchair, standing position (EXCLUDE to/from bath/toilet)	4	3
c. WALK IN ROOM	How resident walks between locations in his/her room	4	2
d. WALK IN CORRIDOR	How resident walks in corridor on unit	4	3
e. LOCOMOTION ON UNIT	How resident moves between locations in his/her room and adjacent corridor on same floor. If in wheelchair, self-sufficiency once in chair	4	2
f. LOCOMOTION OFF UNIT	How resident moves to and returns from off unit locations (e.g., areas set aside for dining, activities, or treatments). If facility has only one floor, how resident moves to and from distant areas on the floor. If in wheelchair, self-sufficiency once in chair	4	2
g. DRESSING	How resident puts on, fastens, and takes off all items of street clothing, including donning/removing prosthesis	4	3
h. EATING	How resident eats and drinks (regardless of skill). Includes intake of nourishment by other means (e.g., tube feeding, total parenteral nutrition)	2	2
i. TOILET USE	How resident uses the toilet room (or commode, bedpan, urinal); transfer on/off toilet, cleanses, changes pad, manages ostomy or catheter, adjusts clothes	4	3
j. PERSONAL HYGIENE	How resident maintains personal hygiene, including combing hair, brushing teeth, shaving, applying makeup, washing/drying face, hands, and perineum (EXCLUDE baths and showers)	4	2

MDS 2.0 September, 2000

Minimum Data Set form (continued)

Resident __Amy J. Gaston__   Numeric Identifier _____

			(A)	(B)
2.	BATHING	How resident takes full-body bath/shower, sponge bath, and transfers in/out of tub/shower (EXCLUDE washing of back and hair.) *Code for most dependent in self-performance and support.* (A) BATHING SELF-PERFORMANCE codes appear below	4	3
		0. Independent—No help provided		
		1. Supervision—Oversight help only		
		2. Physical help limited to transfer only		
		3. Physical help in part of bathing activity		
		4. Total dependence		
		8. Activity itself did not occur during entire 7 days (Bathing support codes are as defined in Item 1, code B above)		

3.	TEST FOR BALANCE (see training manual)	*(Code for ability during test in the last 7 days)* 0. Maintained position as required in test 1. Unsteady, but able to rebalance self without physical support 2. Partial physical support during test; or stands (sits) but does not follow directions for test 3. Not able to attempt test without physical help		
		a. Balance while standing	3	
		b. Balance while sitting—position, trunk control	2	

4.	FUNCTIONAL LIMITATION IN RANGE OF MOTION (see training manual)	*(Code for limitations during last 7 days that interfered with daily functions or placed resident at risk of injury)* (A) RANGE OF MOTION (B) VOLUNTARY MOVEMENT 0. No limitation 0. No loss 1. Limitation on one side 1. Partial loss 2. Limitation on both sides 2. Full loss	(A)	(B)
		a. Neck	/	/
		b. Arm—Including shoulder or elbow	/	/
		c. Hand—Including wrist or fingers	/	/
		d. Leg—Including hip or knee	/	/
		e. Foot—Including ankle or toes	/	/
		f. Other limitation or loss	0	0

5.	MODES OF LOCOMO-TION	*(Check all that apply during last 7 days)*		
		Cane/walker/crutch	a.	Wheelchair primary mode of locomotion	d. X
		Wheeled self	b.		
		Other person wheeled	c.	NONE OF ABOVE	e.

6.	MODES OF TRANSFER	*(Check all that apply during last 7 days)*		
		Bedfast all or most of time	a. X	Lifted mechanically	d.
		Bed rails used for bed mobility or transfer	b.	Transfer aid (e.g., slide board, trapeze, cane, walker, brace)	e.
		Lifted manually	c.	NONE OF ABOVE	f.

7.	TASK SEGMENTA-TION	Some or all of ADL activities were broken into subtasks during last 7 days so that resident could perform them 0. No 1. Yes	0

8.	ADL FUNCTIONAL REHABILITA-TION POTENTIAL	Resident believes he/she is capable of increased independence in at least some ADLs	a.
		Direct care staff believe resident is capable of increased independence in at least some ADLs	b.
		Resident able to perform tasks/activity but is very slow	c.
		Difference in ADL Self-Performance or ADL Support, comparing mornings to evenings	d.
		NONE OF ABOVE	e. 0

9.	CHANGE IN ADL FUNCTION	Resident's ADL self-performance status has changed as compared to status of 90 days ago (or since last assessment if less than 90 days) 0. No change 1. Improved 2. Deteriorated	0

SECTION H. CONTINENCE IN LAST 14 DAYS

1. CONTINENCE SELF-CONTROL CATEGORIES
(Code for resident's PERFORMANCE OVER ALL SHIFTS)

0. CONTINENT—Complete control *[includes use of indwelling urinary catheter or ostomy device that does not leak urine or stool]*

1. USUALLY CONTINENT—BLADDER, incontinent episodes once a week or less; BOWEL, less than weekly

2. OCCASIONALLY INCONTINENT—BLADDER, 2 or more times a week but not daily; BOWEL, once a week

3. FREQUENTLY INCONTINENT—BLADDER, tended to be incontinent daily, but some control present (e.g., on day shift); BOWEL, 2-3 times a week

4. INCONTINENT—Had inadequate control BLADDER, multiple daily episodes; BOWEL, all (or almost all) of the time

a.	BOWEL CONTI-NENCE	Control of bowel movement, with appliance or bowel continence programs, if employed	2
b.	BLADDER CONTI-NENCE	Control of urinary bladder function (if dribbles, volume insufficient to soak through underpants), with appliances (e.g., foley) or continence programs, if employed	2

2.	BOWEL ELIMINATION PATTERN	Bowel elimination pattern regular—at least one movement every three days	a. X	Diarrhea	c.
				Fecal impaction	d.
		Constipation	b.	NONE OF ABOVE	e.

MDS 2.0 September, 2000

3.	APPLIANCES AND PROGRAMS	Any scheduled toileting plan	a.	Did not use toilet room/commode/urinal	f.
		Bladder retraining program	b.	Pads/briefs used	g. X
		External (condom) catheter	c.	Enemas/irrigation	h.
		Indwelling catheter	d.	Ostomy present	i.
		Intermittent catheter	e.	NONE OF ABOVE	j.

4.	CHANGE IN URINARY CONTI-NENCE	Resident's urinary continence has changed as compared to status of 90 days ago (or since last assessment if less than 90 days) 0. No change 1. Improved 2. Deteriorated	0

SECTION I. DISEASE DIAGNOSES

Check only those diseases that have a relationship to current ADL status, cognitive status, mood and behavior status, medical treatments, nursing monitoring, or risk of death. (Do not list inactive diagnoses)

1.	DISEASES	*(If none apply, CHECK the NONE OF ABOVE box)*			
		ENDOCRINE/METABOLIC/NUTRITIONAL		Hemiplegia/Hemiparesis	v.
				Multiple sclerosis	w.
		Diabetes mellitus	a.	Paraplegia	x.
		Hyperthyroidism	b.	Parkinson's disease	y.
		Hypothyroidism	c. X	Quadriplegia	z.
		HEART/CIRCULATION		Seizure disorder	aa.
		Arteriosclerotic heart disease (ASHD)	d.	Transient ischemic attack (TIA)	bb.
		Cardiac dysrhythmias	e.	Traumatic brain injury	cc.
		Congestive heart failure	f.	**PSYCHIATRIC/MOOD**	
		Deep vein thrombosis	g.	Anxiety disorder	dd.
		Hypertension	h.	Depression	ee.
		Hypotension	i.	Manic depression (bipolar disease)	ff.
		Peripheral vascular disease	j. X	Schizophrenia	gg.
		Other cardiovascular disease	k.	**PULMONARY**	
		MUSCULOSKELETAL		Asthma	hh.
		Arthritis	l.	Emphysema/COPD	ii.
		Hip fracture	m.	**SENSORY**	
		Missing limb (e.g., amputation)	n.	Cataracts	jj.
		Osteoporosis	o.	Diabetic retinopathy	kk.
		Pathological bone fracture	p.	Glaucoma	ll.
		NEUROLOGICAL		Macular degeneration	mm.
		Alzheimer's disease	q.	**OTHER**	
		Aphasia	r.	Allergies	nn.
		Cerebral palsy	s.	Anemia	oo.
		Cerebrovascular accident (stroke)	t.	Cancer	pp.
		Dementia other than Alzheimer's disease	u. X	Renal failure	qq.
				NONE OF ABOVE	rr.

2.	INFECTIONS	*(If none apply, CHECK the NONE OF ABOVE box)*			
		Antibiotic resistant infection (e.g., Methicillin resistant staph)	a.	Septicemia	g.
				Sexually transmitted diseases	h.
		Clostridium difficile (c. diff.)	b.	Tuberculosis	i.
		Conjunctivitis	c. X	Urinary tract infection in last 30 days	j.
		HIV infection	d.	Viral hepatitis	k.
		Pneumonia	e.	Wound infection	l.
		Respiratory infection	f.	NONE OF ABOVE	m.

3.	OTHER CURRENT OR MORE DETAILED DIAGNOSES AND ICD-9 CODES	a. *Hypertension* 402.11								
		b.					.		
		c.					.		
		d.					.		
		e.					.		

List other diagnoses here.

Identify other health problems here.

SECTION J. HEALTH CONDITIONS

1.	PROBLEM CONDITIONS	*(Check all problems present in last 7 days unless other time frame is indicated)*			
		INDICATORS OF FLUID STATUS		Dizziness/Vertigo	f.
				Edema	g.
		Weight gain or loss of 3 or more pounds within a 7 day period	a.	Fever	h.
				Hallucinations	i.
		Inability to lie flat due to shortness of breath	b.	Internal bleeding	j.
				Recurrent lung aspirations in last 90 days	k.
		Dehydrated; output exceeds input	c.	Shortness of breath	l.
				Syncope (fainting)	m.
		Insufficient fluid; did NOT consume all/almost all liquids provided during last 3 days	d.	Unsteady gait	n.
				Vomiting	o.
		OTHER		NONE OF ABOVE	p. X
		Delusions	e.		

(continued)

Minimum Data Set form (continued)

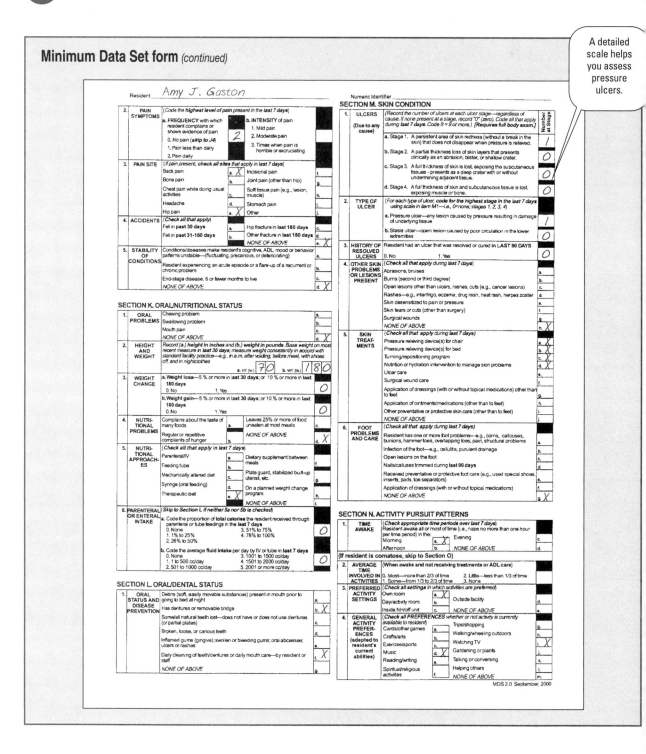

A detailed scale helps you assess pressure ulcers.

Minimum Data Set form *(continued)*

Resident **Amy J. Gaston**

Numeric Identifier _____

5.	PREFERS CHANGE IN DAILY ROUTINE	*Code for resident preferences in daily routines* 0. No change 1. Slight change 2. Major change a. Type of activities in which resident is currently involved b. Extent of resident involvement in activities	

SECTION O. MEDICATIONS

1.	NUMBER OF MEDICA-TIONS	*(Record the number of different medications used in the last 7 days; enter "0" if none used)*	4
2.	NEW MEDICA-TIONS	*(Resident currently receiving medications that were initiated during the last 90 days)* 0. No 1. Yes	0
3.	INJECTIONS	*(Record the number of DAYS injections of any type received during the last 7 days; enter "0" if none used)*	0
4.	DAYS RECEIVED THE FOLLOWING MEDICATION	*(Record the number of DAYS during last 7 days; enter "0" if not used. Note—enter "1" for long-acting meds used less than weekly)* a. Antipsychotic d. Hypnotic b. Antianxiety e. Diuretic c. Antidepressant	X

SECTION P. SPECIAL TREATMENTS AND PROCEDURES

1.	SPECIAL TREAT-MENTS, PROCE-DURES, AND PROGRAMS	a. SPECIAL CARE—*Check treatments or programs received during the last 14 days*	

TREATMENTS			PROGRAMS	
Chemotherapy	a.		Alcohol/drug treatment program	m.
Dialysis	b.		Alzheimer's/dementia special care unit	n. X
IV medication	c.		Hospice care	o.
Intake/output	d.		Pediatric unit	p.
Monitoring acute medical condition	e.		Respite care	q.
Ostomy care	f.		Training in skills required to return to the community (e.g., taking medications, house work, shopping, transportation, ADLs)	r.
Oxygen therapy	g.			
Radiation	h.			
Suctioning	i.			
Tracheostomy care	j.		NONE OF ABOVE	s.
Transfusions	k.			
Ventilator or respirator	l.			

b. THERAPIES - *Record the number of days and total minutes each of the following therapies was administered (for at least 15 minutes a day) in the last 7 calendar days (Enter 0 if none or less than 15 min. daily)*
[Note—count only post admission therapies]
(A) = # of days administered for 15 minutes or more
(B) = total # of minutes provided in last 7 days

	DAYS (A)	MIN (B)
a. Speech - language pathology and audiology services	0	
b. Occupational therapy		
c. Physical therapy	1	
d. Respiratory therapy	0	
e. Psychological therapy (by any licensed mental health professional)	0	

2.	INTERVEN-TION PROGRAMS FOR MOOD, BEHAVIOR, COGNITIVE LOSS	*(Check all interventions or strategies used in last 7 days—no matter where received)*	
		Special behavior symptom evaluation program	a. X
		Evaluation by a licensed mental health specialist in last 90 days	b.
		Group therapy	c.
		Resident-specific deliberate changes in the environment to address mood/behavior patterns—e.g., providing bureau in which to rummage	d. X
		Reorientation—e.g., cueing	e.
		NONE OF ABOVE	f.

3.	NURSING REHABILITA-TION/ RESTOR-ATIVE CARE	*Record the NUMBER OF DAYS each of the following rehabilitation or restorative techniques or practices was provided to the resident for more than or equal to 15 minutes per day in the last 7 days (Enter 0 if none or less than 15 min. daily)*	

a. Range of motion (passive)		f. Walking	
b. Range of motion (active)		g. Dressing or grooming	
c. Splint or brace assistance		h. Eating or swallowing	
TRAINING AND SKILL PRACTICE IN:		i. Amputation/prosthesis care	
d. Bed mobility		j. Communication	
e. Transfer		k. Other	

4.	DEVICES AND RESTRAINTS	*(Use the following codes for last 7 days:)* 0. Not used 1. Used less than daily 2. Used daily	
		Bed rails	
		a. — Full bed rails on all open sides of bed	0
		b. — Other types of side rails used (e.g., half rail, one side)	0
		c. Trunk restraint	0
		d. Limb restraint	0
		e. Chair prevents rising	0
5.	HOSPITAL STAY(S)	Record number of times resident was admitted to hospital with an overnight stay **in last 90 days** (or since last assessment if less than 90 days). *(Enter 0 if no hospital admissions)*	0
6.	EMERGENCY ROOM (ER) VISIT(S)	Record number of times resident visited ER without an overnight stay **in last 90 days** (or since last assessment if less than 90 days). *(Enter 0 if no ER visits)*	0
7.	PHYSICIAN VISITS	In the **LAST 14 DAYS** (or since admission if less than 14 days in facility) how many days has the physician (or authorized assistant or practitioner) examined the resident? *(Enter 0 if none)*	1
8.	PHYSICIAN ORDERS	In the **LAST 14 DAYS** (or since admission if less than 14 days in facility) how many days has the physician (or authorized assistant or practitioner) changed the resident's orders? *Do not include order renewals without change. (Enter 0 if none)*	
9.	ABNORMAL LAB VALUES	Has the resident had any abnormal lab values during the **last 90 days** (or since admission)? 0. No 1. Yes	0

SECTION Q. DISCHARGE POTENTIAL AND OVERALL STATUS

1.	DISCHARGE POTENTIAL	a. Resident expresses/indicates preference to return to the community 0. No 1. Yes	0
		b. Resident has a support person who is positive towards discharge 0. No 1. Yes	0
		c. Stay projected to be of a short duration— discharge projected within 90 days (do not include expected discharge due to death) 0. No 2. Within 31-90 days 1. Within 30 days 3. Discharge status uncertain	0
2.	OVERALL CHANGE IN CARE NEEDS	Resident's overall self sufficiency has changed significantly as compared to status of 90 days ago (or since last assessment if less than 90 days) 0. No change 1. Improved—receives fewer supports, needs less restrictive level of care 2. Deteriorated—receives more support	2

SECTION R. ASSESSMENT INFORMATION

1.	PARTICIPA-TION IN ASSESS-MENT	a. Resident	0. No	1. Yes		1
		b. Family:	0. No	1. Yes	2. No family	0
		c. Significant other:	0. No	1. Yes	2.	0

2. SIGNATURE OF PERSON COORDINATING THE ASSESSMENT:

Christine Saslo, RN, MSN

a. Signature of RN Assessment Coordinator (sign on above line)

b. Date RN Assessment Coordinator signed as complete	0 2	–	0 7	–	2 0 0 9
	Month		Day		Year

This section covers special treatments and procedures that may affect patient care.

MDS 2.0 September, 2000

(continued)

Minimum Data Set form *(continued)*

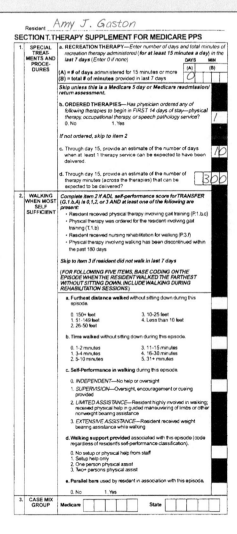

Resident _Amy J. Gaston_   Numeric Identifier _____

SECTION T. THERAPY SUPPLEMENT FOR MEDICARE PPS

1.	SPECIAL TREAT-MENTS AND PROCE-DURES	

a. RECREATION THERAPY—Enter number of days and total minutes of recreation therapy administered (**for at least 15 minutes a day**) in the **last 7 days** (Enter 0 if none)

	DAYS (A)	MIN (B)
(A) = # of days administered for 15 minutes or more		
(B) = total # of minutes provided in last 7 days	0	

Skip unless this is a Medicare 5 day or Medicare readmission/ return assessment.

b. ORDERED THERAPIES—*Has physician ordered any of following therapies to begin in FIRST 14 days of stay—physical therapy, occupational therapy, or speech pathology service?* | 1 |
0. No   1. Yes

If not ordered, skip to item 2

c. Through day 15, provide an estimate of the number of days when at least 1 therapy service can be expected to have been delivered. | 10 |

d. Through day 15, provide an estimate of the number of therapy minutes (across the therapies) that can be expected to be delivered? | 300 |

2.	WALKING WHEN MOST SELF SUFFICIENT	

Complete item 2 if ADL self-performance score for TRANSFER (G.1.b.A) is 0,1,2, or 3 AND at least one of the following are present:
- Resident received physical therapy involving gait training (P.1.b.c)
- Physical therapy was ordered for the resident involving gait training (T.1.b)
- Resident received nursing rehabilitation for walking (P.3.f)
- Physical therapy involving walking has been discontinued within the past 180 days

Skip to item 3 if resident did not walk in last 7 days

(FOR FOLLOWING FIVE ITEMS, BASE CODING ON THE EPISODE WHEN THE RESIDENT WALKED THE FARTHEST WITHOUT SITTING DOWN. INCLUDE WALKING DURING REHABILITATION SESSIONS.)

a. Furthest distance walked without sitting down during this episode.

0. 150+ feet	3. 10-25 feet
1. 51-149 feet	4. Less than 10 feet
2. 26-50 feet	

b. Time walked without sitting down during this episode.

0. 1-2 minutes	3. 11-15 minutes
1. 3-4 minutes	4. 16-30 minutes
2. 5-10 minutes	5. 31+ minutes

c. Self-Performance in walking during this episode.

0. *INDEPENDENT*—No help or oversight
1. *SUPERVISION*—Oversight, encouragement or cueing provided
2. *LIMITED ASSISTANCE*—Resident highly involved in walking; received physical help in guided maneuvering of limbs or other nonweight bearing assistance
3. *EXTENSIVE ASSISTANCE*—Resident received weight bearing assistance while walking

d. Walking support provided associated with this episode (code regardless of resident's self-performance classification).

0. No setup or physical help from staff
1. Setup help only
2. One person physical assist
3. Two+ persons physical assist

e. Parallel bars used by resident in association with this episode.

0. No   1. Yes

3.	CASE MIX GROUP	Medicare [ ][ ][ ][ ][ ] State [ ][ ][ ][ ][ ]

MDS 2.0 September, 2000

Minimum Data Set form *(continued)*

SECTION V. RESIDENT ASSESSMENT PROTOCOL SUMMARY   Numeric Identifier _____

Resident's Name: *Amy J. Gaston*   Medical Record No.: *MM0009922681*

1. Check if RAP is triggered.
2. For each triggered RAP, use the RAP guidelines to identify areas needing further assessment. Document relevant assessment information regarding the resident's status.

 • Describe:
  — Nature of the condition (may include presence or lack of objective data and subjective complaints).
  — Complications and risk factors that affect your decision to proceed to care planning.
  — Factors that must be considered in developing individualized care plan interventions.
  — Need for referrals/further evaluation by appropriate health professionals.

 • Documentation should support your decision-making regarding whether to proceed with a care plan for a triggered RAP and the type(s) of care plan interventions that are appropriate for a particular resident.

 • Documentation may appear anywhere in the clinical record (e.g., progress notes, consults, flowsheets, etc.).
3. Indicate under the Location of RAP Assessment Documentation column where information related to the RAP assessment can be found.
4. For each triggered RAP, indicate whether a new care plan, care plan revision, or continuation of current care plan is necessary to address the problem(s) identified in your assessment. The Care Planning Decision column must be completed within 7 days of completing the RAP (MDS and RAPs).

The RAP summary lists identified problem areas and documents the existence of a corresponding care plan.

A. RAP PROBLEM AREA	(a) Check if triggered	Location and Date of RAP Assessment Documentation	(b) Care Planning Decision—check if addressed in care plan
1. DELIRIUM			
2. COGNITIVE LOSS	X	*progress notes*	X
3. VISUAL FUNCTION			
4. COMMUNICATION	X	*progress notes*	X
5. ADL FUNCTIONAL/ REHABILITATION POTENTIAL			
6. URINARY INCONTINENCE AND INDWELLING CATHETER			
7. PSYCHOSOCIAL WELL-BEING			
8. MOOD STATE			
9. BEHAVIORAL SYMPTOMS			
10. ACTIVITIES			
11. FALLS			
12. NUTRITIONAL STATUS			
13. FEEDING TUBES			
14. DEHYDRATION/FLUID MAINTENANCE			
15. DENTAL CARE			
16. PRESSURE ULCERS	X	*progress notes*	X
17. PSYCHOTROPIC DRUG USE			
18. PHYSICAL RESTRAINTS			

B.   *James Shaw, RN, BSN*
1. Signature of RN Coordinator for RAP Assessment Process   2. `0 2 - 0 7 - 2 0 0 9` Month Day Year

   Christine Saslo, RN, MSN
3. Signature of Person Completing Care Planning Decision   4. `0 2 - 0 7 - 2 0 0 9` Month Day Year

MDS 2.0 September, 2000

Source: Centers for Medicare & Medicaid Services.

status assessment and documents it on a PASARR form. (See *PASARR form.*)

Initial nursing assessment

This required form is similar to the initial assessment form used in other settings. When documenting your initial assessment in a long-term care setting, place special emphasis on the patient's:
- activity level
- hearing and vision
- bowel and bladder control
- nutrition and hydration status
- ability to communicate
- safety
- need for adaptive devices to assist dexterity and mobility
- family relationships
- transition from home or hospital to the long-term care facility.

Nursing summaries

Care and status updates must be completed regularly in long-term care facilities. Usually, you must complete a standard nursing care summary at least once every 2 to 4 weeks for patients with specific problems, such as pressure ulcers, who are receiving skilled care. A summary addressing the specific problems must be done weekly. For patients receiving intermediate care, a standard nursing care summary is usually required every 4 weeks.

Summing it up

The nursing summary describes:
- the patient's ability to perform ADLs
- nutrition and hydration
- safety measures, such as bed rails, restraints, or adaptive devices
- medications and other treatments
- problems the patient has adjusting to the long-term care facility.
    In addition, you must complete a nursing assessment summary at least monthly to comply with Medicare and Medicaid standards.

ADL checklists and flow sheets

ADL checklists and flow sheets are forms that are usually completed by a nursing assistant or a restorative nurse on each shift; then you review and sign them. These forms tell the health care team members about the patient's abilities, degree of

(Text continues on page 308.)

Art of the chart

PASARR form

Before a patient covered by Medicare or Medicaid enters a long-term care facility, he must undergo an evaluation of mental status, using the Preadmission Screening and Annual Resident Review (PASARR) form shown here.

SECTION A. IDENTIFYING INFORMATION FOR APPLICANT/RESIDENT

Last name: Perrone

First Name: Joseph

MI: R

Sex: M   M = Male   F = Female

Date of birth: 08/03/33

Social security number: 012345678

Medicaid Recipient? N
Y = Yes
N = No
P = Pending

SECTION B: REASON FOR SCREENING

Enter code: 1

Preadmission Screening Codes
1-Nursing Facility Applicant
2-PASSPORT Waiver Applicant

Annual RESIDENT REVIEW CODES
3-Expired Time Limit for Convalescent Stay
4-Expired Time for Emergency Admission
5-Expired Time Limit for Respite Admission
6-Significant Change in Condition
7-No Previous PASARR Records
8-ODMH Use Only
9-Other

SECTION C: DEMENTIA QUESTIONS

Yes [ ] No [✓] (1) Does the individual have a documented PRIMARY diagnosis of dementia, Alzheimer's disease, or some other organic mental disorder as defined in *DSM-IV-TR*? If YES, the individual does not have indications of serious MI, go to Section E. If NO, go to the next question.

Yes [ ] No [✓] (2) Does the individual have a SECONDARY diagnosis of dementia, Alzheimer's disease, or some other organic mental disorder as defined in *DSM-IV-TR*? If YES, go to the next question. If NO, go to Section D.

Yes [ ] No [✓] (3) Does the individual have a PRIMARY diagnosis of one of the mental disorders listen in Question D (1) below? If YES, go to Section D. If NO, and the individual does not have indications of serious MI, go to Section E.

SECTION D: INDICATIONS OF SERIOUS MENTAL ILLNESS

Yes [ ] No [ ] (1) Does the individual have a diagnosis of any of the mental disorders listed below? Check all that apply.

a. [ ] Schizophrenic Disorder
b. [ ] Mood Disorder
c. [ ] Delusional (Paranoid) Disorder
d. [ ] Panic or Other Severe Anxiety Disorder
e. [ ] Somatoform Disorder
f. [ ] Personality Disorder
g. [ ] Other Psychotic Disorder
h. [ ] Another Mental Disorder Other Than MR That May Lead to a Chronic Disability
Describe:_____

> If the patient is diagnosed as having a serious mental disorder, document the diagnosis here.

(2) Within the past 2 years, DUE TO THE MENTAL DISORDER, has the individual:

Yes [ ] No [ ] (a) Utilized intensive psychiatric services more than once? Indicate the number of times the individual utilized each service over the last 2 years (e.g., 0,1, 2, 7 times).

a. [ ] Ongoing case management from a MH agency? ("1" if continuously receiving over the last 2 years.)
b. [ ] Emergency mental health services?
c. [ ] Number of admissions to inpatient hospital settings for psychiatric reasons?
d. [ ] Number of admissions to partial hospitalization treatment programs for psychiatric reasons?
e. [ ] Number of admissions to Residential Care Facilities (RCFs) providing MH services or operated by an MH agency?
f. [ ] TOTAL SCORE: If total score equals 2 or more, answer YES to Question D(2). Regardless of score, answer Question D(2)(b).

OR

Yes [ ] No [ ] (b) Had a disruption to his/her usual living arrangement (e.g., arrest, eviction, inter- or intra-facility transfer, locked seclusion)? If YES, answer YES to Question D(2).

(continued)

PASARR form *(continued)*

SECTION D: INDICATIONS OF SERIOUS MENTAL ILLNESS *(continued)*

Yes | No

(3) Within the past 6 months, DUE TO THE MENTAL DISORDER, has the individual experienced one or more of the following functional limitations on a continuing or intermittent basis? Check all that apply.

a. Maintaining Personal Hygiene
b. Dressing Self
c. Walking or Getting Around
d. Maintaining Adequate Diet
e. Preparing or Obtaining Own Meals
f. Maintaining Prescribed Medication Regimen
g. Performing Household Chores
h. Going Shopping
i. Using Available Transportation
j. Managing Available Funds
k. Securing Necessary Support Services
l. Verbalizing Needs

Yes | No

(4) Within the past 2 years, has the individual received SSI or SSDI due to a mental impairment?

Yes | No

(5) Does the individual have indications of serious mental illness?
The individual has indications of serious mental illness if the individual received:
•*Yes to AT LEAST 2 of Questions D(1), D(2), or D(3); OR*
•*Yes to Question D(4).*

> Fill out this section if the patient has mental retardation or a related condition.

SECTION E: INDICATIONS OF MR OR RELATED CONDITION

Yes | No [✓]

(1) Does the individual have a diagnosis of mental retardation (mild, moderate, severe, or profound as described in the *American Association of Mental Retardation's Manual on Classification in Mental Retardation*, 1989)?

Yes | No [✓]

(2) Does the individual have a severe, chronic disability that is attributable to a condition other than mental illness but is closely related to MR because this condition results in impairment of general intellectual functioning or adaptive behavior similar to that of a person with MR and requires treatment or services similar to those required for persons with MR? If YES, specify:_____

Yes | No

If NO, go to question E(6).

(3) Did the disability manifest symptoms before the individual's 22nd birthday?

Yes | No

(4) Is the disability likely to continue indefinitely?

Yes | No

(5) Did the disability result in functional limitations, prior to age 22, in 3 or more of the following major life activities? Check all that apply:

a. Self Care
b. Mobility
c. Economic Self Sufficiency
d. Understanding and Use of Language
e. Self Direction
f. Learning
g. Capacity for Independent Living

Yes | No [✓]

(6) Does the person currently receive services from the County Board of MR/DD?

Yes | No [✓]

(7) Does the person have indications of MR or a related condition?
The individual has indications of MR or a related condition if the individual received:
•*Yes to Question E(1); OR*
•*Yes to all of the following in this Section; Questions 2, 3, 4 AND 5; OR*
•*Yes to Question E(6).*

SECTION F: SUBMITTER INFORMATION/CERTIFICATION

In order to process the screen, the submitter must provide his/her name and address and sign below. If the individual has indications of serious MI (YES to D[5]) and/or MR or a related condition (YES to E[7]), submitters must also complete Section G (next page). If the individual has indications of neither, submitters do not have to complete Section G. The NF may not admit or retain individuals with indications of serious MI and/or MR or a related condition without further review by ODMH and/or ODMR/DD (OAC Rules 5101:3-3-151 and 5101:3-3-152).

Last name: B r o w n

First Name: L i s a

PASARR form *(continued)*

Street address 456 Main Street

City Springhouse   State PA   Zip 19477   Telephone Number (214) 999-9900

I understand that this screening information may be relied upon in the payment of claims that will be from Federal and State funds, and that any willful falsification, or concealment of a material fact, may be prosecuted under Federal and State laws. I certify that to the best of my knowledge the foregoing information is true, accurate, and complete.

Signature *Lisa Brown*   Title *RN*   Date 03-10-09
Employer Gunnyside Care Facility   Month Day Year

PASARR IDENTIFICATION SCREEN

SECTION G: MAILING ADDRESSES

Complete this section ONLY if the individual has indications of serious MI, MR, or a related condition.

(1) What address should be used for mailing results of the PASARR evaluation to the applicant/resident?

In care of

Street address

City   **State**   **Zip**   **Telephone Number**
( )

(2) Please provide the following information about the individual's attending physician:

Last name   **First Name**

Street address

City   **State**   **Zip**   **Telephone Number**
( )

(3) If the individual has a legal representative, please provide the following information about the representative:

Last name   **First Name**

Street address

City   **State**   **Zip**   **Telephone Number**
( )

(continued)

PASARR form *(continued)*

(4) If the individual is an applicant to or resident of an NF, please provide the name and address of the NF:

Name of NF

Street address

City

State

Zip

First 4 letters of county

(5) If the individual is being discharged from a hospital, and the submitter is not employed by the discharging hospital, please provide the name of a contact person and the name and address of the discharging hospital:

Last name

First Name

Discharging hospital

Street address

City

State

Zip

Telephone Number
(   )

---

independence, and special needs so they can determine the type of assistance he requires.

The following tools are examples of checklists and flow sheets that can be used to assess ADLs:

- Katz index
- Lawton scale
- Barthel index and scale.

Katz index

The Katz index ranks the patient's ability in six areas:

- bathing
- dressing
- toileting
- moving from wheelchair to bed and returning
- continence
- feeding.

It describes his functional level at a specific time and rates his performance of each function on three levels: performing without help, needing some help, or having complete disability. (See *Rating ability to perform basic tasks.*)

Art of the chart

Rating ability to perform basic tasks

The Katz index, shown below, is used to assess six basic activities of daily living.

ACTIVITIES	INDEPENDENCE:	DEPENDENCE:
Points (1 or 0)	(1 POINT) NO supervision, direction, or personal assistance	(0 POINTS) WITH supervision, direction, personal assistance, or total care
BATHING Points: _____0_____	(1 POINT) Bathes self completely or needs help in bathing only a single part of the body such as the back, genital area, or disabled extremity.	(0 POINTS) Needs help with bathing more than one part of the body, getting in or out of the tub or shower. Requires total bathing.
DRESSING Points: _____1_____	(1 POINT) Gets clothes from closets and drawers and puts on clothes and outer garments complete with fasteners. May have help tying shoes.	(0 POINTS) Needs help with dressing self or needs to be completely dressed.
TOILETING Points: _____0_____	(1 POINT) Goes to toilet, gets on and off, arranges clothes, cleans genital area without help.	(0 POINTS) Needs help transferring to the toilet, cleaning self or uses bedpan or commode.
TRANSFERRING Points: _____1_____	(1 POINT) Moves in and out of bed or chair unassisted. Mechanical transferring aides are acceptable.	(0 POINTS) Needs help in moving from bed to chair or requires a complete transfer.
CONTINENCE Points: _____0_____	(1 POINT) Exercises complete self-control over urination and defecation.	(0 POINTS) Is partially or totally incontinent of bowel or bladder.
FEEDING Points: _____1_____	(1 POINT) Gets food from plate into mouth without help. Preparation of food may be done by another person.	(0 POINTS) Needs partial or total help with feeding or requires parenteral feeding.

TOTAL POINTS = ___3___ 6 = High (patient independent) 0 = Low (patient very dependent)

Adapted with permission from the Gerontological Society of America. Katz, S., et al. "Progress in the Development of the Indexes of ADL," *The Gerontologist* 10:20-30, 1970.
Adapted version © 2000 by the Hartford Institute for Geriatric Nursing, College of Nursing, New York University. Used with permission.

Lawton scale

The Lawton scale of instrumental activities evaluates the patient's ability to perform complex personal care activities necessary for independent living. Activities include:

- using the telephone
- housekeeping
- shopping
- doing laundry
- managing finances
- taking medications
- preparing meals
- transportation.

Activities are rated on a three-point scale, ranging from without help (3), to needing some help (2), to complete disability (1). (See *Rating ability to perform complex tasks*.)

Barthel index and scale

The Barthel index and scale is used to evaluate:

- feeding
- moving from wheelchair to bed and returning
- performing personal hygiene
- getting on and off the toilet
- bathing
- walking on a level surface or propelling a wheelchair
- going up and down stairs
- dressing and undressing
- maintaining bowel continence
- controlling the bladder.

Each item is scored according to the amount of assistance needed. Over time, results reveal improvement or decline. Another scale, the Barthel self-care rating scale, evaluates function in more detail. (See *Getting better or worse?* pages 312 to 314.)

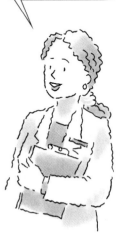

Assess your patient's ability to perform ADLs with the Katz index, Lawton scale, and Barthel index and scale.

Care plans

Standards for care plans are developed by individual long-term care facilities. When a patient is admitted to a facility, an interim care plan is used until there's an interdisciplinary care conference regarding the patient. The interim care plan should be in place within 24 hours of admission. After the interim plan, a full care plan is developed for the patient. The interdisciplinary care plan should be completed within 7 days of the completion of the MDS. A documented review of the plan must be completed every 3 months or when the patient's status changes.

(Text continues on page 315.)

Art of the chart

Rating ability to perform complex tasks

The Lawton scale of instrumental activities (shown below) provides information about a patient's ability to perform more sophisticated tasks than basic activities of daily living.

Name _John Shapiro_   Rated by _James Mott, RN_   Date _2/12/09_

Patient's name → Your name

1. Can you use the telephone?
   without help .... ③
   with some help 2
   completely unable 1

2. Can you get to places beyond walking distance?
   without help 3
   with some help .... ②
   not without special arrangements 1

3. Can you go shopping for groceries?
   without help 3
   with some help .... ②
   completely unable 1

4. Can you prepare your own meals?
   without help .... ③
   with some help 2
   completely unable 1

5. Can you do your own housework?
   without help .... ③
   with some help 2
   completely unable 1

6. Can you do your own handyman work?
   without help 3
   with some help .... ②
   completely unable 1

7. Can you do your own laundry?   Date
   without help .... ③
   with some help 2
   completely unable 1

8a. Do you take or use any medications?
   Yes (If yes, answer question 8b.) .... ①
   No (If no, answer question 8c.) 2

8b. Do you take your own medication?
   without help (in the right doses at the right times) .... ③
   with some help (if someone prepares it for you or reminds you to take it) 2
   completely unable 1

8c. If you had to take medication, could you do it?
   without help (in the right doses at the right time) 3
   with some help (if someone prepared it for you or reminded you to take it) 2
   completely unable 1

9. Can you manage your own money?
   without help .... ③
   with some help 2
   completely unable 1

Activities are rated on a 3-point scale.

Questions may need to be modified for individual patients.

The first answer in each case — except for 8a — indicates independence; the second indicates capability with assistance; and the third, dependence. In this version the maximum score is 29, although scores have meaning only for a particular patient, such as when declining scores over time reveal deterioration.

Adapted with permission from Lawton, M.P., and Brody, E.M. "Assessment of Older People: Self-Maintaining and Instrumental Activities of Daily Living," *The Journal of Gerontology* 9(3):179-86, Autumn 1969.

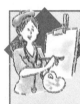

Art of the chart

Getting better or worse?

The Barthel index and scale (shown below) is used to assess the patient's ability to perform 10 activities of daily living, document findings for other health care team members, and reveal improvement or decline.

Patient Name: _Jack Boyd_

Evaluator: _Kate Roth, RN_

Date: _2/14/09_

Activity	Score
FEEDING 0 = unable 5 = needs help cutting, spreading butter, etc., or requires modified diet 10 = independent	10
BATHING 0 = dependent 5 = independent (or in shower)	5
GROOMING 0 = needs to help with personal care 5 = independent face/hair/teeth/shaving (implements provided)	5
DRESSING 0 = dependent 5 = needs help but can do about half unaided 10 = independent (including buttons, zippers, laces, etc.)	5
BOWELS 0 = incontinent (or needs to be given enemas) 5 = occasional accident 10 = continent	5
BLADDER 0 = incontinent, or catheterized and unable to manage alone 5 = occasional accident 10 = continent	5
TOILET USE 0 = dependent 5 = needs some help, but can do some things alone 10 = independent (on and off, dressing, wiping)	5

Getting better or worse? *(continued)*

Activity	Score
TRANSFERS (BED TO CHAIR AND BACK)	*10*
0 = unable, no sitting balance	
5 = major help (one or two people, physical), can sit	
10 = minor help (verbal or physical)	
15 = independent	
MOBILITY (ON LEVEL SURFACES)	*5*
0 = immobile or < 50 yards	
5 = wheelchair independent, including corners, > 50 yards	
10 = walks with help of one person (verbal or physical) > 50 yards	
15 = independent (but may use any aid; for example, stick) > 50 yards	
STAIRS	*5*
0 = unable	
5 = needs help (verbal, physical, carrying aid)	
10 = independent	

TOTAL SCORE
(0–100)

60

DEFINITION AND DISCUSSION OF SCORING

A patient scoring 100 is continent, feeds himself, dresses himself, gets up out of bed and chairs, bathes himself, walks at least a block, and can ascend and descend stairs. This does not mean that he is able to live alone: he may not be able to cook, keep house, and meet the public, but he is able to get along without attendant care.

Feeding

    10 = Independent. The patient can feed himself a meal from a tray or table when someone puts the food within his reach. He must put on an assistive device if this is needed, cut up the food, use salt and pepper, spread butter, etc. He must accomplish this in a reasonable time.

    5 = Some help is necessary (with cutting up food, etc., as listed above).

Bathing

    5 = Patient may use a bathtub or a shower, or take a complete sponge bath. He must be able to do all the steps involved, in whichever method is employed, without another person being present.

Grooming

    5 = Patient can wash hands and face, comb hair, clean teeth, and shave. He may use any kind of razor but he must put in blade or plug in razor without help as well as get it from drawer or cabinet. Female patient must put on her own makeup, if used, but need not braid or style hair.

Dressing

    10 = Patient is able to put on and remove and fasten all clothing (including any prescribed corset or braces), and tie shoe laces (unless patient requires adaptations for this). Such special clothing as suspenders, loafer shoes, or dresses that open down the front may be used when necessary.

    5 = Patient needs help in putting on and removing or fastening any clothing. He must do at least half the work himself and must accomplish this in a reasonable time. Female patient need not be scored on use of a brassiere or girdle unless these are prescribed garments.

(continued)

Getting better or worse? *(continued)*

Bowels

    10 = Patient is able to control his bowels without accidents. He can use a suppository or take an enema when necessary (as in spinal cord injury patients who have had bowel training).

    5 = Patient needs help in using a suppository or taking an enema or has occasional accidents.

Bladder

    10 = Patient is able to control his bladder day and night. Spinal cord injury patients who wear an external device and leg bag must put them on independently, clean and empty bag, and stay dry day and night.

    5 = Patient has occasional accidents or cannot wait for the bedpan or get to the toilet in time or needs help with an external device.

Toilet use

    10 = Patient is able to get on and off toilet, fasten and unfasten clothes, prevent soiling of clothes, and use toilet paper without help. He may use a wall bar or other stable object for support if needed. If he needs a bedpan instead of a toilet, he must be able to place it on a chair, empty it, and clean it.

    5 = Patient needs help to overcome imbalance, handle clothes, or use toilet paper.

Transfers (bed to chair and back)

    15 = Independent in all phases of this activity. Patient can safely approach the bed in his wheelchair, lock brakes, lift footrests, move safely to bed, lie down, come to a sitting position on the side of the bed, change the position of the wheelchair if necessary to transfer back into it safely, and return to the wheelchair.

    10 = Either the patient needs some minimal help in some step of this activity, or needs to be reminded or supervised for safety in one or more parts of this activity.

    5 = Patient can come to a sitting position without the help of a second person but needs to be lifted out of bed, or if he transfers with a great deal of help.

Mobility (on level surfaces)

    15 = Patient can walk at least 50 yards without help or supervision. He may wear braces or prostheses and use crutches, a cane, or a walkerette but not a rolling walker. He must be able to lock and unlock braces if used, get the necessary mechanical aides into position for use, stand up and sit down, and dispose of them when he sits. (Putting on and taking off braces is scored under dressing.)

    10 = Patient needs help or supervision in any of the above but can walk at least 50 yards with a little help.

    5 = If a patient cannot ambulate but can propel a wheelchair independently, he must be able to go around corners, turn around, maneuver the chair to a table, bed, toilet, etc. He must be able to push a chair at least 50 yards. Do not score this item if the patient gets scored for walking.

Stairs

    10 = Patient is able to go up and down a flight of stairs safely without help or supervision. He may and should use handrails, canes, or crutches when needed. He must be able to carry canes or crutches as he ascends or descends stairs.

    5 = Patient needs help with or supervision of any one of the above items.

Adapted with permission from the Maryland State Medical Society. Mahoney, F.I., and Barthel, D.W. "Functional Evaluation: The Barthel Index," *Maryland State Medical Journal* 14:56-61, 1965.

In long-term care settings, care plans usually evolve from an interdisciplinary approach to care, with contributions by the patient, members of his family, and other health care providers.

As always, base your care plan on the patient's health problems, nursing diagnoses, and expected treatment outcomes. Include measurable patient outcomes with reasonable time frames and specific interventions to achieve them.

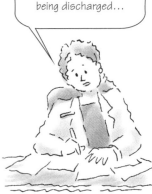

My patient is being discharged...

Discharge and transfer forms

When the facility discharges a patient to home or to a hospital, you must document the reason for discharge, the patient's destination, his mode of transportation, and the person or staff member accompanying him, if appropriate.

Guidelines drawn up by The Joint Commission emphasize the need to assess and summarize the patient's condition at transfer time. (See *Transfer and personal belongings forms,* page 316.)

Other important data to include in this document are a list of prescribed medications, skin assessment findings, overall condition, the disposition of personal belongings, and teaching topics that you covered (such as diet, medications, skin care, and other areas).

Documentation guidelines

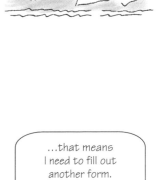

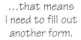

...that means I need to fill out another form.

In long-term care facilities, consider the following points when updating your records:

• When writing nursing summaries, address specific patient problems noted in the care plan.

• When writing progress notes, confirm that the patient's progress is being evaluated and reevaluated in relation to the goals or outcomes in the care plan. If goals aren't met, address this. Also, describe and document additional actions.

• Record transfers and discharges according to facility protocol.

• Document changes in the patient's condition, and report them to the doctor and the family within 24 hours.

• Document follow-up interventions or other measures taken in response to a change in the patient's condition.

• Keep a record of visits from family or friends and of phone calls about the patient. State or federal regulators may fine your facility if these aren't charted.

• If an incident occurs, such as a fall or a treatment error, fill out an incident report and write follow-up notes for at least 48 hours after the incident (or follow your facility's policy).

• During the patient's first week of residence, keep detailed records on each shift.

(Text continues on page 318.)

Art of the chart

Transfer and personal belongings forms

Patients in long-term care facilities may be admitted to the hospital, discharged to home, or transferred to other facilities. The forms below are used during this process.

1. PATIENT'S LAST NAME _Clark_	FIRST NAME _Robert_	MI _T_	2. SEX _Male_	3. SOCIAL SECURITY NUMBER _144-44-4444_

4. PATIENT'S ADDRESS (Street, City, State, Zip Code) _1 Wise street Springhouse, PA 19411_	5. DATE OF BIRTH _2-8-28_	6. RELIGION _unknown_

7. DATE OF THIS TRANSFER _2/28/09_

8. FACILITY NAME AND ADDRESS TRANSFERRING TO _Seniors Care Facility 22 Elderly Way Phila., PA_

9. PHYSICIAN IN CHARGE AT TIME OF TRANSFER _Dr. W. Nicholas_
Will this physician care for patient after admission to new facility? ❑ YES ☒ NO

10. DATES OF STAY AT FACILITY
TRANSFERRING FROM

ADMISSION _1/14/09_   DISCHARGE _2/28/09_

11. PAYMENT SOURCE FOR CHARGES TO PATIENT

A. ☒ SELF OR FAMILY
B. ❑ PRIVATE INSURANCE

C. ❑ BLUE CROSS BLUE SHIELD
D. ❑ EMPLOYER OR UNION

E. ❑ PUBLIC AGENCY (Give name)
F. ❑ OTHER (Explain)

12-A. NAME AND ADDRESS OF FACILITY TRANSFERRING FROM _Community Hospital 3000 Medical Way, Phila., PA_

12-B. NAMES AND ADDRESSES OF ALL HOSPITALS AND EXTENDED CARE FACILITIES FROM WHICH PATIENT WAS DISCHARGED IN PAST 60 DAYS.

13. CLINIC APPOINTMENT   DATE   TIME   CLINIC APPOINTMENT CARD ATTACHED

14. DATE OF LAST PHYSICAL EXAMINATION _2/26/09_

15. RELATIVE OR GUARDIAN: Name _Katherine Clark_   Address _1 Wise street Springhouse, PA 19411_   Phone number _1-215-999-9000_

16. DIAGNOSES AT TIME OF TRANSFER
(a) Primary _Stroke_
(b) Secondary _Type 1 diabetes_

EMPLOYMENT RELATED:
❑ YES
☒ NO

VITALS AT TIME OF TRANSFER
T _98°_   P _68_   R _20_   B/P _140/82_

ADVANCE DIRECTIVES ❑ YES ☒ NO ❑ COPY ATTACHED
CODE STATUS _Full code_

CHECK ALL THAT APPLY
Disabilities
❑ Amputation
☑ Paralysis _(L) side_
❑ Contracture
❑ Pressure Ulcer
Impairments
❑ Mental

☑ Speech
❑ Hearing
☑ Vision
❑ Sensation
Incontinence
☑ Bladder
☑ Bowel
☑ Saliva

Activity Tolerance Limitations
❑ None
☑ Moderate
❑ Severe
Patient knows diagnosis?
☑ Yes
❑ No

Potential for Rehabilitation
❑ Good
☑ Fair
❑ Poor
IMPORTANT MEDICAL INFORMATION
(State allergies if any)
PCN

DIET, DRUGS, AND OTHER THERAPY at time of discharge
-Mechanical soft diet (2,000 cal)
-Megace 4 tabs 6 h
-Lasix 40 mg P.O. b.i.d.
-Aspirin 81 mg P.O. daily
-Humulin 70/30 20 units daily in a.m. & at bedtime

(Physician, please sign below)

SUGGESTIONS FOR ACTIVE CARE
BED
Position in good body alignment and change position every _2_ hrs.
Avoid _flat supine_ position
Prone position _2_ time/day as tolerated.
SITTING
_4_ hr _3_ times/day

WEIGHT BEARING
❑ Full
☑ Partial
❑ None
on_____Leg

EXERCISES
Range of motion _3_ times/day.
to _(L) extremities_ by
❑ patient ❑ nurse ❑ family
Stand _3_ min. _2_ times/day.

LOCOMOTION
Walk _unable_ times/day.

SOCIAL ACTIVITIES
Encourage (☑ Group ❑ Individual) activities (☑ within ❑ outside) home.
❑ Transportation: ☑ Ambulance
❑ Car ❑ Car for handicapped
❑ Bus

Signature of Physician or Nurse _John Brown, RN_   Date _2 / 28 / 09_

Transfer and personal belongings forms *(continued)*

Any articles of clothing or other belongings left at the hospital will be held for 30 days after discharge. Items remaining after this period will be disposed of by the hospital.

			COMMENTS
Date: 2/28/09			
Initials: CR			
VALUABLES DESCRIBE			
Wallet:		✔	1 brown leather wallet
Money (Amount): $25.00		✔	1-$20.00 bill 5 $1 bills
Watch:			
Jewelry:			
Glasses/Contacts: Glasses		✔	Wire rim-gold
Hearing Aids:			
Dentures:		✔	
Partial			
Complete		✔	Container labeled
Keys			
ARTICLE DESCRIBE			
Ambulatory Aids:			
Cane, Walker, Etc.			
Bedclothes		✔	1 pair plaid pajamas
Belt			
Dress			
Outer Wear			
Pants			
Pocketbook			
Shirt			
Shoes			
Sweater			
Undergarments			
Other			

All belongings were sent home with patient's family: YES   (NO)

Patient's Signature _____

Witnessed by Hospital Personnel Mary Jones, RN _____

• Flag a new patient by putting a red dot on the chart, bed, or door or by using a similar system so that all staff members are aware of the new resident and become familiar with him. (Remember, however, to be sensitive to each patient's need for confidentiality and dignity.)

• Keep reimbursement in mind when documenting. For a facility to qualify for payment, its records must clearly reflect the level of care given to the patient.

• Make sure that your records accurately reflect skilled services the patient receives.

• Always record a doctor's verbal and telephone orders, and have the doctor countersign them within 48 hours.

• Document visits by the doctor to the patient. Generally accepted standards require one visit after admission, another after the first 30 days, and at least one every 60 days thereafter. However, the resident's condition ultimately guides the frequency of doctor's visits.

Overwhelmed by all the documentation? Then take the quick quiz after the chapter review on the next page.

That's a wrap!

Long-term care documentation review

The basics

• Documentation isn't done as often for patients in long-term care.

• It can be extensive because of the long government forms involved.

Regulatory agencies

• *Medicare* provides reimbursement for patients requiring skilled care if minimum daily documentation is done to prove need.

• *Medicaid* provides reimbursement for patients who receive skilled care. To ensure reimbursement, document care once per day.

• The *CMS* requires staff members of long-term care facilities to complete the MDS, review the patient's status every 3 months, and perform a comprehensive reassessment annually.

• *OBRA* was enacted by Congress in 1987 to protect the rights of patients. Regulations include specifics for patient assessments and care plans.

• The Joint Commission accredits long-term care facilities.

Forms used in long-term care

• *MDS* is a multidisciplinary form that's mandated by OBRA and must be completed for every long-term care patient.

• *RAP* includes the patient's primary problems and documents the corresponding care plan.

• *PASARR* documents complete assessment of the patient's mental status.

• The *initial assessment form* is similar to the initial assessment form used in other settings

Long-term care documentation review (continued)

but places greater emphasis on activity, hearing and vision, bowel and bladder control, communication, safety, assistive devices, family relationships, and transition.

• The *nursing summary* must be completed once per month and describes the patient's ability to perform ADLs, his nutrition and hydration status, safety measures, treatments, and problems adjusting to the long-term care facility.

• *ADL checklists and flow sheets* indicate the patient's abilities, degree of independence, and special needs to determine the type of assistance he requires.

• *Care plans* usually evolve from an interdisciplinary approach to care and should always be based on the patient's health problems, nursing diagnoses, and expected outcomes.

• *Discharge and transfer forms* must include the reason for discharge as well as the patient's destination and mode of transportation.

Documentation guidelines

• In nursing summaries, address patient problems.

• In progress notes, evaluate progress.

• Record transfers and discharges.

• Document changes in the patient's condition and follow-up information.

• Keep a record of family and friend visits and phone calls.

• If an incident occurs, fill out an incident report and write follow-up notes for 48 hours.

• Keep detailed records during the patient's first week.

• Make sure records clearly reflect the level of care for reimbursement purposes.

• Record the doctor's verbal and telephone orders, and have them signed within 48 hours.

• Document visits by the doctor.

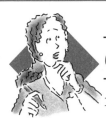

Quick quiz

1. The two levels of care in long-term care settings are:
- A. skilled and intermediate.
- B. acute and critical.
- C. geriatric and special need.
- D. primary and secondary.

Answer: A. Skilled and intermediate care, the two levels of care in long-term care settings, differ in the amount and type of nursing skills provided.

2. The MDS is required by:
- A. Medicare.
- B. Medicaid.
- C. OBRA.
- D. The Joint Commission.

Answer: C. Under the federal law known as OBRA, an initial assessment must be documented on an MDS form.

3. In a long-term care facility, you must write an interdisciplinary care plan within:
    A.   14 days of the completion of the MDS.
    B.   7 hours of the completion of the MDS.
    C.   24 hours of the completion of the MDS.
    D.   7 days of the completion of the MDS.

Answer: D. You must complete the care plan within 7 days of the completion of the MDS and update and review it every 3 months.

4. A tool for assessing the patient's mental status is:
    A.   Katz index.
    B.   Lawton scale.
    C.   PASARR form.
    D.   RAP summary.

Answer: C. A Preadmission Screening and Annual Resident Review (PASARR) form documents the patient's mental status and is required by Medicare and Medicaid for reimbursement.

5. Medicare and Medicaid require nursing assessment summaries to be completed:
    A.   weekly.
    B.   monthly.
    C.   daily.
    D.   biweekly.

Answer: B. In addition, nursing care summaries must be completed at least once per week for patients receiving skilled care and every 2 weeks for those receiving intermediate care.

6. Patients in long-term care facilities must be seen by the doctor at least once:
    A.   every 60 days.
    B.   per month.
    C.   every 6 months.
    D.   per week.

Answer: A. Patients are seen by doctors on an as-needed basis; however, they must be seen at least every 60 days.

Scoring

☆☆☆   If you answered all six questions correctly, outasight! You're PASARR (Perfectly Amazing, Stupendous, and Artful at Records and Reports).

☆☆   If you answered four or five questions correctly, unreal! No doubt about it, you're the RAP (Really Awesome Paperwork) expert.

☆   If you answered fewer than four questions correctly, keep plugging! You're an ADL (Admirably Dedicated Learner).

Appendices and index

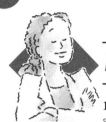

Practice makes perfect

1. A 68-year-old patient was just admitted to your unit. She's tired and wants to know why she has to answer so many questions. You explain to her that nursing documentation is necessary because:

    A.   it's a state-mandated requirement.

    B.   it's a mode of communication.

    C.   the nurse-manager told you to do it.

    D.   the doctor wants it done.

2. A 67-year-old patient on your unit recently had abdominal surgery and requires several dressing changes per day. He expresses concern about whether Medicare will pay for all the supplies being used. You explain to him that:

    A.   he doesn't have to worry because Medicare pays for everything.

    B.   the government has plenty of money to pay for supplies.

    C.   you'll try and cut back on the number of dressing changes.

    D.   nurses accurately document the number of supplies used, which aids reimbursement.

3. One of your patients overheard facility personnel discussing the facility's recent accreditation. He wants to know how a facility becomes accredited. You explain that to receive accreditation the facility must:

    A.   maintain accurate records that reflect standards of care.

    B.   provide quality of care in intensive care units.

    C.   maintain accurate doctor documentation only.

    D.   maintain accurate nursing documentation only.

4. You tell your patient that you must attend your facility's performance improvement committee meeting and that another nurse will be caring for her while you're gone. The patient wants to know what performance improvement is. Which description is most appropriate?

    A.   A committee in which the members are chosen based on the quality of care they deliver

    B.   A method used to develop, implement, and evaluate quality measures in your facility

    C.   A method used to identify problems that occur within the facility

    D.   A committee that tracks nursing and medical errors

5. A 65-year-old patient is admitted to your unit with an exacerbation of chronic obstructive pulmonary disease. After the patient is settled into bed, you begin asking about his health history. What information should be included in a health history?

    A.   Medical diagnosis
    B.   The patient's cultural information
    C.   Your best advice on the patient's illness
    D.   Your opinion of the patient's chief complaint

6. A 72-year-old patient is admitted to your unit with a fever of un-known origin. You complete the health history and the admission assessment. From this data, you begin making your nursing diagnosis. Which components should be included in the nursing diagnosis?
    A.   Human response or problem
    B.   Medical diagnosis
    C.   Expected outcome
    D.   Evaluation

7. The nurse caring for your patient on the previous shift identified *Impaired physical mobility* as a nursing diagnosis for the patient. One of the expected outcomes states, "The patient will ambulate unassisted by 3/12/09." Which element of the outcome hasn't been included?
    A.   Behavior
    B.   Time
    C.   Condition
    D.   Measure

8. A 68-year-old patient with type 2 diabetes mellitus is admitted to your unit with a diagnosis of unstable angina. Which type of care plan would best meet this patient's needs?
    A.   Standardized
    B.   Traditional
    C.   Both standardized and traditional
    D.   Computerized

9. You need to develop a medication teaching plan for a patient with angina and type 2 diabetes mellitus. You must include instructions about when to take each medication. Which type of learning outcome is required for this patient?
    A.   Cognitive domain
    B.   Affective domain
    C.   Psychomotor domain
    D.   Effective domain

10. During an admission assessment, the patient states that she enjoys reading. You observe numerous books and magazines at her bedside. Based on this information, which type of learning materials are most appropriate for this patient?
    A.   Videotapes
    B.   Brochures and pamphlets
    C.   Computers
    D.   Closed-circuit television

11. You're developing a teaching plan for a patient with coronary artery disease. Which learning outcome is in the psychomotor domain?

    A.   The patient will state when to take each prescribed medication.

    B.   The Pt will demonstrate willingness to comply with lifestyle changes.

    C.   The patient will demonstrate how to measure his heart rate.

    D.   The patient will describe the symptoms of heart failure.

12. A 45-year-old patient comes to the short procedure unit for a hernia repair; his stay is uneventful. Which charting method is best for this patient?

    A.   Narrative

    B.   Problem-oriented medical record

    C.   FOCUS charting

    D.   Charting by exception

13. When using narrative charting, you document the following statements for a patient who recently underwent exploratory abdominal surgery: *Pt states that incisional pain is unrelieved 30 min. after administration of analgesic. He's grimacing and holding incision site.* This documented observation is an example of:

    A.   a change in the patient's condition.

    B.   the patient's response to teaching.

    C.   a lack of improvement in the patient's condition.

    D.   the patient's response to a treatment or medication.

14. A 52-year-old patient was admitted 3 days ago with acute myocardial infarction. One of the problems on her problem-oriented medical record (POMR) problem list has been resolved. This should be indicated by:

    A.   assigning a different number to the problem.

    B.   placing the problem at the bottom of the list.

    C.   retiring the problem number.

    D.   using that number for a different problem.

15. A patient underwent colon resection 2 days ago. During his dressing change, you notice an increase in serosanguineous drainage from his incision. Because this is a deviation from written guidelines, you document this observation on the nursing and medical order flow sheet. This type of charting system is called:

    A.   charting by exception.

    B.   problem-intervention-evaluation.

    C.   narrative.

    D.   POMR.

16. You've been teaching a patient with recently diagnosed diabetes about monitoring his blood glucose. To document this in the progress notes, you record the data, action, and evaluation of his response to the teaching. This type of charting format is called:

    A.   POMR.
    B.   Core.
    C.   FACT.
    D.   PIE.

17. A 29-year-old patient is admitted to your unit after sustaining a femur fracture in a motor vehicle accident. You're performing your admission assessment and compiling the data on a form that contains a checklist. Which type of form are you using?

    A.   Open-ended
    B.   Closed-ended
    C.   Integrated
    D.   Traditional

18. Because of your patient's deteriorating condition, you were unable to complete the admission database form. You report this information at change of shift. The Joint Commission requires an initial admission assessment to be completed within how many hours after admission?

    A.   8 hours
    B.   12 hours
    C.   24 hours
    D.   48 hours

19. You withhold your patient's blood pressure medication because his blood pressure is below the specified parameters needed to administer the medication. You circle the omitted dose on the medication Kardex; however, there's no space on the medication Kardex to document why the dose was withheld, so you must also document this information:

    A.   on the graphic form.
    B.   in the patient care Kardex.
    C.   in the care plan.
    D.   in the progress notes.

20. Your patient has an oral temperature of 103.2° F (39.6° C). You document this finding on the graphic flow sheet. Which other step is necessary?

    A.   Document this finding on the patient care Kardex.
    B.   Document this finding and your interventions in narrative form in the progress notes.
    C.   None; you only need to document on the graphic flow sheet.
    D.   Document this finding in the care plan.

21. An 82-year-old patient admitted with heart failure is scheduled for discharge. Your facility combines discharge summaries and patient instructions in one form. The patient receives one copy and the other remains with the medical record. Which trait is an advantage of this form?

    A.   It eliminates the need for additional teaching.

    B.   It establishes compliance with The Joint Commission requirements.

    C.   It's a narrative discharge summary.

    D.   It prevents malpractice accusations.

22. A 73-year-old patient is referred to your home health agency. As you assess his condition, using the OASIS form, he states, "Why do you have to ask so many questions?" What is an appropriate response?

    A.   "The government requires this paperwork."

    B.   "My agency is required by the Centers for Medicare and Medicaid Services to complete this form for reimbursement purposes."

    C.   "My agency has always required this paperwork."

    D.   "Because all patients over the age of 18, including women receiving maternal-child services, must have a completed copy of this form in their records."

23. A patient is admitted to your long-term care facility. Her son, who's with her, asks you what the difference is between a skilled care unit and an intermediate care unit. What's your best response?

    A.   "It depends on what part of the country you live in."

    B.   "A skilled facility provides specialized nursing skills and an intermediate facility provides less-complex care."

    C.   "A skilled facility provides less-complex care and an intermediate facility provides specialized nursing skills."

    D.   "Both provide specialized and less-complex care."

24. An 86-year-old patient is being admitted to your skilled care facility. Her son asks, "How does Medicare know how to reimburse for my mother's care?" You reply that Medicare requires:

    A.   bimonthly documentation.

    B.   weekly documentation.

    C.   monthly documentation.

    D.   daily documentation.

25. You're completing a nursing summary for a patient who's receiving skilled nursing care. How often must you complete this summary?

    A.   Every 3 months

    B.   Every 2 to 4 weeks

    C.   Once, on admission only

    D.   Every week

26. A patient who sustained a closed head injury in a motor vehicle accident is admitted to your skilled care facility. You're now working on this patient's interim care plan. This care plan should be completed:

    A.   within 7 days of admission.

    B.   within 48 hours of admission.

    C.   within 24 hours of admission.

    D.   within 3 days of admission.

27. A patient needs to be assessed for his ability to perform activities of daily living (ADLs). Which assessment tool helps evaluate six basic ADLs?

    A.   Katz index

    B.   Lawton scale

    C.   Barthel index and scale

    D.   Conner's rating scale

28. While documenting in your patient's progress notes, you notice that you've made a mistake. How should you proceed?

    A.   Cross out the error completely.

    B.   Use white-out and continue to document.

    C.   Draw a single line through the entry.

    D.   Pull out that progress note and start on a new sheet.

29. You're concerned about your patient's sleeping patterns. How should you document your findings?

    A.   *Pt sleeps a lot.*

    B.   *Pt appears to sleep a lot.*

    C.   *Pt sleeps deeply.*

    D.   *Pt appears to have slept from 10 p.m. to 12 N.*

30. Your facility has started to use military time. Your patient received a one-time dose of furosemide 40 mg I.V. at 3 p.m. How should you document the administration time?

    A.   *Pt received furosemide 40 mg I.V. at 1500 hours.*

    B.   *Pt received furosemide 40 mg I.V. at 0300 hours.*

    C.   *Pt received furosemide 40 mg I.V. at 2300 hours.*

    D.   *Pt received furosemide 40 mg I.V. at 1300 hours.*

31. A nursing assistant was assigned to give morning care to your patient. How should you document the care he received from the assistant?

    A.   *Morning care given by Nancy Jones, NA.*

    B.   *Morning care given.*

    C.   *Morning care given by nurse's aide.*

    D.   *Morning care given by NJ.*

32. A doctor gives you a verbal order for digoxin 0.25 mg P.O. stat for your patient with heart failure. How should you handle documenting this verbal order?

    A.   Record the order on the doctor's order sheet and read it back.

    B.   Include the doctor's prescriber number in the order.

    C.   Sign the doctor's name.

    D.   Don't record anything; wait for the doctor to come by later and supply a written order.

33. Your patient told you that he isn't happy with the care he has been receiving at your facility and that he's thinking of suing. How should you proceed?

    A.   Notify the patient's family members and discuss the problem.

    B.   Fill out an incident report.

    C.   Chart factually and defensively.

    D.   Document in the chart that you filed an accident report.

34. An 83-year-old patient fell while getting himself out of bed. What information should you include in your documentation?

    A.   Mention that an incident report was completed.

    B.   Describe what you saw and heard and the actions you took when you arrived at the patient's bedside.

    C.   Describe what you think occurred.

    D.   Describe another staff member's suggestions about how to prevent falls.

35. A patient is to undergo surgery in the morning and the doctor asks you to witness the patient's signing of the consent form. What should you do?

    A.   Sign the form if the doctor asks you to even if you don't have access to the patient.

    B.   Make sure that the doctor explained the procedure.

    C.   Console the patient because patients are typically anxious before surgery.

    D.   Make sure the patient is competent, awake, and alert before he signs the consent form.

36. A 19-year-old patient who was recently diagnosed with diabetes mellitus asks to see his chart. What should you do first?

    A.   Immediately allow the patient to view his chart.

    B.   Ask the patient if he has questions about his treatment.

    C.   Check with your nurse-manager.

    D.   Check with the doctor.

37. Your patient refuses to take his 10 a.m. medication. How should you document this on his medication administration record?

    A.   Cross out the time the drug was to be administered.

    B.   Circle the time the drug was to be administered.

    C.   Leave the space blank where you would typically sign your initials.

    D.   White out the time the drug was to be administered.

38. An 81-year-old patient admitted with dehydration requires I.V. therapy. After establishing I.V. access, you must document:

    A.   the number of venipuncture attempts made.

    B.   the date, time, and venipuncture site; type and gauge of the catheter; and number of venipuncture attempts made.

    C.   the name of the catheter used.

    D.   only the date and time I.V. access was established.

39. A patient diagnosed with lower GI bleeding is ordered a transfusion of 1 unit of packed red blood cells. What information should you document about this procedure?

    A.   Confirmation that you alone verified the blood label information

    B.   Patient's vital signs before the transfusion

    C.   Patient's vital signs before, during, and after the transfusion as well as the total volume of blood transfused

    D.   Patient's vital signs before and after the transfusion

40. When assisting the doctor with a bone marrow aspiration, what should you document in the patient's chart?

    A.   The patient's comments during the procedure

    B.   Teaching provided

    C.   What the doctor thinks the patient's prognosis is

    D.   The approach the doctor used for the procedure

41. A 49-year-old patient is admitted for a colon resection. You're documenting his admission assessment using a computerized nursing information system. What's one advantage of computerized systems?

    A   Information storage and retrieval is slow.

    B.   Patient confidentiality is assured.

    C.   The quality of nursing care is difficult to track.

    D.   Communication between health care disciplines is increased.

42. Which abbreviations are on The Joint Commission "Do not use list"? Select all that apply.

    A. MSO_4

    B.   D/C

    C.   ml

    D.   sq

    E.   I.V.

    F.   HS

43. A nurse is taking a verbal order from a doctor. In what order should the nurse perform the following tasks to follow standard procedure for taking a verbal order?

A. Sign your name.

B. Record the order verbatim.

C. On the first line of the note, write "verbal order."

D. Write the doctor's name and your name as the nurse who received the order.

E. Make sure the doctor countersigns the order within the time limits set by your facility.

44. Which characteristics describe the critical pathway charting method? Select all that apply.

A. Promotes professional nursing documentation

B. Promotes decreased nursing documentation

C. Promotes achievement of expected patient and family outcomes

D. Reduces the cost and length of stay

E. Provides complete documentation for complex situations with unpredictable outcomes

F. Establishes a framework for instituting and monitoring continuous quality improvement

45. When documenting medication administration, which procedures should you follow? Select all that apply.

A. After administering the first dose, sign your full name and write your licensure status and your initials in the appropriate space.

B. If a medication was skipped, cross out the time on the medication administration record.

C. Immediately document the drug's abbreviation, dose, and frequency; the number of doses ordered or the stop date; and the administration time for doses given.

D. Use only standard abbreviations.

E. After withholding a medication, document the reason it was omitted and which dose wasn't given.

F. Include the date and administration time as well as the medication dose, route, and frequency.

46. A 63-year-old man is admitted to your medical-surgical unit for a colon resection and you start documenting his admission assessment. Which statement about this form is true?

A. It's used to document the patient's continued assessment.

B. It must be completed within 48 hours of admission.

C. It can't be integrated with nursing and medical assessments.

D. It contains physiologic, psychosocial, and cultural information that's used throughout hospitalization.

47. You're a home health care nurse who's visiting a patient for the first time. Which forms do you need to give the patient to read and sign? Select all that apply.

    A.   Equipment acceptance

    B.   OASIS

    C.   Consent for services

    D.   Privacy statement

    E.   Advance directives, including a do-not-resuscitate option

    F.   Medical update and patient information

48. Which agency is a branch of the Department of Health and Human Services that regulates compliance with federal Medicare and Medicaid standards?

    A.   Centers for Medicare and Medicaid Services (CMS)

    B.   The Joint Commission

    C.   Commission on Accreditation for Rehabilitation Facilities (CARF)

    D.   American Association of Retired People (AARP)

49. Which actions characterize nursing information system software programs? Select all that apply.

    A.   Collect information

    B.   Transmit information

    C.   Format information

    D.   Make suggestions about information

    E.   Display and print information

    F.   Store information

50. When releasing information to the media regarding a patient's status, which term should be used to describe a patient's condition when it's unstable with indicators that are questionable?

    A.   Good

    B.   Fair

    C.   Serious

    D.   Critical

Answers

1. B. The medical record is the main source of information and communication among nurses, doctors, physical therapists, social workers, and other caregivers. It helps provide the patient with better care.

2. D. Reimbursement from Medicare depends heavily on accurate nursing documentation.

3. A. The medical orders and progress notes of doctors and nursing personnel in a patient's medical record are evaluated by accrediting organizations to assess standards of care.

4. B. Individual states and The Joint Commission require all health care facilities to regularly monitor, evaluate, and seek ways to improve the quality of care for their patients.

5. B. The health history should include the patient's cultural information.

6. A. A nursing diagnosis usually has three components — the human response or problem, related factors, and signs and symptoms.

7. D. The four elements of an outcome statement are behavior, measure, condition, and time. Measure should include criteria for measuring the behavior and should specify how much, how long, or how far.

8. C. A standardized plan (especially one classified by medical diagnosis or diagnosis-related groups [DRGs]), which takes into account the patient's multiple diagnoses, and a traditional plan, which allows for a more individualized care plan for a patient with multiple diagnoses, would both meet this patient's needs.

9. A. Cognitive learning outcomes are related to understanding.

10. B. When choosing learning materials, you should focus on which material is best for the individual patient. Be sure to keep the patient's abilities and limitations in mind as you chose learning materials.

11. C. The psychomotor domain involves manual skills; therefore, demonstrating heart rate measurement is within the psychomotor domain.

12. C. FOCUS charting works best in acute care settings and on units where the same care and procedures are frequently repeated; this is the case in a short procedure unit.

13. D. When documenting a patient's response to a treatment or medication in a narrative note, be sure to include the patient's stated response and your observations.

14. C. After you've resolved a problem, show that it's inactive by retiring the problem number and highlighting the problem with a colored felt-tip pen. Don't use that number again for the same patient.

15. A. The charting by exception (CBE) format requires documentation of abnormal findings only. Guidelines for each body system are printed on CBE forms.

16. B. In the Core system, which focuses on the nursing process, the progress notes are recorded using DAE: data (D), action (A), and evaluation (E).

17. B. A closed-ended admission database form comes with preprinted headings, checklists, and questions with specific responses. To use it, simply check off the appropriate response.

18. C. The Joint Commission requires an initial nursing assessment to be completed within 24 hours of admission. Check your facility's policy, however, because your facility may require the form to be completed in a shorter time.

19. D. If your medication administration record or medication Kardex doesn't have space to explain why a dose was omitted, you need to document the reason in the progress notes.

20. B. Using flow sheets doesn't exempt you from narrative charting, in which you should describe your observations, patient teaching performed, patient responses, detailed interventions, and any unusual circumstances.

21. B. A narrative-style discharge summary is similar to a progress note; it contains the patient's status at admission and discharge, significant information about the patient's stay, and instructions given to the patient and his family members.

22. B. Explaining government regulations and reimbursement to the patient will increase his knowledge and cooperation.

23. B. Skilled patient care includes I.V. therapy, parenteral nutrition, respiratory care, and mechanical ventilation. Intermediate care includes care of patients who have chronic illnesses and those who need less complex care such as assistance with activities of daily living.

24. D. Medicare provides reimbursement for patients who require skilled care, such as chemotherapy and tube feedings. They require daily documentation to justify that the service is needed.

25. B. Usually, you must complete a standard nursing summary at least once every 2 to 4 weeks for patients with specific problems who are receiving skilled nursing care.

26. C. The interim care plan must be in place within 24 hours of admission.

27. A. The Katz index ranks the patient's ability in six basic ADLs— bathing, dressing, toileting, moving from wheelchair to bed and returning, continence, and feeding.

28. C. When you make a mistake in charting, correct it immediately by drawing a single line through the entry and writing "error" above or beside it, along with your initials, the date, and the time.

29. D. Record just the facts, exactly what you see, hear, and do—not your opinions or assumptions.

30. A. Most facilities require the nurse to chart in military time, which expresses time as a continuous 24-hour period.

31. A. If you need to chart the actions of nursing assistants or technicians, write the caregiver's full name, not just her initials.

32. A. When documenting a verbal order, first write V.O. on the first line (indicating that it's a verbal order), then write the doctor's name and your name as the nurse who received the order, and then write the order verbatim. It's the doctor's responsibility to countersign this order within your facility's time limit.

33. C. Document the patient's complaints using his own words, and record the specific care given to the patient in direct response to his complaints. When a patient threatens to sue, notify your nurse-manager or nursing supervisor immediately. She'll contact the risk management department, which may be able to offer advice about how to handle this difficult situation.

34. B. When a patient falls, document what you saw and heard. Also document the accounts given by witnesses. Avoid documenting what you think may have occurred. Documenting that an incident report was completed may open up you and the facility to a lawsuit.

35. D. Before witnessing a patient's consent, make sure that the patient is competent, awake, and alert and is aware of what he's doing. Also make sure that the patient understands the procedure and the associated risks. Simply giving the patient an explanation doesn't ensure that he understands. Notify your nurse-manager and the doctor immediately if you suspect that that patient has doubts about the procedure or his condition. Performing a procedure without voluntary consent may be considered battery.

36. B. Your patient has a legal right to see his chart. However, if he asks to see it, you should first ask him if he has any questions about his treatment and try to clear up any confusion. The patient may just be confused about his care.

37. B. Circle the time and document the reason for omission.

38. B. When documenting I.V. catheter insertion, document the date, time, and venipuncture site. Also document the type and gauge of the catheter and the number of venipuncture attempts made.

39. C. Proper documentation of a blood transfusion includes the patient's vital signs before, during, and after the transfusion as well as the total volume of blood transfused. Before administering blood or blood components, the bag must be identified by two health care professionals who verify that the information on the label is correct.

40. B. When assisting a doctor during a procedure, you must always document the date, time, and name of the procedure; the doctor who performed it; how it was performed; how the patient tolerated it; adverse reactions; and teaching provided.

41. D. One advantage of computerized nursing information systems is that they increase communication among health care providers from different disciplines.

42. A, B, D, F. The abbreviations MSO_4, D/C, sq, and HS are all on The Joint Commission's "Do not use list."

43. CDBAE. The appropriate sequence for recording a verbal order is write "verbal order" on the note, write the doctor's name and your name, record the verbal order verbatim, sign your name, and make sure the doctor countersigns the verbal order.

44. A, C, D, F. Critical pathways promote professional nursing documentation, promote achievement of expected patient and family outcomes, reduce the cost and length of stay, and establish a framework for instituting and monitoring continuous quality improvement. They also ensure continuity of care and appropriate use of resources.

45. A, D, E, F. After administering the first dose of a medication, sign your full name and write your licensure status and your initials in the appropriate space. You should use only standard abbreviations. When in doubt, write out the word or phrase. After withholding a medication, document the reason it was omitted and which dose wasn't given. Include the date and administration time as well as the medication dose, route, and frequency.

46. D. The admission assessment contains physiologic, psychosocial, and cultural information that's used throughout hospitalization. It can be integrated with nursing and medical assessment and must be completed within 24 hours of admission.

47. A, C, D, E. Examples of documentation that must be signed by a home health care patient include equipment acceptance documentation (must include equipment given to the patient as well as his acceptance of the equipment), consent for services, a privacy statement, and any advance directives or do-not-resuscitate orders.

48. A. The CMS regulates compliance with federal Medicare and Medicaid standards, including completion of the Minimum Data Set and other forms.

49. A, B, C, E, F. Nursing information system software programs collect, format, and transmit patient information. They can also display, print, and store this information.

50. C. A patient who's listed as unstable with questionable indicators would be reported as *serious*.

Glossary

Accountability: obligation to accept responsibility for or account for one's actions

Accreditation: official recognition from a professional or government organization that a health care facility meets relevant standards

Advance directive: document used as a guideline for life-sustaining medical care of a patient with an advanced disease or disability, who's no longer able to indicate his own wishes; includes living wills and durable powers of attorney for health care

Barthel index and scale: functional assessment tool used to evaluate an older patient's overall well-being and self-care abilities; evaluates the ability to perform 10 self-care activities

Case management: model for management of health care facilities in which one professional — usually a nurse or a social worker — assumes responsibility for coordinating care so that patients move through the health care system in the shortest time and at the lowest possible cost

Charting by exception (CBE): charting system that departs from traditional systems by requiring documentation of only significant or abnormal findings

Core charting: charting system that focuses on the nursing process; components include a database, care plan, flow sheets, progress notes, and discharge summary

Critical pathway: documentation tool used in managed care and case management in which a time line is defined for the patient's condition and for the achievement of expected outcomes; used by caregivers to determine on any given day where the patient should be in his progress toward optimal health

Database: subjective and objective patient information collected during your initial assessment of the patient; includes information obtained by taking your patient's health history, performing a physical examination, and analyzing laboratory test results

Diagnosis-related group (DRG): system of classifying or grouping patients according to medical diagnosis for purposes of reimbursement of hospitalization costs under Medicare

Durable power of attorney for health care: legal document whereby a patient authorizes another person to make medical decisions for him should he become incompetent to do so

FOCUS charting: charting system that uses assessment data, first to evaluate patient-centered topics (or foci of concern) and then to document precisely and concisely

Health history: summary of a patient's health status that includes physiologic, psychological, cultural, and psychosocial data

Health maintenance organization (HMO): organization that provides an agreed-upon health service to voluntary enrollees who prepay a fixed, periodic fee that's set without regard to the amount or kind of services received (people who belong to an HMO are cared for by member doctors with limited referrals to outside specialists)

Incident report: formal written report that informs facility administrators (and the facility's insurance company) about an incident and that serves as a contemporary factual statement in the event of a lawsuit

Incremental record: record kept according to time and occurrences

Independent practice association (IPA) model HMO: health maintenance organization that contracts with an association of doctors to provide doctor services to its members while the doctors maintain their independent practices

Informed consent: permission obtained from a patient to perform a specific test or procedure after the patient has been fully informed about the test or procedure

Interventions: nursing actions taken to meet a patient's health care needs; should reflect nurse's agreement with the patient on how to meet defined goals or expected outcomes

The Joint Commission: private, nongovernmental agency that establishes guidelines for the operation of hospitals and other health care facilities, conducts accreditation programs and surveys, and encourages the attainment of high standards of institutional medical care; members include representatives from the American Medical Association, American College of Physicians, and American College of Surgeons

Katz index: assessment tool used to evaluate a patient's ability to perform the basic functions of bathing, dressing, toileting, transfer, continence, and feeding

Lawton scale: assessment tool used to evaluate a patient's ability to perform relatively complex tasks, such as using a telephone, cooking, managing finances, and taking medications

Learning outcomes: outcomes developed as part of a patient-teaching plan that identify what a patient needs to learn, how you'll teach him, and how you'll evaluate what he has learned

Living will: witnessed document indicating a patient's desire to be allowed to die a natural death, rather than be kept alive by life-sustaining measures; applies to decisions that will be made after a terminally ill patient is incompetent and has no reasonable possibility of recovery

Minimum Data Set (MDS): standardized assessment tool that must be filled out for every patient admitted to a long-term care facility as mandated by the federal government

North American Nursing Diagnosis Association International (NANDA-I): organization responsible for developing and categorizing nursing diagnoses and examining applications of nursing diagnoses in clinical practice, education, and research

Nursing diagnosis: clinical judgment made by a nurse about a patient's responses to actual or potential health problems or life processes; describes a patient problem that the nurse can legally solve; may apply to families and communities as well as individual patients

Nursing process: systematic approach to identifying a patient's problems and then taking nursing actions to address them; steps include assessing the patient's problems, forming a diagnostic statement, identifying expected outcomes, creating a plan to achieve expected outcomes and solve the patient's problems, implementing the plan or assigning others to implement it, and evaluating the plan's effectiveness

Occurrence reporting: reporting by doctors, nurses, or other staff of incidents, either when they're observed or shortly after; also called *incident reporting*

Occurrence screening: identification of adverse events through a review of medical records

Outcome criteria: standards by which measurable goals, or outcomes, are objectively evaluated

Outcome documentation: charting that focuses on patient behaviors and responses to nursing care; documents the patient's condition in relation to predetermined outcomes included in the care plan

Peer review organization (PRO): basic component of a performance improvement program in which the results of health care given to a specific patient population are evaluated according to outcome criteria established by peers of the professionals delivering the care; promoted by professional organizations as a means of maintaining standards of care

Practice guidelines: sequential instructions for treating patients with specific health problems

Preadmission screening annual resident review (PASARR): form used to assess the mental status of a patient before admission to a long-term care facility; required for Medicare or Medicaid reimbursement

Problem-intervention-evaluation (PIE) charting: charting system that organizes patient information according to patient's problems; integrates the patient's care plan into the progress notes in order to simplify the documentation process

Problem-oriented medical record (POMR): method of organizing the medical record; consists of baseline data, a problem list, and a care plan for each problem

Performance improvement: commitment on the part of a health care facility or several health disciplines to work together to achieve an optimal degree of excellence in the services rendered to every patient (state regulatory and accrediting agencies may re-

quire health care facilities to regularly monitor, evaluate, and seek ways to improve the quality of care)

Resident assessment protocol (RAP): form required by federal mandate for use in long-term care facilities that identifies the patient's primary problems and care needs and documents the existence of a care plan

Risk management: identification, analysis, evaluation, and elimination or reduction of risks to patients, visitors, or employees; involves loss prevention and control and the handling of all incidents, claims, and other insurance- and litigation-related tasks.

SOAP charting: structured method of recording progress notes in which data are organized into four categories: Subjective, Objective, Assessment, and Planning

SOAPIE charting: structured method of recording progress notes in which data are organized into six categories: Subjective, Objective, Assessment, Planning, Implementation, and Evaluation

SOAPIER charting: structured method of recording progress notes in which data are organized into seven categories: Subjective, Objective, Assessment, Planning, Implementation, Evaluation, and Revision

Source-oriented narrative record: method of organizing the medical record in which each discipline records information in a separate section of the medical record

Utilization review: program, initiated by reimbursing agents to maintain control over health care providers, that may focus on length of stay, treatment regimen, validation of tests and procedures, and verification of the use of medical supplies and equipment

Selected references

American Nurses Association. "Principles for Documentation," 2005. Available: www.NursingWorld.org.

Austin, S. "Seven Legal Tips for Safe Nursing Practice," *Nursing2008* 38(3):34-9; quiz 39-40, March 2008.

Carpenito-Moyett, L.J. *Nursing Care Plans and Documentation: Nursing Diagnosis and Collaborative Problems*, 5th ed. Philadelphia: Lippincott Williams & Wilkins, 2008.

"Charting Checkup: Charting Tips for Long-Term Care," *LPN2006* 2(1):9-11, January-February 2006.

Cheevakasemsook, A., et al. "The Study of Nursing Documentation Complexities," *International Journal of Nursing Practice* 12(6):366-74, December 2006.

Complete Guide to Documentation. Philadelphia: Lippincott Williams & Wilkins, 2008.

Ferrell, K.G. "Documentation, Part 2: The Best Evidence of Care," *AJN*, 107(7):61-64, July 2007.

Hakes, B., and Whittington, J. "Assessing the Impact of an Electronic Medical Record on Nurse Documentation Time," *Computers, Informatics, Nursing* 26(4):234-41, July-August 2008.

Helleso, R. "Information Handling in the Nursing Discharge Note," *Journal of Clinical Nursing* 15(1):11-21, January 2006.

The Joint Commission. *Comprehensive Accreditation Manual for Hospitals: The Official Handbook*. Oakbrook Terrace, Il. 2009.

Martin, K. *60 Essential Forms for Long-Term Care Documentation*, Marblehead, Mass.: HCPro, 2006.

Nursing Know-How: Charting Patient Care. Philadelphia: Lippincott Williams & Wilkins, 2009.

Smith, L.S. "Chart Smart: Documenting with photographs," *Nursing* 37(8):20, August 2007.

Strople, B., and Ottani, P. "Can Technology Improve Intershift Report? What the Research Reveals," *Journal of Professional Nursing* 22(3):197-204, May-June 2006.

Index

i refers to an illustration; t refers to a table.

i refers to an illustration; t refers to a table.

i refers to an illustration; t refers to a table.